Nada Tawfig Hashim, Rasha Babiker, Muhammed Mustahsen Rahman,
and Bakri Gobara Gismalla (Eds.)
Periodontal Medicine

Periodontal Medicine

Biomarkers, Bioengineering, and the Periodontal Microbiome

Edited by
Nada Tawfig Hashim, Rasha Babiker, Muhammed Mustahsen Rahman, and Bakri Gobara Gismalla (Eds.)

DE GRUYTER

Editors
Dr Nada Tawfig Hashim
RAK College of Dental Sciences
RAK Medical & Health Sciences University
Al Qusaidat
Ras Al Khaimah
United Arab Emirates
nada.tawfig@rakmhsu.ac.ae

Prof. Muhammed Mustahsen Rahman
RAK College of Dental Sciences
RAK Medical & Health Sciences University
Al Qusaidat
Ras Al Khaimah
United Arab Emirates
mustahsen@rakmhsu.ac.ae

Dr Rasha Babiker
RAK College of Medical Sciences
RAK Medical & Health Sciences University
Al Qusaidat
Ras Al Khaimah
United Arab Emirates
rashababiker@rakmhsu.ac.ae

Prof. Bakri Gobara Gismalla
Faculty of Dentistry
University of Khartoum
Khartoum
Sudan
bakrigobara10@gmail.com

ISBN 978-3-11-914338-7
e-ISBN (PDF) 978-3-11-221990-4
e-ISBN (EPUB) 978-3-11-222001-6

Library of Congress Control Number: 2025946932

Bibliographic information published by the Deutsche Nationalbibliothek
The Deutsche Nationalbibliothek lists this publication in the Deutsche Nationalbibliografie;
detailed bibliographic data are available on the Internet at http://dnb.dnb.de.

© 2026 Walter de Gruyter GmbH, Berlin/Boston, Genthiner Straße 13, 10785 Berlin
Cover image: Mohammed Haneefa Nizamudeen/iStock/Getty Images Plus
Typesetting: Integra Software Services Pvt. Ltd.

www.degruyterbrill.com
Questions about General Product Safety Regulation:
productsafety@degruyterbrill.com

Preface

Periodontal medicine has emerged as a discipline that redefines our understanding of oral health and its systemic implications. Far beyond a localized inflammatory condition, periodontitis is now recognized as a disease with profound effects on cardiovascular health, metabolic regulation, pregnancy outcomes, and immune function. This book was conceived to explore these connections and highlight the scientific advances that are reshaping diagnosis and therapy.

The volume is organized around three interrelated themes: biomarkers that improve detection and prognosis; bioengineering strategies that open new horizons for regenerative therapy; and the periodontal microbiome, which serves as a central player in oral-systemic crosstalk. Together, these perspectives reflect the rapid evolution of periodontology into a multidisciplinary field at the interface of dentistry, medicine, and biotechnology.

The text is intended for clinicians, researchers, and students alike, offering both foundational knowledge and forward-looking insights. By addressing molecular mechanisms, translational approaches, and emerging therapeutic innovations, the chapters aim to bridge science with clinical practice and stimulate dialogue across disciplines.

This book represents the collective contributions of colleagues, co-authors, and mentors whose insights and encouragement have been invaluable. I hope it will serve not only as a reference but also as an inspiration for future research and innovation in the pursuit of personalized and integrative periodontal care.

https://doi.org/10.1515/9783112219904-202

Contents

List of Authors

Nada Tawfig Hashim
Department of Periodontics
RAK College of Dental Sciences
RAK Medical & Health Sciences University
Al Qusaidat
Ras Al Khaimah
United Arab Emirates
And
Department of Oral Rehabilitation
Faculty of Dentistry
University of Khartoum
Khartoum
Sudan
nada.tawfig@rakmhsu.ac.ae
Chapters 1, 2, 3, 4, 5, 6, 7, 8, 9, 10, 11, 12

Rasha Babiker
RAK College of Medical Sciences
RAK Medical & Health Sciences University
Al Qusaidat
Ras Al Khaimah
United Arab Emirates
And
Faculty of Medicine
National University
Sudan
rashababiker@rakmhsu.ac.ae
Chapters 1, 2, 3, 4, 5, 6, 9, 10

Nallan C. S. K. Chaitanya
RAK College of Dental Sciences
RAK Medical & Health Sciences University
Al Qusaidat
Ras Al Khaimah
United Arab Emirates
krishna.chytanya@rakmhsu.ac.ae
Chapter 1, 11

Muhammed Mustahsen Rahman
Department of Periodontics
RAK College of Dental Sciences
RAK Medical & Health Sciences University
Al Qusaidat
Ras Al Khaimah
United Arab Emirates
mustahsen@rakmhsu.ac.ae
Chapters 1, 4, 6, 10

Riham Mohammed
RAK College of Dental Sciences
RAK Medical & Health Sciences University
Al Qusaidat
Ras Al Khaimah
United Arab Emirates
riham.abdelraouf@rakmhsu.ac.ae
Chapters 2, 3, 4

Md Sofiqul Islam
RAK College of Dental Sciences
RAK Medical & Health Sciences University
Al Qusaidat
Ras Al Khaimah
United Arab Emirates
sofiqul.islam@rakmhsu.ac.ae
Chapters 5, 7, 8

Sivan Padma Priya
RAK College of Dental Sciences
RAK Medical & Health Sciences University
Al Qusaidat
Ras Al Khaimah
United Arab Emirates
sivan.padma@rakmhsu.ac.ae
Chapter 7

Vivek Padmanabhan
RAK College of Dental Sciences Padmanabhan
RAK Medical & Health Sciences University
Al Qusaidat
Ras Al Khaimah
United Arab Emirates
vivek.padmanabhan@rakmhsu.ac.ae
Chapters 7, 12

https://doi.org/10.1515/9783112219904-204

Bakri Gobara
Department of Oral Rehabilitation
Faculty of Dentistry
University of Khartoum
Khartoum, Sudan
And
Faculty of Dentistry
National University
Sudan
bakrigobara10@gmail.com
Chapters 8, 10

Mariam Elsheikh
Faculty of Dentistry
University of Khartoum
Khartoum, Sudan
mariam.elhadi@uofk.edu
Chapter 9

Nada Tawfig Hashim, Rasha Babiker, Nallan C. S. K. Chaitanya, and Muhammed Mustahsen Rahman

1 Periodontal Microbiome and Systemic Crosstalk: Unraveling the Oral-Systemic Axis

1.1 Introduction

The human oral cavity contains approximately 700 bacterial species which form a complex microbial community. Periodontal dysbiosis, which occurs when oral microbiota becomes unbalanced, results in periodontitis. This is a chronic inflammatory condition affecting tooth-supporting structures [1, 2]. Research has shown that periodontal dysbiosis causes various systemic health problems including cardiovascular disease and diabetes mellitus and adverse pregnancy outcomes and neurodegenerative disorders such as Alzheimer's disease [3, 4]. The newly discovered oral-systemic link demonstrates complex relationships between microbial virulence and host immune response and systemic inflammatory pathways. The scientific and clinical implications of this interaction are profound [5, 6]. The reframing of periodontitis as a systemic risk factor instead of a local condition has led to the expansion of dental treatment into preventive and interdisciplinary healthcare [7]. This chapter explains how periodontal dysbiosis affects systemic health through immunological responses and microbiological and molecular processes while clarifying the bidirectional relationship between oral infection and inflammatory diseases. The chapter emphasizes the need for interprofessional collaboration in healthcare delivery because of periodontitis's complex nature and its widespread systemic effects.

1.2 The Periodontal Microbiome in Health and Disease

The oral health depends on a healthy periodontal microbiome which maintains both microbial diversity and ecological stability [8]. *Streptococcus sanguinis* (*S. sanguinis*) along with *Actinomyces naeslundii* (*A. naeslundii*) and *Capnocytophaga* spp. are commensal organisms that maintain the ecological balance of the oral cavity [9]. The ecological niches these organisms occupy prevent pathogen growth by generating inhibitory metabolites such as hydrogen peroxide and promote the immune system to develop tolerance instead of inflammation [10]. The maintenance of this balance stands essential for achieving oral health [11]. Periodontal dysbiosis represents a concerning condition because it develops when the oral microbiota shifts toward patho-

https://doi.org/10.1515/9783112219904-001

genic inflammation-promoting communities [12]. Disease progression is marked by anaerobic gram-negative overgrowth, particularly red complex members including *Porphyromonas gingivalis* (*P. gingivalis*), *Treponema denticola* (*T. denticola*), *Tannerella forsythia* (*T. forsythia*), and *Fusobacterium nucleatum* (*F. nucleatum*) [13]. These microorganisms express their pathogenicity through a series of virulence factors [14] (Figure 1.1). For instance, lipopolysaccharides (LPS), particularly those of *P. gingivalis*, stimulate toll-like receptor (TLR) pathways – mainly TLR2 and TLR4 – leading to breaking of the epithelial barrier and release of pro-inflammatory cytokines including IL-1β and tumor necrosis factor-alpha (TNF-α) [15]. Adhesins and fimbriae facilitate attachment to the host cell and coaggregation with other microbes for successful biofilm formation [16]. Proteolytic enzymes, such as gingipains (arginine-specific and lysine-specific proteases), hydrolyze structural and immune molecules such as collagen, immunoglobulins, complement proteins, and cytokines, thus critically disrupting tissue integrity and host immune response [17]. Outer membrane vesicles (OMVs) also facilitate targeted delivery of virulence molecules into host cells for bacterial survival, immune evasion, and chronic inflammation [18].

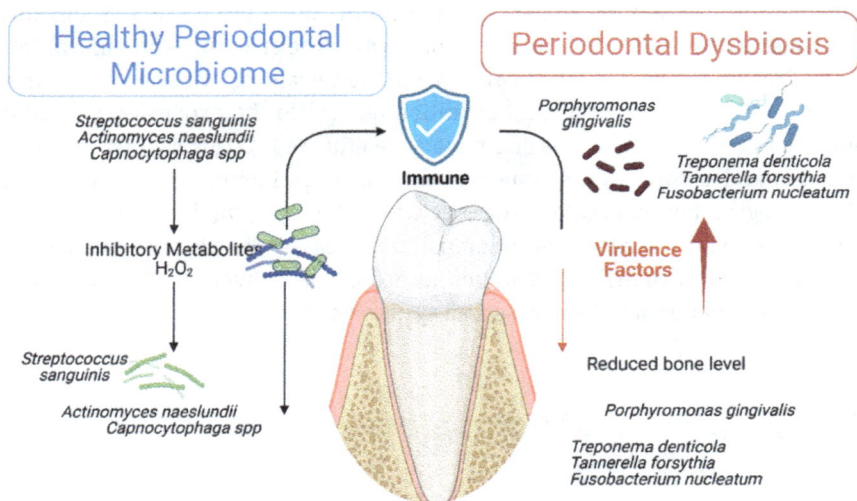

Figure 1.1: Healthy periodontal microbiome versus dysbiosis. Protective commensals maintain immune balance, whereas pathogens and virulence factors drive inflammation and bone loss. The figure is created with Biorender.com.

A unique feature of *P. gingivalis* is its role as a keystone pathogen, a term that reflects its significant impact on the microbiome despite its low population numbers [19]. Even in minimal quantities, *P. gingivalis* can alter the microbial environment by breaking down innate immune responses, primarily through manipulating complement-TLR interactions [19]. This immunological interference leads to diminished neutrophil clearance, persistent inflammation, and the recruitment of other pathogenic species, perpetuating a pro-dysbiotic and pro-inflammatory environment [20]. Understanding the role of *P. gingivalis* as a keystone pathogen is a fascinating area of research.

Periodontal pathogens can evade the immune system in different ways, such as the modulation of TLR signaling to inhibit the release of antimicrobial peptides which includes [21]:

– The downregulation of TLR expression and the interference with TLR signaling pathways effectively dampened the host immune response [21].
– Suppression of complement activation by the cleavage of C3 and C5 components [22].
– Modulation of inflammasome pathways to either attenuate or exploit host cytokine synthesis [23].

These bacteria along with their metabolites distribute systemically through transitory bacteremia which occurs when patients perform routine activities like brushing teeth or flossing or chewing in infected areas [24]. Upon entering the circulation, these microorganisms may spread to distant tissues, where they have been associated with the development of systemic illnesses, including cardiovascular plaques, pancreatic islets, placental tissue, and the central nervous system [25, 26]. For instance, the presence of periodontal pathogens in atherosclerotic plaques indicates their possible contribution to cardiovascular disease development [27]. The collective capacity of periodontal pathogens to modify microbial ecology, avoid immune elimination, and spread systemically is the essence of the oral-systemic axis, demonstrating the systemic risk presented by localized periodontal inflammation [28].

1.3 Mechanisms of Oral-Systemic Crosstalk

The link between periodontal disease and systemic conditions arises through multiple interrelated pathways.

1.3.1 Bacteremia and Microbial Translocation

The primary pathway linking periodontal infections to systemic diseases is bacteremia, through which periodontal pathogens disperse from the oral cavity to secondary body sites. Periodontal pockets with inflamed and ulcerated epithelium during tooth brushing, flossing, mastication, or dental procedures allow entry of bacteria into the blood [29]. After becoming systemic, the microorganisms use their virulence factors, adhesins, invasins, and immune eavesdropping molecules, to attach to and potentially impair target organs [5] (Figure 1.2). Among these microorganisms, *P. gingivalis* is the most extensively researched with respect to its systemic effect [30]. Upon entering the bloodstream, it selectively targets endothelial cells, and this is due to its fimbriae and OMVs. Its gingipains – a series of cysteine proteases – also degrade host protein and influence vascular permeability, which facilitates its invasion of vascular tissues [31]. *P. gingivalis* proteins and DNA have also been detected in atherosclerotic plaques on many occasions, suggesting its involvement in cardiovascular disease [32]. Its detection in hepatic tissue is also associated with metabolic alteration, and detection in placental and amniotic fluid suggests its role in causing adverse pregnancy outcomes [33, 34]. Additionally, in the central nervous system, *P. gingivalis* and its gingipains are demonstrated to exist in brain tissue of Alzheimer's disease patients, and they are also implicated in tau protein cleavage and in the promotion of chronic neuroinflammation [35]. Another prevalent periodontal pathogen is *F. nucleatum*, which has a high affinity for placental and colorectal tissues [36]. The surface adhesin FadA present in this bacterium facilitates its adherence to and invasion of endothelial cells, and subsequent translocation to sites outside the oral cavity [37]. *F. nucleatum* has been detected in the placenta, amniotic fluid, and fetal tissues of pregnant women, often with incidences of preterm birth and fetal loss. It was also detected in colorectal cancer tissues and may affect the tumor microenvironment, immune evasion, and metastatic properties [36, 38]. *T. denticola* is a flagellated spirochete with the ability to spread to neural tissue through its flagellar motility and dentilisin proteolytic activity [39]. Through this particular protease, degradation of extracellular matrix components is enabled, hence allowing trans-endothelial migration. *T. denticola* DNA has already been detected in cerebrospinal fluid and brain tissue samples, demonstrating a potential contribution to neurodegeneration [40]. Moreover, a synergistic interaction between *P. gingivalis* and *T. Denticola* can worsen systemic inflammatory responses and promote joint colonization in autoimmune diseases, such as rheumatoid arthritis (RA) [41, 42]. Another key member of the dysbiotic community with systemic implications is *T. forsythia* [43]. The organism produces virulence factors, including BspA, a leucine-rich repeat protein that promotes epithelial invasion, and sialidases that enable mucosal breakdown [43]. These features enable *T. forsythia* to avoid immune detection and perpetuate low-grade chronic inflammation. Its DNA has been detected in pancreatic tissues, establishing a connection between its occurrence and insulin resistance, thereby causing the onset of metabolic syndrome and type 2 diabetes [44, 45]. Though *Aggregatibacter actinomycetemcomitans*

(*A. actinomycetemcomitans*) does not belong to the red complex category, it is a notable pathogen in systemic dissemination with its extremely powerful leukotoxin (LtxA) being specifically targeted against host leukocytes and causing immune suppression [46]. This microbe has been recovered from endocardial surfaces and heart valves and is considered one of the principal etiologic agents of infective endocarditis, especially in patients who have underlying cardiac disease [47]. This microorganism has also been associated with joint inflammation, and both its antigens and nucleic acids have been detected in synovial tissues, which has been found to be associated with arthritis-like symptoms in vulnerable patients [48]. In summary, the fact that these pathogens can migrate from the periodontal habitat to distal anatomical locations is a testament to their advanced pathogenic mechanisms. Not only do they establish themselves in extraoral habitats by endothelial attachment, immunomodulation, and proteolytic functions, but they are also directly implicated in the pathogenesis of intricate systemic disease [49]. This insight into microbial pathways explains the systemic relevance of periodontal health and reinforces the increasing acceptance of periodontitis as a modifiable risk factor for noncommunicable diseases, highlighting the interconnectedness of these pathogens and the complexity of the issue [50].

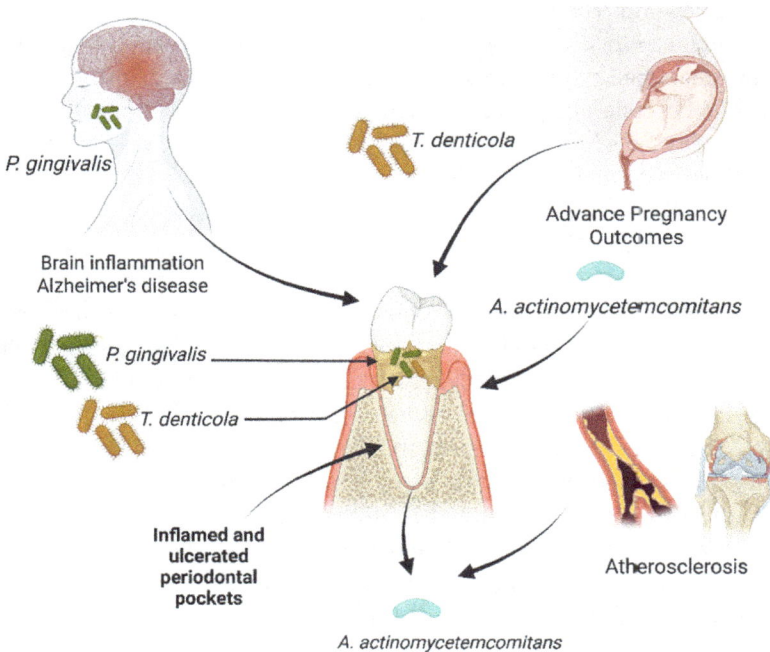

Figure 1.2: Systemic impact of periodontal pathogens. Oral bacteria disseminate from periodontal pockets and contribute to brain inflammation, adverse pregnancy outcomes, and atherosclerosis. The figure is created with Biorender.com.

1.3.2 Systemic Inflammation

Periodontitis is a chronic infectious inflammatory systemic disease that generates systemic inflammatory mediators, which circulate in the body and are involved in the pathogenesis of systemic diseases. CRP, IL-6, TNF-α, and MMPs are found to be key players among them [51] (Figure 1.3). These molecules are secreted by activated immune cells such as macrophages, dendritic cells, neutrophils, and gingival fibroblasts of inflamed periodontal tissue [51, 52]. Endotoxins secreted by the bacterium *P. gingivalis*, such as LPS, activate these cells via TLRs TLR2 and TLR4, resulting in a chronic and severe inflammatory response. After release into the local periodontal environment, these cytokines and enzymes move across the highly vascularized epithelial tissue of ulcerated periodontal pockets into the systemic bloodstream [53].

IL-6, a pleiotropic cytokine with diverse actions, is the major orchestrator of acute phase responses. It is the protein CRP, which rises in the blood during inflammation that is not only an inflammatory biomarker, but also a functional mediator because IL-6 causes the liver hepatocytes to produce this molecule [54]. Patients with periodontitis have elevated circulating concentrations of inflammatory biomarkers, including C-reactive protein (CRP), and are linked with endothelial dysfunction and vascular damage through mechanisms involving monocyte adhesion and low-density lipoprotein (LDL) uptake [51, 55]. The cytokine TNF-α, a signaling protein that participates in systemic inflammatory responses, plays a key role as it leads to insulin resistance, destabilizes atherosclerotic plaques, which are fatty deposits in arterial walls, and induces the expression of adhesion molecules and chemokines on vascular endothelium [56, 57]. This interaction of IL-6 with TNF-α is a feedback loop that augments systemic low-grade inflammation and hence worsens conditions like cardiovascular disease, type 2 diabetes, and RA, highlighting the urgent necessity to determine their effect [58].

MMP-8 and MMP-9, proteolytic enzymes released during periodontal disease remodeling, are important in the degradation of vascular connective tissues [59]. Their over-release systemically can cause atherosclerotic plaque instability and breakdown of joint cartilage, indicating the seriousness of their impact [60].

The pathophysiology of systemic diseases and periodontitis is due to the ongoing release of immuno-inflammatory mediators into the systemic circulation, as opposed to microbial transmission. Periodontal microbes infiltrate the circulation to reach distant tissues and create an inflammatory milieu that exacerbates pre-existing diseases and accelerates the course of disorders associated with endothelial dysfunction, insulin resistance, and connective tissue breakdown [28, 51].

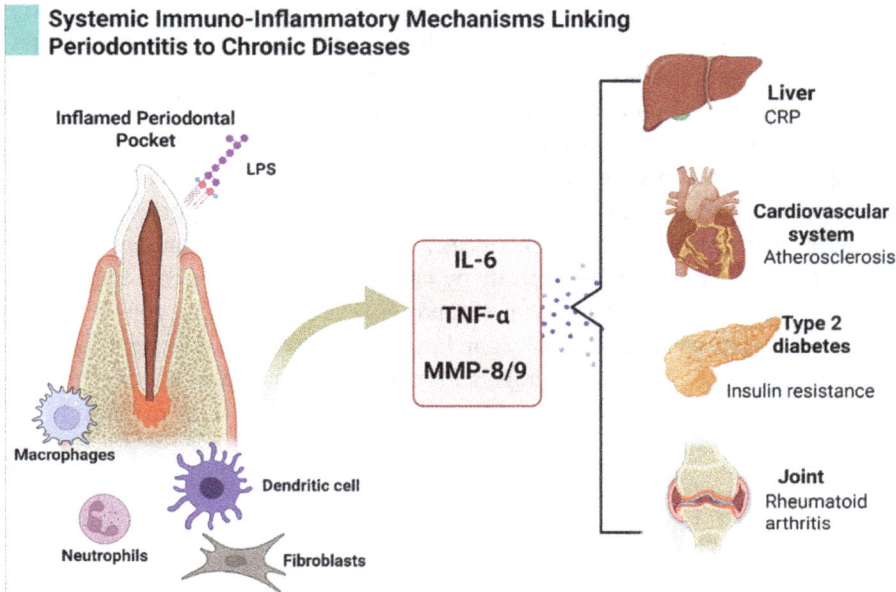

Systemic Immuno-Inflammatory Mechanisms Linking Periodontitis to Chronic Diseases

Figure 1.3: Systemic immunoinflammatory mechanisms linking periodontitis to chronic diseases. Periodontal inflammation drives IL-6, TNF-α, and MMP-8/9 release, contributing to systemic disorders. The figure is created with Biorender.com.

1.3.3 Molecular Mimicry and Immune Cross-Reactivity

Periodontal infections cause systemic disease via molecular mimicry mechanisms [28]. The unique enzyme peptidylarginine deiminase (PPAD), produced by *P. gingivalis*, plays a role in this process. The enzyme converts arginine residues in bacterial and host proteins to citrulline, creating a post-translational modification that results in citrullinated peptides (Figure 1.4). These peptides have similar sequences to citrullinated human tissue antigens and are presented by epitope-sharing alleles of HLA-DRB1 [61, 62].

This genetic element in genetically predisposed individuals enhances the ability of antigen-presenting cells to display citrullinated epitopes, thereby stimulating T-helper cells to generate anti-citrullinated protein antibodies (ACPAs) [63]. These ACPAs form immunological complexes that tend to accumulate in joints and other tissues, activate complement pathways, and trigger chronic inflammation. Importantly, a number of bacterial citrullinated proteins, such as citrullinated enolase and heat-shock proteins contain epitopes that are identical to host structural proteins in synovial tissue [61, 64].

The process of molecular mimicry subverts immunologic tolerance and thus triggers the initiation of systemic autoimmunity. In RA, this type of immunologic disequilibrium is expressed in terms of synovial membrane hyperplasia, neutrophil and macrophage infiltrate, and sequential cartilage and bone destruction [64]. Clinical and serological studies have suggested that patients with RA also possess elevated levels of both *P. gingivalis* DNA in subgingival plaque and circulating ACPAs, with longitudinal studies reporting a temporal relationship between the onset of periodontitis and ACPA seroconversion [65, 66]. Not only does *P. gingivalis* cause inflammation, but it also creates autoimmune disease directly by producing neoantigens that impair host immune regulation [67, 68]. This has profound implications in that it redefines periodontitis not merely as a localized infection but also as a potential etiology of systemic inflammatory disease [28, 51]. It highlights the cooperative nature of systemic disease prevention, making the audience feel the need for teamwork and cooperation in the process.

1.3.4 Dysregulated Innate Immunity

Periodontal infections greatly affect host immunity by regulating TLR signaling, an important part of the innate immune response [69]. The TLRs are pattern recognition receptors (PRRs) on the surfaces of epithelial cells, dendritic cells, macrophages, and neutrophils. They recognize conserved microbial structures called pathogen-associated molecular patterns (PAMPs) [70]. In periodontitis, TLR 2 and TLR 4 are mainly involved in recognizing bacterial components like LPS of *P. gingivalis*, lipoproteins of *T. denticola*, and other microbial patterns [71]. This recognition initiates NF-κB signaling and the release of pro-inflammatory cytokines like IL-1β, IL-6, and TNF-α for pathogen elimination. Periodontal pathogens have adapted mechanisms, however, to inhibit or suppress TLR signaling for their survival [72].

A prime example is the remarkable versatility of *P. gingivalis*, which is mirrored in the unusual composition of its LPS. The structure can stimulate or inhibit TLR 4 in a variable fashion, depending on the phosphorylation pattern of its lipid A [73, 74]. This extraordinary feature enables *P. gingivalis* to be a 'stealth pathogen,' suppressing antimicrobial activities when it is convenient and promoting inflammation when it is conducive to its ecological dominance [75]. Furthermore, *P. gingivalis* may also activate the TLR 2-TLR 1 heterodimer signaling pathway, contrasting with the classical TLR 4 pathways, and thereby orient subsequent signaling towards chronic, low-grade inflammation instead of efficacious bacterial clearance [76]. This ongoing activation results in a sustained release of inflammatory mediators into the systemic circulation, which cause insulin resistance, endothelial dysfunction, and acute-phase responses in the liver, and thus establish an association between oral infections and systemic metabolic dysregulation [77, 78].

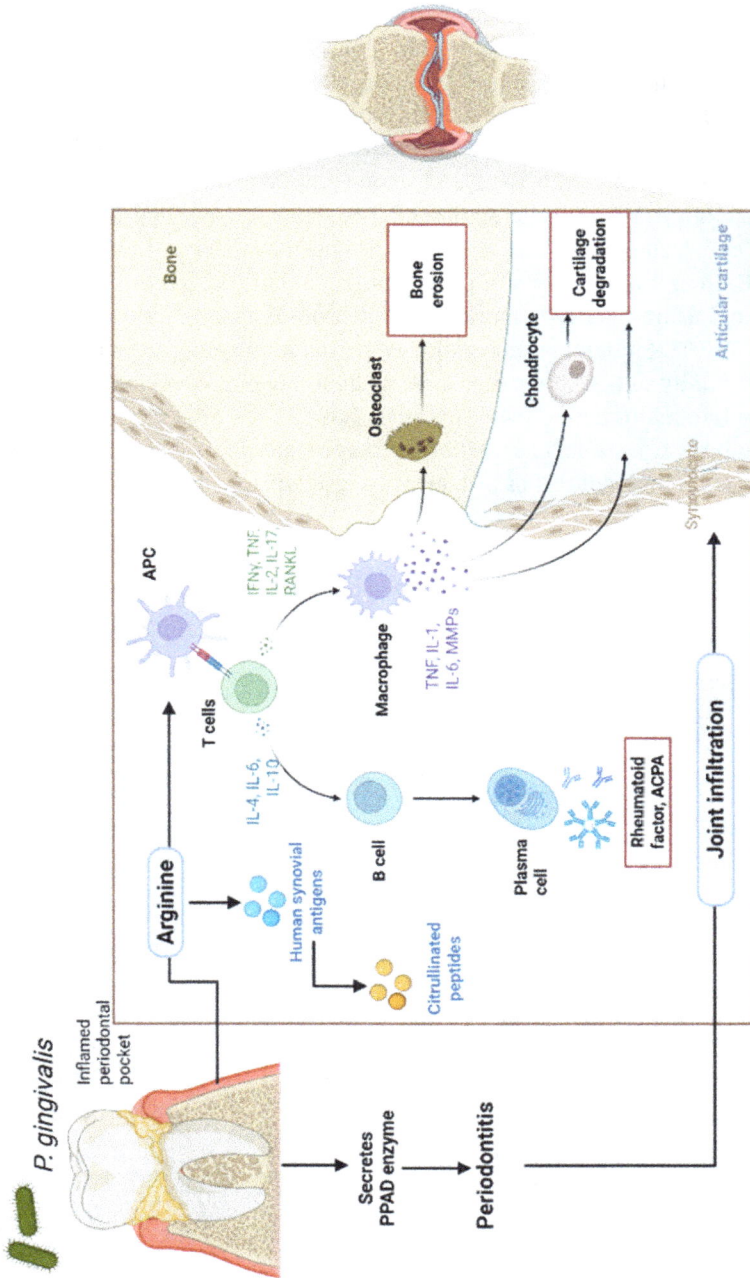

Figure 1.4: Pathogenic link between periodontitis and rheumatoid arthritis. *P. gingivalis* PAD enzyme activity promotes immune dysregulation, joint infiltration, and cartilage degradation. The figure is created with Biorender.com.

At the same time, these microbial signals trigger the activation of inflammasomes, more specifically the NLRP3 inflammasome, and a cytosolic sensor of danger signals [79]. NLRP3, when stimulated by bacterial products and metabolic stress, causes the maturation of pro-IL-1β and pro-IL-18 to active forms via caspase-1, thereby amplifying the inflammatory response [80] (Figure 1.5). Chronic stimulation of the inflammasome in periodontitis leads to local tissue destruction and systemic low-grade inflammation, which is implicated in a plethora of diseases such as type 2 diabetes, atherosclerosis, and Alzheimer's disease [23, 81]. Studies have shown increased systemic levels of IL-1β and IL-18 in severe periodontitis patients, which are associated with high levels of insulin resistance markers and neuroinflammatory events [82, 83]. By hijacking the TLR-TLR-inflammasome pathway, periodontal pathogens take advantage of innate immunity to keep their ecological niche in the oral cavity and promote a systemic pro-inflammatory state [84]. This issue has serious repercussions in advancing periodontitis from a local infection to a systemic disease, hence lending weight to the notion of periodontitis as a gateway to systemic inflammatory burden.

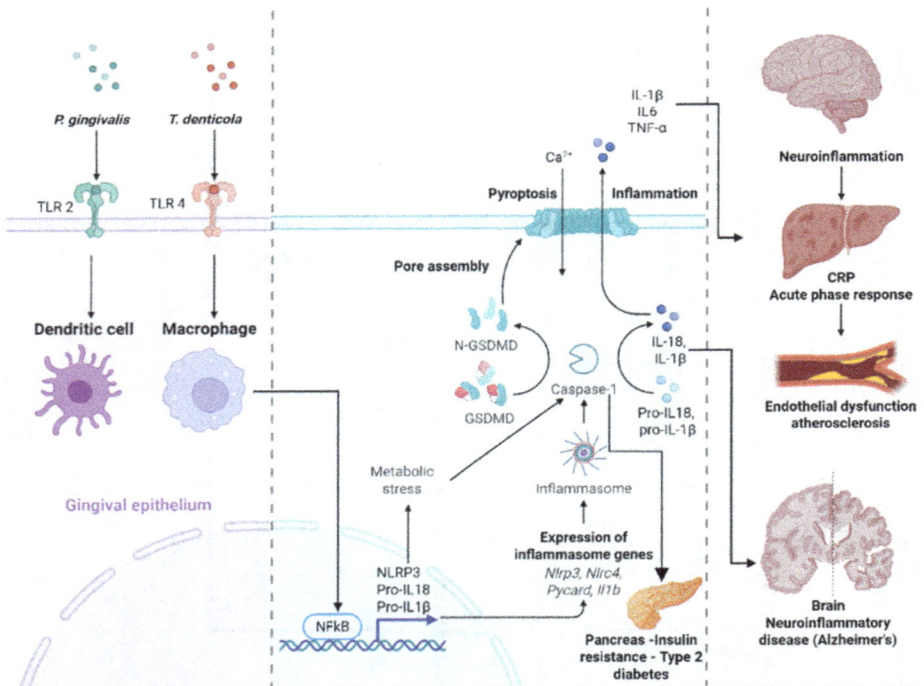

Figure 1.5: Molecular mechanisms linking periodontal pathogens with systemic inflammation. *P. gingivalis* and *T. denticola* activate TLR signaling, inflammasomes, and pyroptosis, contributing to neuroinflammation, liver CRP release, atherosclerosis, and metabolic dysfunction. The figure is created with Biorender.com.

1.4 Conclusion

This chapter delineates the complex role of periodontal dysbiosis in not only facilitating local tissue destruction but also as a contributing factor to systemic disease processes. Rather than a mere localized oral disease, periodontitis represents a biological pathway through which pathogenic bacteria and their virulence factors affect distant organs via mechanisms such as microbial translocation, systemic inflammation, immune mimicry, and dysregulated innate immunity. The systemic-oral link, once a theoretical concept, is now supported by molecular and clinical evidence, highlighting the far-reaching implications of maintaining periodontal health. Prominent pathogens, such as *P.gingivalis*, *F. nucleatum*, and *T. denticola*, have demonstrated effects that reach beyond the oral cavity, causing vascular impairment, neuroinflammatory events, adverse pregnancy outcomes, and autoimmune responses. Microbial components' interaction with host immune response not only sustains chronic inflammation but also constructs molecular environments favorable to disease onset in individuals with genetic susceptibility. Knowledge of these pathways transforms the conventional paradigm of periodontal treatment, altering it from a solely mechanical process to one in which the discipline demands the incorporation of systemic disease prevention strategies. This necessitates a more integrated model of health in which dental clinicians operate in close collaboration with medical practitioners to screen for risk patients and implement early interventions. Through the now more evident link between periodontitis and systemic disease, periodontal treatment has been regarded as an important component of overall health care, emphasizing its central position in preventive dentistry and public health policy.

References

[1]   Butera, A., & Scribante, A. (2025). Editorial for oral microbes and human health. Microorganisms, 13(4), 922.

[2]   Jiao, Y., Hasegawa, M., & Inohara, N. (2014). The role of oral pathobionts in dysbiosis during periodontitis development. Journal of Dental Research, 93(6), 539.

[3]   Cui, Z., Wang, P., & Gao, W. (2025). Microbial dysbiosis in periodontitis and peri-implantitis: Pathogenesis, immune responses, and therapeutic. Frontiers in Cellular Infection and Microbiology, 15, 1517154.

[4]   Chandra Nayak, S., Latha, P., & Kandanattu, B. et al. (2025). The oral microbiome and systemic health: Bridging the gap between dentistry and medicine. Cureus, 17(2), e78918.

[5]   Rajasekaran, J. J., Krishnamurthy, H. K., Bosco, J., Jayaraman, V., Krishna, K., Wang, T., & Bei, K. (2024). Oral microbiome: a review of its impact on oral and systemic health. Microorganisms, 12(9), 1797.

[6]   Liu, Y., Qv, W., Ma, Y., Zhang, Y., Ding, C., Chu, M., & Chen, F. (2022). The interplay between oral microbes and immune responses. Frontiers in Microbiology, 13, 1009018.

[7]   Isola, G., Santonocito, S., Lupi, S. M., Polizzi, A., Sclafani, R., Patini, R., & Marchetti, E. (2023). Periodontal health and disease in the context of systemic diseases. Inflammatory Mediators, 2023, 9720947.

[8]   Di Stefano, M., Polizzi, A., Santonocito, S., Romano, A., Lombardi, T., & Isola, G. (2022). Impact of oral microbiome in periodontal health and periodontitis: a critical review on prevention and treatment. International Journal of Molecular Sciences, 23(9), 5142.

[9]   Ezaura, E., Nicu, E. A., Krom, B. P., & Keijser, B. J. F. (2014). Acquiring and maintaining a normal oral microbiome: Current perspective. Frontiers in Cellular Infection and Microbiology, 4, 85.

[10] Khan, I., Bai, Y., Zha, L., Ullah, N., Ullah, H., Hussain Shah, S. R., Sun, H., & Zhang, C. (2021). Mechanism of the gut microbiota colonization resistance and enteric pathogen infection. Frontiers in Cellular Infection and Microbiology, 11, 716299.

[11] Bhatnagar, D. M. (2021). Oral health: a gateway to overall health. Contemporary Clinical Dentistry, 12(3), 211–212.

[12] Radaic, A., & Kapila, Y. L. (2020). The oralome and its dysbiosis: New insights into oral microbiome-host interactions. Computational and Structural Biotechnology Journal, 19, 1335–1360.

[13] Mohanty, R., Asopa, S. J., Joseph, M. D., Singh, B., Rajguru, J. P., Saidath, K., & Sharma, U. (2019). Red complex: Polymicrobial conglomerate in oral flora: a review. Journal of Family Medicine and Primary Care, 8(11), 3480.

[14] Kendlbacher, F. L., Bloch, S., Hager-Mair, F. F., Bacher, J., Janesch, B., Thurnheer, T., Andrukhov, O., & Schäffer, C. (2023). Multispecies biofilm behavior and host interaction support the association of *Tannerella serpentiformis* with periodontal health. Molecular Oral Microbiol, 38(2), 115–133.

[15] Xu, W., Zhou, W., Wang, H., & Liang, S. (2020). Roles of *Porphyromonas gingivalis* and its virulence factors in periodontitis. Advances in Protein Chemistry and Structural Biology, 120, 45.

[16] Kreve, S., & Reis, A. C. D. (2021). Bacterial adhesion to biomaterials: What regulates this attachment? A review. Japanese Dental Science Review, 57, 85–96.

[17] Chow, Y. C., Yam, H. C., Gunasekaran, B., Lai, W. Y., Wy, W., Agarwal, T., Ong, Y. Y., Cheong, S. L., & Tan, S. (2022). Implications of *Porphyromonas gingivalis* peptidyl arginine deiminase and gingipain R in human health and diseases. Frontiers in Cellular Infection and Microbiology, 12, 987683.

[18] Magaña, G., Harvey, C., Taggart, C. C., & Rodgers, A. M. (2023). Bacterial outer membrane vesicles: Role in pathogenesis and host-cell interactions. Antibiotics, 13(1), 32.

[19] Olsen, I., Lambris, J. D., & Hajishengallis, G. (2017). *Porphyromonas gingivalis* disturbs host-commensal homeostasis by changing complement function. Journal of Oral Microbiology, 9(1), 1340085.

[20] Maekawa, T., Krauss, J. L., Abe, T., Jotwani, R., Triantafilou, M., Triantafilou, K., Hashim, A., Hoch, S., Curtis, M. A., Nussbaum, G., Lambris, J. D., & Hajishengallis, G. (2014). *Porphyromonas gingivalis* manipulates complement and TLR signaling to uncouple bacterial clearance from inflammation and promote dysbiosis. Cell Host & Microbe, 15(6), 768.

[21] Coutinho-Silva, R. (2019). Immunological pathways triggered by *Porphyromonas gingivalis* and *Fusobacterium nucleatum*: Therapeutic possibilities?. Inflammatory Mediators, 2019, 7241312.

[22] Hajishengallis, G., Kajikawa, T., Hajishengallis, E., Maekawa, T., Reis, E. S., Mastellos, D. C., Yancopoulou, D., Hasturk, H., & Lambris, J. D. (2019). Complement-dependent mechanisms and interventions in periodontal disease. Frontiers Immunol, 10, 406.

[23] Hashim, N., Babiker, R., Mohammed, R., Rehman, M. M., & Gobara, B. (2023). The role of inflammasomes in periodontal disease and pathogenesis. Journal of Population Therapeutics and Clinical Pharmacology, 30(6), 226–238.

[24] Olsen, I. (2008). Update on bacteraemia related to dental procedures. Transfusion and Apheresis Science, 39(2), 173–178.

[25] Zachary, J. F. (2017). Mechanisms of microbial infections. In: Pathologic Basis of Veterinary Disease, 6th ed., Elsevier: St Louis, 132.

] Rocca, P., Fornaini, C., Wang, Z., Tan, L., & Merigo, E. (2020). Focal infection and periodontitis: a narrative report and new possible approaches. International Journal of Microbiology, 2020, 8875612.

[27] Czerniuk, M. R., Surma, S., Romańczyk, M., Nowak, J. M., Wojtowicz, A., & Filipiak, K. J. (2022). Unexpected relationships: Periodontal diseases, atherosclerosis-plaque destabilization? From the teeth to a coronary event. Biology (Basel), 11(2), 272.

[28] Hajishengallis, G. (2015). Periodontitis: from microbial immune subversion to systemic inflammation. Nature Reviews Immunology, 15(1), 30–44.

[29] Li, X., Kolltveit, K. M., Tronstad, L., & Olsen, I. (2000). Systemic diseases caused by oral infection. Clinical Microbiology Reviews, 13(4), 547–558.

[30] Mei, F., Xie, M., Huang, X., Long, Y., Lu, X., Wang, X., & Chen, L. (2020). Porphyromonas gingivalis and its systemic impact: Current status. Pathogens, 9(11), 944.

[31] Bikker, F. J., Gibbs, S., & Krom, B. P. (2023). Mechanisms of *Porphyromonas gingivalis* to translocate over the oral mucosa and other tissue barriers. Journal of Oral Microbiology, 15(1), 2205291.

[32] Ruan, Q., Guan, P., Qi, W., Li, J., Xi, M., Xiao, L., Zhong, S., Ma, D., & Ni, J. (2023). Porphyromonas gingivalis regulates atherosclerosis through an immune pathway. Frontiers Immunol, 14, 1103592.

[33] Ahn, S., Yang, J. W., Oh, J., Shin, Y. Y., Kang, J., Park, H. R., Seo, Y., & Kim, S. (2021). *Porphyromonas gingivalis* exacerbates the progression of fatty liver disease via CD36-PPARγ pathway. BMB Reports, 54(6), 323.

[34] León, R., Silva, N., Ovalle, A., Chaparro, A., Ahumada, A., M,, Martinez, M., & Gamonal, J. (2007). Detection of *Porphyromonas gingivalis* in the amniotic fluid in pregnant women with a diagnosis of threatened premature labor. Journal of Periodontol, 78(7), 1249–1255.

[35] Dominy, S. S., Lynch, C., Ermini, F., Benedyk, M., Marczyk, A., Konradi, A., Nguyen, M., Haditsch, U., Raha, D., Griffin, C., Holsinger, L. J., Arastu-Kapur, S., Kaba, S., Lee, A., Ryder, M. I., Potempa, B., Mydel, P., Hellvard, A., & Adamowicz, K. et al. (2019). *Porphyromonas gingivalis* in Alzheimer's disease brains: Evidence for disease causation and treatment with small-molecule inhibitors. Science Advances, 5(1), eaau3333.

[36] Sun, C., Li, B., Wang, B., Zhao, J., Zhang, X., Li, T., Li, W., Tang, D., Qiu, M., Wang, X., Zhu, C., & Qian, Z. (2019). The role of *Fusobacterium nucleatum* in colorectal cancer: From carcinogenesis to clinical management. Chronic Diseases and Translational Medicine, 5(3), 178–187.

[37] Fardini, Y., Wang, X., Temoin, S., Nithianantham, S., Lee, D., Shoham, M., & Han, Y. W. (2011). *Fusobacterium nucleatum* adhesin FadA binds vascular endothelial cadherin and alters endothelial integrity. Molecular Microbiology, 82(6), 1468–1480.

[38] Vander Haar, E. L., So, J., Gyamfi-Bannerman, C., & Han, Y. W. (2018). *Fusobacterium nucleatum* and adverse pregnancy outcomes: Epidemiological and mechanistic evidence. Anaerobe, 50, 55–59.

[39] Dashper, S. G., Seers, C. A., Tan, K. H., & Reynolds, E. C. (2011). Virulence factors of the oral spirochete *Treponema denticola*. Journal of Dental Research, 90(6), 691–703.

[40] Pisani, F., Pisani, V., Arcangeli, F., Harding, A., & Singhrao, S. K. (2023). *Treponema denticola* has the potential to cause neurodegeneration in the midbrain via the periodontal route of infection – a narrative review. International Journal of Environmental Research and Public Health, 20(11), 6049.

[41] Zhu, Y., Dashper, S. G., Chen, Y. Y., Crawford, S., Slakeski, N., & Reynolds, E. C. (2013). *Porphyromonas gingivalis* and *Treponema denticola* synergistic polymicrobial biofilm development. PLoS One, 8(8), e71727.

[42] Lu, J., Wang, Y., Wu, J., Duan, Y., Zhang, H., & Du, H. (2025). Linking microbial communities to rheumatoid arthritis: Focus on gut, oral microbiome and their extracellular vesicles. Frontiers Immunol, 16, 1503474.

[43] Schäffer, C., & Andrukhov, O. (2024). The intriguing strategies of *Tannerella forsythia*'s host interaction. Frontiers in Oral Health, 5, 1434217.

[44] Sekot, G., Posch, G., Messner, P., Matejka, M., Rausch-Fan, X., Andrukhov, O., & Schäffer, C. (2011). Potential of the *Tannerella forsythia* S-layer to delay the immune response. Journal of Dental Research, 90(1), 109–114.

[45] Ogrendik, M. (2015). Oral bacteria in pancreatic cancer: Mutagenesis of the p53 tumour suppressor gene. International Journal of Clinical & Experimental Pathology, 8(9), 11835–11836.

[46] Talapko, J., Juzbasic, M., Mestrovic, T., Matijevic, T., Mesaric, D., & Katalinic, D. et al. (2024). *Aggregatibacter actinomycetemcomitans*: from the oral cavity to the heart valves. Microorganisms, 12(7), 1451.

[47] Norskov-Lauritsen, N., Claesson, R., Birkeholm Jensen, A., Aberg, C. H., & Haubek, D. (2019). *Aggregatibacter actinomycetemcomitans*: Clinical significance of a pathobiont subjected to ample changes in classification and nomenclature. Pathogens, 8(4), 243.

[48] Looh, S. C., Soo, Z. M. P., Wong, J. J., Yam, H. C., Chow, S. K., & Hwang, J. S. (2022). *Aggregatibacter actinomycetemcomitans* as the aetiological cause of rheumatoid arthritis: What are the unsolved puzzles? Toxins (Basel), 14(1), 50.

[49] Elgreu, T., Lee, S., Wen, S., Elghadafi, R., Tangkham, T., & Ma, Y. et al. (2022). The pathogenic mechanism of oral bacteria and treatment with inhibitors. Clinical and Experimental Dental Research, 8(1), 439–448.

[50] Hashim, N. T., Babiker, R., Priya, S. P., Mohammed, R., Chaitanya, N. C., & Padmanabhan, V. et al. (2024). Microbial dynamics in periodontal regeneration: Understanding microbiome shifts and the role of antifouling and bactericidal materials – a narrative review. Current Issues in Molecular Biology, 46(11), 12196–12213.

[51] Martinez-Garcia, M., & Hernandez-Lemus, E. (2021). Periodontal inflammation and systemic diseases: An overview. Frontiers in Physiology, 12, 709438.

[52] Huang, N. (2014). Immuno-pathogenesis of periodontal disease: Current and emerging paradigms. Current Oral Health Reports, 1(2), 124.

[53] Marcano, R., Rojo, M. A., Cordoba-Diaz, D., & Garrosa, M. (2021). Pathological and therapeutic approach to endotoxin-secreting bacteria involved in periodontal disease. Toxins, 13(8), 533.

[54] Tanaka, T., Narazaki, M., & Kishimoto, T. (2014). IL-6 in inflammation, immunity, and disease. Cold Spring Harbor Laboratory Press, 6(10), a016295.

[55] Hajishengallis, G., & Chavakis, T. (2021). Local and systemic mechanisms linking periodontal disease and inflammatory comorbidities. Nature Reviews Immunology, 21(7), 426–440.

[56] Da Costa, R. M., Neves, K. B., & Mestriner, F. L. et al. (2016). TNF-α induces vascular insulin resistance via positive modulation of PTEN and decreased Akt/eNOS/NO signaling in high fat diet-fed mice. Cardiovascular Diabetology, 15, 119.

[57] Yuan, T., Yang, T., Chen, H., Fu, D., Hu, Y., & Wang, J. et al. (2018). New insights into oxidative stress and inflammation during diabetes mellitus-accelerated atherosclerosis. Redox Biology, 20, 247–260.

[58] Tylutka, A., & Walas, L. (2024). Level of IL-6, TNF, and IL-1β and age-related diseases: a systematic review and meta-analysis. Frontiers Immunol, 15, 1330386.

[59] Luchian, I., Goriuc, A., Sandu, D., & Covasa, M. (2022). The role of matrix metalloproteinases (MMP-8, MMP-9, MMP-13) in periodontal and peri-implant pathological processes. International Journal of Molecular Sciences, 23(3), 1806.

[60] Wang, X., & Khalil, R. A. (2018). Matrix metalloproteinases, vascular remodeling, and vascular disease. Advanced Pharmacology, 81, 241–330.

[61] Krutyholowa, A., Strzelec, K., Dziedzic, A., Bereta, G. P., Potempa, J., & Gawron, K. (2022). Host and bacterial factors linking periodontitis and rheumatoid arthritis. Frontiers Immunol, 13, 980805.

[62] Gawron, K., Bereta, G., Nowakowska, Z., Lazarz, M., Szmigielski, B., & Mizgalska, D. et al. (2014). Peptidylarginine deiminase from *Porphyromonas gingivalis* (PPAD) contributes to infection of gingival fibroblasts and induction of PGE2-signaling pathway. Molecular Oral Microbiol, 29(6), 321.

[63] Nguyen, H., & James, E. A. (2016). Immune recognition of citrullinated epitopes. Immunology, 149(2), 131.

[64] Kurowska, W., Kuca-Warnawin, E. H., Radzikowska, A., & Maslinski, W. (2017). The role of anti-citrullinated protein antibodies (ACPA) in the pathogenesis of rheumatoid arthritis. Central European Journal of Immunology, 42(4), 390.

[65] Westra, J., Vissink, A., & Brouwer, E. (2012). Periodontitis in established rheumatoid arthritis patients: a cross-sectional clinical, microbiological and serological study. Arthritis Res Ther, 14(5), R222.

[66] Astuti, L., Masulili, S. L., Gunardi, I., Sulijaya, B., & Soeroso, Y. (2025). Periodontal pathogens correlate with rheumatoid arthritis disease parameters: a systematic review based on clinical studies. Journal of Dentistry, 13(5), 214.

[67] Tracy, A., Buckley, C. D., & Raza, K. (2017). Pre-symptomatic autoimmunity in rheumatoid arthritis: When does the disease start? Seminars in Immunopathology, 39, 423–435.

[68] Quirke, A. M., Lugli, E. B., & Wegner, N. et al. (2014). Heightened immune response to autocitrullinated *Porphyromonas gingivalis* peptidylarginine deiminase: a potential mechanism for breaching immunologic tolerance in rheumatoid arthritis. Annals of the Rheumatic Diseases, 73, 263–269.

[69] Gu, Y., & Han, X. (2020). Toll-like receptor signaling and immune regulatory lymphocytes in periodontal disease. International Journal of Molecular Sciences, 21(9), 3329.

[70] Wicherska-Pawlowska, K., Wrobel, T., & Rybka, J. (2021). Toll-like receptors (TLRs), NOD-like receptors (NLRs), and RIG-I-like receptors (RLRs) in innate immunity: TLRs, NLRs, and RLRs ligands as immunotherapeutic agents for hematopoietic diseases. International Journal of Molecular Sciences, 22(24), 13397.

[71] Marchesan, J., Jiao, Y., Schaff, R. A., Hao, J., Morelli, T., & Kinney, J. S. et al. (2015). TLR4, NOD1 and NOD2 mediate immune recognition of putative newly identified periodontal pathogens. Molecular Oral Microbiol, 31(3), 243.

[72] Su, G., Peng, Y., Ruan, H., Cheng, J., Deng, T., & Zhang, Y. (2025). Regulating periodontal disease with smart stimuli-responsive systems: Antimicrobial activity, immunomodulation, periodontium regeneration. Materials Today Bio, 32, 101863.

[73] Xiao, X., Sankaranarayanan, K., & Khosla, C. (2017). Biosynthesis and structure–activity relationships of the lipid A family of glycolipids. Current Opinion in Chemical Biology, 40, 127–137.

[74] Garcia-Vello, P., Di Lorenzo, F., Zucchetta, D., Zamyatina, A., De Castro, C., & Molinaro, A. (2022). Lipopolysaccharide lipid A: a promising molecule for new immunity-based therapies and antibiotics. Pharmacology and Therapeutics, 230, 107970.

[75] Chopra, A., Bhat, S. G., & Sivaraman, K. (2020). *Porphyromonas gingivalis* adopts intricate and unique molecular mechanisms to survive and persist within the host: a critical update. Journal of Oral Microbiology, 12(1), 1801090.

[76] Pandi, K., Angabo, S., Gnanasekaran, J., Makkawi, H., Eli-Berchoer, L., Glaser, F., & Nussbaum, G. (2023). *Porphyromonas gingivalis* induction of TLR2 association with vinculin enables PI3K activation and immune evasion. PLOS Pathogens, 19(4), e1011284.

[77] Wielento, A., Bereta, G. P., Lagosz-Cwik, K. B., Eick, S., Lamont, R. J., Grabiec, A. M., & Potempa, J. (2022). TLR2 activation by *Porphyromonas gingivalis* requires both PPAD activity and fimbriae. Frontiers Immunol, 13, 823685.

[78] Maekawa, T., Krauss, J. L., Abe, T., Jotwani, R., Triantafilou, M., & Triantafilou, K. et al. (2014). *Porphyromonas gingivalis* manipulates complement and TLR signaling to uncouple bacterial clearance from inflammation and promote dysbiosis. Cell Host & Microbe, 15(6), 768–778.

[79] Swanson, K. V., Deng, M., & Ting, Y. (2019). The NLRP3 inflammasome: Molecular activation and regulation to therapeutics. Nature Reviews Immunology, 19(8), 477.

[80] Paik, S., Kim, J. K., Silwal, P., Sasakawa, C., & Jo, E. (2021). An update on the regulatory mechanisms of NLRP3 inflammasome activation. Cellular and Molecular Immunology, 18(5), 1141–1160.

[81] Hashim, N., Babiker, R., Mohammed, R., Rehman, M. M., Ncsk, C., & Gobara, B. (2024). NLRP3 inflammasome in autoinflammatory diseases and periodontitis: advances in management. Journal of Pharmacy and Bioallied Sciences, 16(Suppl 2), S1110–9.

[82] Alarcon-Sanchez, M. A., Romero-Castro, N. S., Becerra-Ruiz, J. S., Romero-Servin, S., & Heboyan, A. (2024). Increased IL-18 levels are associated with periodontitis: a systematic review and meta-analysis. BMC Oral Health, 24, 981.

[83] Su, Y., Ye, L., Hu, C., Zhang, Y., Liu, J., & Shao, L. (2023). Periodontitis as a promoting factor of T2D: Current evidence and mechanisms. International Journal of Oral Science, 15(1), 1–12.

[84] Abdulkareem, A. A., Al-Taweel, F. B., Al-Sharqi, A. J. B., Gul, S. S., Sha, A., & Chapple, I. L. C. (2023). Current concepts in the pathogenesis of periodontitis: From symbiosis to dysbiosis. Journal of Oral Microbiology, 15(1) 2197779.

Nada Tawfig Hashim, Rasha Babiker, and Riham Mohammed
2 Periodontitis and Systemic Diseases

2.1 Introduction

Periodontitis has evolved from a merely localized oral infection to a chronic inflammatory disease of greater systemic importance [1]. Increasing evidence from the fields of molecular biology, immunology, and clinical epidemiology has transformed our knowledge regarding its importance as an etiologic agent in a variety of systemic diseases [2]. The dynamic interaction between periodontal pathogens and host immune mechanisms not only leads to local tissue damage but also initiates a cascade of inflammatory, microbial, and metabolic events with extraoral consequences [3]. The delivery of microbial constituents, systemic increase in pro-inflammatory mediators, molecular mimicry, and reprogramming of the immune responses are all part of the biological process by which periodontitis affects distant organs [4]. These processes are now associated with the initiation and development of a range of chronic diseases, such as cardiovascular disease (CVD), diabetes mellitus, adverse pregnancy outcomes, neurodegenerative disease (e.g., Alzheimer's disease (AD)), rheumatoid arthritis (RA), and chronic obstructive pulmonary disease (COPD) [3, 5].

This chapter discusses the mechanistic links of periodontitis to various systemic diseases, incorporating recent advances in microbial genomics, host-pathogen interaction, and translational medicine. By shedding light on the common pathways of inflammation, immune dysregulation, and microbial translocation, this chapter emphasizes the systemic importance of periodontal health. Furthermore, it addresses the clinical significance of such associations and promotes a more integrated model of health care involving both dental and medical care in chronic disease prevention and management.

2.2 Periodontitis and Cardiovascular Disease (CVD)

The association of periodontitis with CVD extends beyond epidemiological correlation and suggests mechanistically linked pathobiology on the grounds of chronic inflammation, microbial translocation, and endothelial dysfunction [6, 7]. Recent evidence based on high-throughput sequencing and proteomic analysis validates that periodontal pathogens, notably *Porphyromonas gingivalis* (*P. gingivalis*), *Aggregatibacter actinomycetemcomitans* (*A. Actinomycetemcomitans*), and *Fusobacterium nucleatum* (*F. nucleatum*), possess the potential for hematogenous spread during mastication or dental intervention, with concomitant presence of bacterial DNA and live species in human atheromatous plaques [8, 9]. This implies not merely association but even di-

https://doi.org/10.1515/9783112219904-002

rect microbial colonization and causality in atherogenesis [10]. *P. gingivalis* has been demonstrated to infect endothelial cells, and trigger TLR2 – and TLR4 – TLR2/TLR4-dependent signaling, inducing eNOS (endothelial Nitric Oxide Synthase) downregulation and compromised nitric oxide (NO) bioavailability – features of early endothelial dysfunction [11]. Pathogen-induced nuclear factor kappa B (NF-κB) and MAPK pathway activation, on the contrary, upregulates adhesion molecules VCAM-1 (Vascular Cell Adhesion Molecule-1) and ICAM-1 (Vascular Cell Adhesion Molecule-1) to promote monocyte adhesion and transmigration into the intima. Besides structural vascular damage, periodontal inflammation leads to a pro-thrombotic state [12, 13]. Systemic elevation of cytokines interleukin-6 (IL-6), tumor necrosis factor-alpha (TNF-α) instigates hepatic synthesis of acute-phase reactants, such as fibrinogen and C-reactive protein (CRP), while bacterial virulence factors, such as gingipains in *P. gingivalis* directly activate platelets through protease-activated receptor (PAR) signaling to induce aggregation, thrombin generation, and fibrin clot [14] (Figure 2.1).

A. Actinomycetemcomitans secretes leukotoxin A (LtxA), which causes leukocyte lysis and formation of neutrophil extracellular traps (NETosis) and thus enhances vascular inflammation and thrombogenesis [15]. Recent translational research has also highlighted the role of immune-metabolic cross-talk, where *P. gingivalis* modulates lipid metabolism by upregulating oxidized low-density lipoprotein (LDL) receptors (CD36 and LOX-1), and induces foam cell formation [16, 17]. Additionally, periodontitis also appears to activate bone marrow-derived myeloid progenitor cells to differentiate into a pro-inflammatory phenotype (trained immunity) that persists systemically even after periodontal treatment. Such changes not only augment the progression of atherosclerosis but also predispose the subject to plaque rupture and acute coronary events [18, 19].

Therapeutically, periodontal treatment – scaling and root planing, adjunctive antimicrobials, and host-modulation therapy – has been linked to improvement in flow-mediated dilation, CRP and IL-6 suppression, and endothelial biomarker stabilization [20–22]. More recent investigations highlight the influence of timing, disease severity, and host susceptibility (e.g., diabetics or apolipoprotein E (ApoE) variant subjects) on cardiovascular benefit [23–25]. Future directions will likely include CRISPR-mediated manipulation of bacterial virulence, keystone pathogen vaccine targeting, and application of biologic agents (e.g., interleukin-1 beta (IL-1β) inhibitors) in high-risk periodontitis-CVD individuals.

Periodontitis and CVD are linked by microbial, inflammatory, thrombotic, and metabolic pathways. Understanding these processes not only strengthens oral health as one of the determinants of systemic disease prevention but also gives a scientific basis for periodontal treatment as a measure to alter cardiovascular risk [26, 27].

2.3 Periodontitis and Diabetes Mellitus

The relationship between periodontitis and diabetes mellitus is now recognized as a strong, bidirectional relationship, based on shared pathophysiology through chronic inflammation, immune dysregulation, and tissue destruction [28] (Figure 2.1). Hyperglycemia in diabetes leads to the deposition of advanced glycation end-products (AGEs) in periodontal tissues. These AGEs bind to their receptor (RAGE) on endothelial cells and macrophages, inducing NF-κB-mediated pro-inflammatory cytokine transcription of IL-1β, IL-6, and TNF-α that perpetuate and exacerbate periodontal inflammation [29, 30]. Meanwhile, hyperglycemia impairs neutrophil chemotaxis and phagocytosis, increases oxidative stress, and inhibits collagen synthesis and cross-linking, leading to defective wound healing and accelerated periodontal destruction [31-33]. These host-modulated alterations create a dysbiotic microenvironment that supports keystone pathogens such as *P. gingivalis* and *Tannerella forsythia* (*T. forsythia*) [34]. However, it is important to consider that periodontitis has systemic metabolic consequences that adversely impact insulin resistance and glycemic control to a significant degree. This chronic disease state results in a persistent overproduction of IL-6, TNF-α, and CRP, known to inhibit insulin receptor substrate (IRS) signaling in hepatocytes, adipocytes, and muscle cells [35, 36]. Interestingly, *P. gingivalis* can invade extraoral tissues and directly inhibit GLUT4 translocation via TLR2/TLR4-induced JNK and PI3K/ AKT pathway activation. In hepatocytes, cysteine proteases gingipains secreted by *P. gingivalis* induce lipid accumulation and ER stress, further disrupting metabolism [37, 38]. *F. nucleatum* has also been implicated in destabilizing intestinal barrier function, inducing gut-derived endotoxemia, which can synergize with oral-derived inflammation to exacerbate insulin resistance [39, 40].

Current evidence strongly supports the role of periodontitis in shaping adipokine profiles. It tends to increase leptin and resistin levels while decreasing adiponectin, a profile closely associated with metabolic syndrome and type 2 diabetes [41, 42].

There is strong therapeutic evidence that nonsurgical periodontal treatment results in modest but statistically significant decreases in HbA1c (Hemoglobin A1c) levels (mean difference ~0.4%), especially in individuals with poorly controlled diabetes [43, 44]. These effects are even greater when treatment is supported with adjunctive antimicrobials, host-modulation therapy, or probiotics that replenish microbiome balance and minimize systemic endotoxemia [45-47]. Periodontal therapy also has the added advantage of decreasing systemic markers of oxidative stress and enhancing endothelial function in diabetic patients [48]. Thus, the incorporation of dental and medical care, especially in chronic disease care models, is essential for enhancing both periodontal and metabolic outcomes.

The bidirectional interplay between periodontal disease and derangements in glycemic control requires bidirectional screening, interdisciplinary treatment guidelines, and individualized therapeutic approaches based on patients' immunometabolic profiles. Additional knowledge of shared molecular mechanisms – i.e., TLR signaling pathways, AGE-RAGE axis, and cytokine regulatory networks – can yield novel therapies that address both periodontal and diabetic manifestations concurrently.

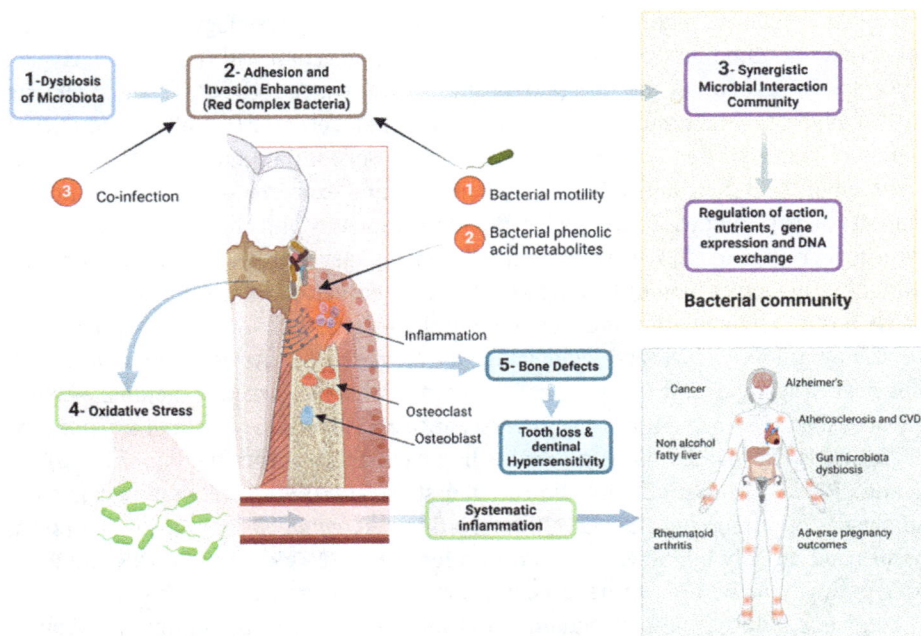

Figure 2.1: Overview of pathways linking oral microbiota to systemic diseases. Pathogenic bacteria adhere to and invade oral tissues, interact within biofilms, and trigger oxidative stress, enhancing virulence and immune modulation. These events facilitate bacterial dissemination and inflammatory mediator release into circulation, contributing to chronic inflammation and extraoral conditions, such as CVD, diabetes, and adverse pregnancy outcomes. Created with Biorender.com.

2.4 Periodontitis and Adverse Pregnancy Outcomes

The link between periodontitis during pregnancy and adverse pregnancy outcomes – preterm birth, low birth weight, preeclampsia, and intrauterine growth restriction – has been the subject of much interest over the past two decades [49]. While early epidemiological research suggested a strong association, subsequent molecular and mechanistic research has identified the pathways by which periodontal disease potentially contributes to complications in pregnancy, including microbial translocation, systemic inflammation, and placental immune activation [50–52].

During pregnancy, hormonal and immunological changes increase gingival vascularity and impair local immune surveillance, exacerbating gingival inflammation and facilitating microbial invasion of subepithelial tissues [53, 54]. *F. nucleatum, P. gingivalis,* and

Treponema denticola have been recovered in placental tissue, amniotic fluid, and fetal membranes in most instances of pregnancy complicated by premature rupture of membranes, preterm labor, or stillbirth [50, 55, 56]. *F. nucleatum*, indeed, bears FadA adhesin, which binds to VE-cadherin in endothelial cells to promote hematogenous dissemination across the feto-maternal barrier [57]. Upon translocation, microbes are capable of directly stimulating TLR4 and TLR2 signaling in decidual and trophoblast cells, initiating local inflammation with elevated prostaglandins, TNF-α, and IL-1β – mediators known to cause uterine contractility and cervical ripening and lead to preterm labor [58].

Other than direct microbial effect, systemic dissemination of pro-inflammatory cytokines like IL-6, interleukin-8 (IL-8), CRP, and TNF-α in the course of periodontal inflammation can cross the placental barrier and alter fetal growth [59] (Figure 2.2). These cytokines promote decidual vasoconstriction, deficient trophoblastic invasion, and endothelial dysfunction, mechanisms that are central to the development of pre-eclampsia [60, 61]. Moreover, gram-negative periodontal bacterium lipopolysaccharide (LPS) can disrupt the function of syncytiotrophoblast, reduce placental perfusion, and stimulate the maternal hypothalamic-pituitary-adrenal axis to increase circulating cortisol, thereby inhibiting fetal growth and reducing birth weight [62, 63].

Recent reports also illustrate epigenetic control of placental gene expression by periodontal pathogens. For instance, *P. gingivalis* infection is shown to alter DNA methylation and miRNA (microRNA) expression patterns of angiogenesis genes (e.g., VEGF (Vascular Endothelial Growth Factor), immune regulatory genes, and nutrient transport genes, thereby creating a link between oral infection and long-term developmental programming of the fetus [64–66]. In spite of the clear mechanistic insight, interventional studies aiming at periodontal therapy during pregnancy have provided conflicting results. Some studies show a positive effect of periodontal therapy on reducing preterm birth and low birth weight, while others find no significant benefit, particularly when treatment is initiated late in pregnancy [67–69]. Meta-analyses indicate that interventions – typically scaling and root planing – delivered prior to the 28th week of pregnancy can decrease preterm birth and low birth weight, especially in females with severe periodontitis [70, 71]. The heterogeneity in study settings, diagnostic criteria, microbial profiles, and treatment regimens prevents direct comparisons. In addition, the timing of therapy, the level of pre-existing inflammation, and host genetic determinants can modify therapeutic efficacy [71].

In the future, emerging approaches like probiotic-guided oral home care, modulating host response with anti-inflammatory compounds, and CRISPR-mediated pathogen control hold enormous potential for more precise oral inflammation control in pregnancy. Periodontal evaluation and prevention should be made a part of standard prenatal care protocols, especially in those who are at increased risk, to prevent the inflammatory load on the maternal-fetal interface. Periodontitis affects pregnancy outcomes by direct microbial invasion of fetal tissues and indirect systemic immunoinflammatory mechanisms [61–65]. Understanding these mechanisms points to the importance of early recognition and personalized periodontal disease treatment as an integral component of overall maternal health care.

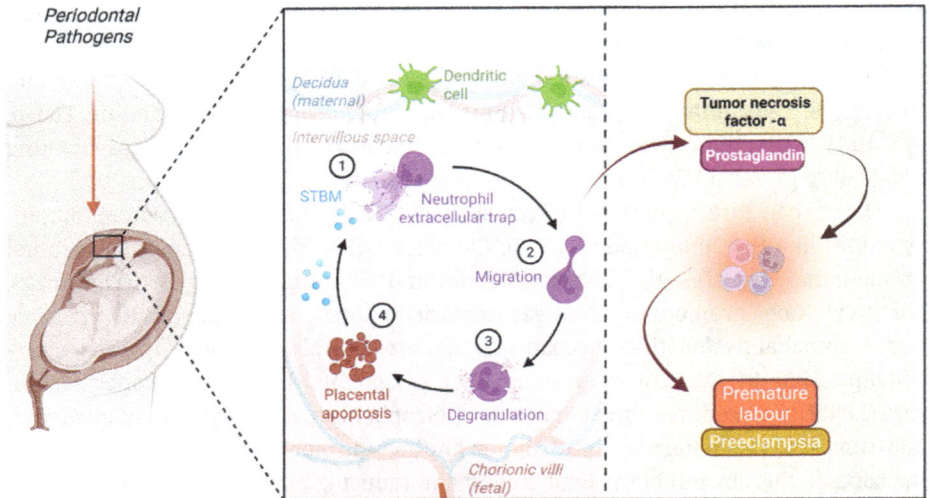

Figure 2.2: Mechanism linking periodontal infection to adverse pregnancy outcomes. Pathogens trigger placental immune activation/NETs, raising TNF-α and prostaglandins that precipitate preeclampsia and preterm labor. Created with Biorender.com.

2.5 Periodontitis and Alzheimer's Disease

The convergence of neurodegeneration and oral health has been increasingly attracting attention with the advent of the oral-brain axis concept [72]. Accumulating evidence supports that periodontitis, may have a significant role in the etiogenesis of AD and other dementias [73]. The connection is based on microbial translocation, priming of neuroinflammation, and direct neurotoxicity, thereby transforming the conventional framework of AD pathogenesis [74, 75] (Figure 2.3). A particular observation has been the presence of *P. gingivalis* DNA, (LPS), and gingipains (prominently Kgp and Rgp proteases) in the hippocampus, cerebral cortex, and cerebrospinal fluid of AD brains [76]. Notably, gingipains have been found to degrade tau protein at selective lysine and arginine residues, thereby promoting the hyperphosphorylation and eventual formation of tau into neurofibrillary tangles – a hallmark of Alzheimer's pathology [77]. Furthermore, gingipains destabilize synaptic integrity and interfere with host proteins of seminal significance in neuronal signaling, including the NMDA (N-Methyl-D-Aspartate) receptor subunit and ApoE, thereby enhancing synaptic loss and damaging memory functions [78–80].

From a mechanistic perspective, *P. gingivalis* has several ways to invade the CNS [1]: hematogenous spread during episodes of transient bacteremia, particularly in patients with severe periodontitis and systemic inflammation [2, 81]; retrograde axonal transport via the trigeminal nerve, providing a direct route for delivery of bacterial components to the brainstem and beyond [3, 82]; and compromised integrity of the blood-brain barrier (BBB) in older or inflamed patients, permitting LPS and other inflammatory mediators to cross and subsequently activate resident microglia [83].

On entry into the brain, *P. gingivalis* LPS binds to TLR2 and TLR4 on microglia and astrocytes to activate the production of IL-1β, IL-6, and TNF-α, and to maintain a low-grade chronic neuroinflammatory state permissive for neuronal injury and glial scarring [84].

In addition, systemic inflammation caused by periodontitis is also involved in the activation of peripheral monocytes and the recruitment of cytokine-producing cells into the CNS. These cytokines have the potential to further upregulate indoleamine 2,3-dioxygenase and kynurenine pathways, which are neurotoxic and are associated with cognitive impairment [85, 86]. In addition, *P. gingivalis* infection breaks the gut-brain axis, influencing the intestinal microbiota and establishing a systemic pro-inflammatory milieu that promotes neurodegenerative disease progression [87]. These findings have been backed by animal model studies: mice infected orally with *P. gingivalis* develop cognitive and memory impairments, Aβ1-42 deposition, and synaptic loss [88, 89]. Blocking gingipains using small-molecule inhibitors (e.g., COR388 or atuzaginstat) has also been demonstrated to decrease neuroinflammation and amyloid burden and improve cognitive function in these experimental models [90]. These encouraging findings have moved forward into early human clinical trials, with active studies underway using gingipain inhibitors as a therapeutic approach for AD.

Beyond *P. gingivalis*, other periodontopathogens like *F. nucleatum* and *T. denticola* may synergize to promote CNS inflammation. Their LPS and outer membrane vesicles (OMVs) were shown to cause microglial activation and reactive oxygen species (ROS) production. Furthermore, polymicrobial biofilm products can increase BBB permeability in concert and accelerate neurodegenerative processes via a "multiple-hit" scenario [91, 92].

Periodontitis – through its microbial virulence factors, systemic inflammation, and neuroimmune modulation – is now a plausible candidate upstream factor in AD pathogenesis [77–80]. As causality is investigated, translational opportunity arises. Future strategies could involve periodontal screening in neurologically at-risk patients, preventive oral care measures, and the identification of oral-derived biomarkers for early detection of neurodegenerative risk. On this basis, periodontitis treatment could be more than oral health, representing a neuroprotective intervention in the elderly.

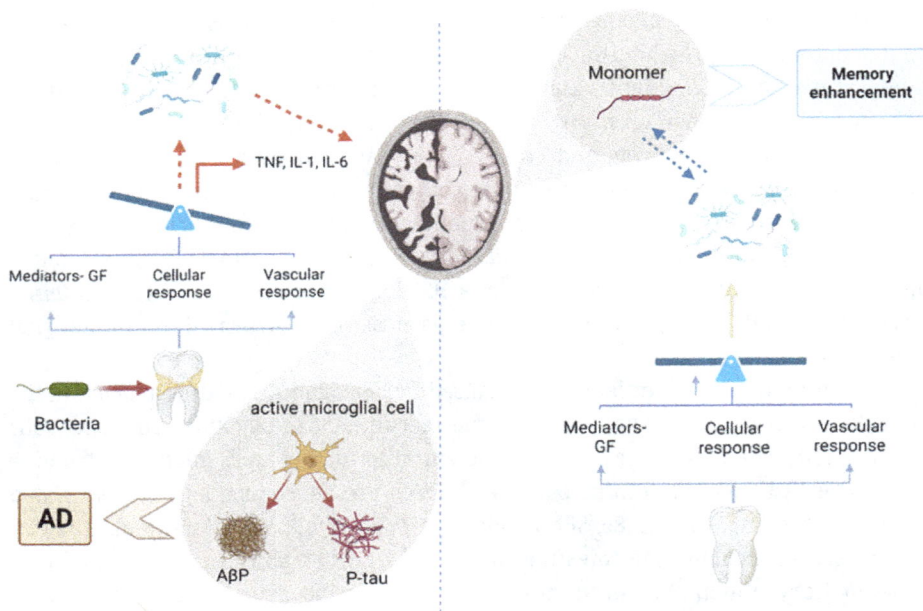

Figure 2.3: Oral-brain axis in Alzheimer's disease. Periodontal pathogens activate microglia and cytokines (TNF-α, IL-1, and IL-6), driving Aβ/pTau pathology; balanced signaling supports memory.

2.6 Periodontitis and Rheumatoid Arthritis

The interaction between RARA and periodontitis is being ever more acknowledged as a consequence of common immunopathogenic processes, such as chronic inflammation, autoantibody formation, and microbiota-induced immune dysregulation [93]. The major periodontal pathogen *P. gingivalis* has a central role through the expression of peptidylarginine deiminase, which catalyzes the citrullination of host and bacterial proteins [94]. This particular biological process is responsible for the generation of neoepitopes that are quite similar to the endogenous antigens present within the synovial tissues [95]. The similarity later gives rise to a robust immune response that results in the production of anti-citrullinated protein antibodies, which are characteristically present in patients suffering from RA [94, 95]. In the same way, the bacterium *A. actinomycetemcomitans* is accountable for promoting hypercitrullination among neutrophils via the action of LtxA [15, 96, 97]. This process also contributes to autoimmune priming that characterizes the underlying pathology [96]. These pathogens, together with chronic periodontal inflammation, play a major role in orchestrating systemic increases in pro-inflammatory mediators, such as IL-1β, IL-6, and most notably, TNF-α, which is recognized as a key effector involved in both joint and periodontal tissue destructive processes [98, 99]. The abundance of TNF-α is a prevalence characteristic of RA pathophysiology, while also accounting for the destruction of periodontal connective tissue and bone resorption. This common inflammatory profile forms the rationale for the therapeutic overlap that exists between these two intertwined diseases [93, 100]. Anti-TNF medications, including infliximab and etanercept, not only proved to be effective in decreasing RA disease activity but also exhibited favorable effects on periodontal inflammation, clinical attachment levels, and bleeding on probing [101, 102]. Such findings highlight the interrelatedness of systemic and oral inflammation and indicate that immunomodulatory therapy in RA can, at the same time, suppress the progression of periodontal disease. Clinically, the higher incidence and severity of periodontitis among RA patients, and the documented improvement of periodontal findings following RA-directed treatment, warrant a bidirectional interaction that necessitates coordinated management approaches [93, 103].

2.7 Periodontitis and Chronic Obstructive Pulmonary Disease

The relationship between periodontitis and COPD has become a leading focus of clinical and mechanistic research interest [104]. Both diseases belong to the group of chronic inflammatory diseases, with features of ongoing immune dysregulation, tissue damage, and the influence of microbes [104, 105]. Epidemiologic investigations have shown that individuals with periodontitis are at higher risk of acquiring COPD, and COPD patients tend to have more severe periodontal disease. This two-way association suggests co-pathogenic processes and potentially shared therapeutic targets [104–107].

The hypothesized biological link aims at systemic and local inflammation, microbial aspiration, and immune stimulation [107]. Periodontitis, characterized by a dysbiotic change in oral microbiota in favor of anaerobic gram-negative bacteria, such as *P. gingivalis*, *F. nucleatum*, and *T. denticola*, results in the chronic release of proinflammatory mediators like IL-1β, TNF-α, IL-6, and matrix metalloproteinases (MMPs) [60, 108, 109]. Such cytokines extend beyond the gingiva into systemic circulation, where they maintain chronic low-grade inflammation, which is a characteristic feature of COPD pathophysiology [110] (Figure 2.4).

Also, the oral cavity serves as a reservoir for respiratory pathogens [110]. Periodontal pockets harbor not just classical periodontal bacteria but also opportunistic infections like *Pseudomonas aeruginosa* (*P. aeruginosa*) and *Haemophilus influenzae* (*H. influenzae*) [111]. Through aspiration of oral secretions, particularly in elderly or hospitalized patients with dysphagia or compromised oral hygiene, these organisms colonize the lower respiratory tract, causing bronchial inflammation, airway remodeling, and COPD exacerbations [112]. *F. nucleatum* has especially been recovered from bronchoalveolar lavage fluid in COPD patients, pointing to its migration from the oral cavity to the pulmonary milieu [113].

One such mechanism involves upregulation of toll-like receptors (TLRs) on airway epithelial cells and alveolar macrophages. Periodontal pathogen-associated molecular patterns like LPS, fimbriae, and OMVs stimulate TLR2 and TLR4, activating NF-κB and MAPK pathways, resulting in mucosal inflammation and oxidative stress within the lung. The resulting cytokine cascade enhances neutrophil infiltration and elastase release, which further accelerates alveolar destruction, a key feature of emphysematous change in COPD [114–116].

In addition, both COPD and periodontitis patients often exhibit dysregulated innate immunity, particularly in neutrophil function. Neutrophils in these patients show delayed apoptosis, hyper-degranulation, and impaired phagocytosis, resulting in protracted tissue injury in the lungs and the periodontium. The systemic neutrophilic phenotype may be reflective of an overlapping inflammatory endotype that links the two conditions [117–119].

Oxidative stress also connects the pathogenesis of COPD and periodontitis. Both conditions generate excessive ROS, which amplify lipid peroxidation, DNA damage, and extracellular matrix degradation. Salivary and serum oxidative stress biomarkers, such as 8-OHdG (8-Hydroxy-2'-Deoxyguanosine) and malondialdehyde are elevated in both disease subjects, suggesting the existence of a shared oxidative-inflammatory cycle [120–122].

Clinically, interventional studies have demonstrated that periodontal treatment can improve respiratory parameters, decrease COPD exacerbations, and lower systemic inflammatory biomarkers like CRP and IL-6. These results are in support of the position of periodontal health as a modifiable risk factor in COPD management [123, 124].

In summary, the link between COPD and periodontitis is based on microbial aspiration, systemic inflammation, shared immune dysregulation, and oxidative stress [119–124]. These mechanistic similarities highlight the need for comorbid models of care in respiratory and oral disease patients. The early identification and treatment of periodontal inflammation can be a valuable adjunctive strategy to avoid pulmonary decline and enhance overall systemic well-being.

2.8 Clinical Implications and Interdisciplinary Integration

The growing recognition of periodontitis as a determinant of systemic disease pathology is a revolution in dental and medical sciences [3]. Periodontal inflammation can no longer be viewed as a localized entity but as a chronic systemic inflammation capable of affecting many organ systems [3, 4]. This new paradigm calls for a transdisci-

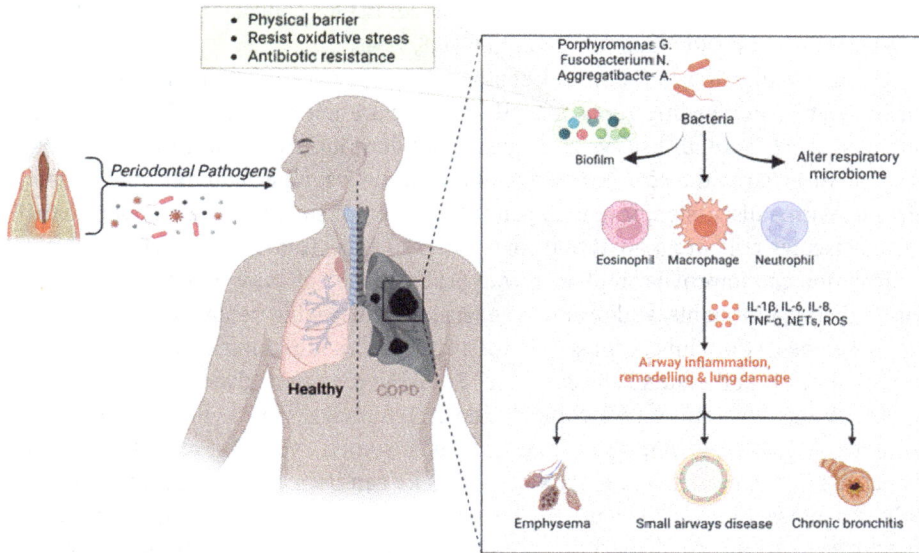

Figure 2.4: Oral-lung axis in COPD. Aspiration of periodontal pathogens (*P. gingivalis*, *F. nucleatum*, *A. actinomycetemcomitans*) activates epithelial/immune responses (IL-1β, IL-6, TNF-α, MMPs, and ROS), driving airway inflammation, remodeling, and lung damage (emphysema, small-airway disease, chronic bronchitis). Created with Biorender.com.

plinary model that includes periodontics as part of the comprehensive prevention, early detection, and treatment of systemic disease.

Periodontal examinations should be made a regular part of total medical examination, especially for the patients having CVD, diabetes mellitus, poor pregnancy outcomes, respiratory infections, and neurodegenerative disorders [125]. Periodontal infection could be detected early through the utilization of clinical markers (e.g., probing bleeding, pocket depth, and attachment loss) along with supportive biomarkers (e.g., salivary IL-6 and MMP-8), and it can act as an early warning of systemic inflammatory burden. Their incorporation into cardiology, endocrinology, and obstetrics clinics may allow risk stratification and initiate referral to dental practitioners [126].

Interprofessional communication and data exchange between dental and medical practitioners hold equal significance. Healthcare professionals frequently lack awareness regarding the seriousness or systemic implications of unmanaged periodontal disease, whereas dentists may neglect the systemic signs presented by their patients [127]. The implementation of interdisciplinary referral systems, collaborative electronic health records, and ongoing education in both medical and dental fields can substantially improve patient outcomes. For example, a patient with poorly controlled diabetes and recurrent periodontal infections would benefit from collaborative case management by an endocrinologist and a periodontist for concurrent treatment of hyperglycemia and periodontal inflammation [128, 129].

Patient education is front and center in this integration. Individuals must be made aware that bleeding gums or tooth mobility are not merely local events but potential signs of more diffuse systemic dysregulation [130]. Public education campaigns must be directed at the bidirectional relationship between periodontitis and systemic disease, with a discussion of how improved oral health can impact metabolic control, cardiovascular risk, pregnancy, and cognitive resilience. Informing patients with such information can improve compliance with oral hygiene behavior, improve attendance for dental appointments, and promote general health-seeking behavior [131].

A key aspect of clinical integration is managing modifiable risk factors common to periodontitis and systemic disease [132]. Smoking cessation, glycemic control, blood pressure management, stress control, and nutritional support must be addressed from an oral-systemic viewpoint [133, 134]. For instance, reduction of systemic oxidative stress or the lowering of dietary sugar intake can improve periodontal and metabolic outcomes. In the same vein, the incorporation of oral hygiene instruction in primary care clinics – particularly in those with pre-existing comorbidities – can be a low-cost preventive measure [135, 136].

Additionally, health systems need to develop to incorporate periodontal status into risk assessment tools for systemic disease, particularly in diabetic and cardiovascular patients. This may include validated scoring systems that take account of periodontal indices in addition to conventional medical parameters like HbA1c or lipid profiles [137].

On the policy level, public health policy needs to prioritize access to preventive dental care within chronic disease management. Insurance policies and clinical guidelines have to speak to the interconnectedness of oral and systemic health and include periodontal care not only for tooth saving alone but as an evidence-based intervention in optimization of systemic health [51, 138].

The incorporation of periodontal treatment within the context of the wider field of systemic medicine is both a clinical imperative and a scholarly responsibility. Through the promotion of interdiscipline alliances, patient education, and synchrony of healing objectives between the medical and dental disciplines, medical practitioners can tackle, collectively, the concomitant issues of oral and systemic disease – the dawn of a new era in personalized, integrated, and biologically compatible healthcare provision [139].

2.9 Conclusion

The interaction between periodontal dysbiosis and systemic disease is one of dynamic, multifaceted interactions governed by microbial virulence, host response, and chronic inflammation. Ongoing research is increasingly revealing the molecular basis of this interaction, and it is increasingly clear that the oral cavity cannot be viewed in isolation from the entire body. Understanding periodontitis as a modifiable risk factor for systemic disease changes the dental practitioner's role and requires an interdisciplinary, collaborative model of healthcare. Associating oral health with systemic health is perhaps one of the most significant developments in medicine today, and the periodontal microbiome is at its core.

References

[1] Foroughi, M., Torabinejad, M., & Angelov, N. et al. (2025). Bridging oral and systemic health: Exploring pathogenesis, biomarkers, and diagnostic innovations in periodontal disease. Infection. doi:10.1007/s15010-02568-y.

[2] Riley, L. W., & Blanton, R. E. (2018). Advances in molecular epidemiology of infectious diseases: Definitions, approaches, and scope of the field. Microbiology Spectrum, 6(6), 1–12, 10.1128/microbiolspec.ame-0001-2018.

[3] Martínez-García, M., & Hernández-Lemus, E. (2021). Periodontal inflammation and systemic diseases: An overview. Frontiers in Physiology, 12, 709438.

[4] Körtési, T., & Anicka, A. (2024). The connection between the oral microbiota and the kynurenine pathway: Insights into oral and certain systemic disorders. Current Issues in Molecular Biology, 46(11), 12641–12657.

[5] Cekici, A., Kantarci, A., Hasturk, H., & Van Dyke, T. E. (2014). Inflammatory and immune pathways in the pathogenesis of periodontal disease. Periodontology 2000, 64(1), 57–80.

[6] Tonetti, M. S., & Van Dyke, T. E. Working group 1 of the joint EFP/AAP workshop. (2013). Periodontitis and atherosclerotic cardiovascular disease: Consensus report of the joint EFP/AAP workshop on periodontitis and systemic diseases. Journal of Clinical Periodontology, 40(Suppl 14), S24–S29.

[7] Sharma, P., Dietrich, T., Ferro, C. J., Cockwell, P., & Chapple, I. L. (2016). Association between periodontitis and mortality in stages 3–5 chronic kidney disease: NHANES III and linked mortality study. Journal of Clinical Periodontology, 43, 104–113.

[8] Reyes, L., Herrera, D., Kozarov, E., Roldan, S., & Progulske-Fox, A. (2013). Periodontal bacterial invasion and infection: Contribution to atherosclerotic pathology. Journal of Clinical Periodontology, 40, S30–S50.

[9] Kozarov, E. V., Dorn, B. R., Shelburne, C. E., Dunn, W. A. Jr, & Progulske-Fox, A. (2005). Human atherosclerotic plaque contains viable invasive *Actinobacillus actinomycetemcomitans* and *Porphyromonas gingivalis*. Arteriosclerosis, Thrombosis & Vascular Biology, 25, e17–e18.

[10] Chukkapalli, S. S., Velsko, I. M., Rivera-Kweh, M. F., Zheng, D., Lucas, A. R., & Kesavalu, L. (2015). Polymicrobial oral infection with four periodontal bacteria orchestrates a distinct inflammatory response and atherosclerosis in ApoE-null mice. PLoS One, 10, e0143291.

[11] Velsko, I. M., Chukkapalli, S. S., Rivera, M. F., Lee, J. Y., Chen, H., Zheng, D., Bhattacharyya, I., Gangula, P. R., Lucas, A. R., & Kesavalu, L. (2014). Active invasion of oral and aortic tissues by *Porphyromonas gingivalis* in mice causally links periodontitis and atherosclerosis. PLoS One, 9, e97811.

[12] Range, H., Labreuche, J., Louedec, L., Rondeau, P., Planesse, C., Sebbag, U., Bourdon, E., Michel, J. B., Bouchard, P., & Meilhac, O. (2014). Periodontal bacteria in human carotid atherothrombosis as a potential trigger for neutrophil activation. Atherosclerosis, 236, 448–455.

[13] Huang, X., Xie, M., Lu, X., Mei, F., Song, W., Liu, Y., & Chen, L. (2022). The roles of periodontal bacteria in atherosclerosis. International Journal of Molecular Sciences, 24(16), 12861.

[14] Uehara, A., Imamura, T., Potempa, J., Travis, J., & Takada, H. (2008). Gingipains from *Porphyromonas gingivalis* synergistically induce the production of proinflammatory cytokines through protease-activated receptors with Toll-like receptor and NOD1/2 ligands in human monocytic cells. Cellular Microbiology, 10(5), 1181–1189.

[15] Vega, B. A., & Kachlany, S. C. (2019). *Aggregatibacter actinomycetemcomitans* leukotoxin (LtxA; Leukothera®): Mechanisms of action and therapeutic applications. Toxins, 11(9), 489.

[16] Afzoon, S., Amiri, M. A., Mohebbi, M., Hamedani, S., & Farshidfar, N. (2023). A systematic review of the impact of *Porphyromonas gingivalis* on foam cell formation: Implications for the role of periodontitis in atherosclerosis. BMC Oral Health, 23, 481.

[17] Ruan, Q., Guan, P., Qi, W., Li, J., Xi, M., Xiao, L., Zhong, S., Ma, D., & Ni, J. (2023). *Porphyromonas gingivalis* regulates atherosclerosis through an immune pathway. Frontiers in Immunology, 14, 1103592.

[18] Hajishengallis, G., & Chavakis, T. (2021). Local and systemic mechanisms linking periodontal disease and inflammatory comorbidities. Nature Reviews Immunology, 21(7), 426–440.

[19] Mitroulis, I., Hajishengallis, G., & Chavakis, T. (2023). Bone marrow inflammatory memory in cardiometabolic disease and inflammatory comorbidities. Cardiovascular Research, 119(18), 2801–2814.

[20] Ramírez, J. H., Arce, R. M., & Contreras, A. (2011). Periodontal treatment effects on endothelial function and cardiovascular disease biomarkers in subjects with chronic periodontitis: Protocol for a randomized clinical trial. Trials, 12, 46.

[21] Saffi, M. A. L., Rabelo-Silva, E. R., Polanczyk, C. A., Furtado, M. V., Montenegro, M. M., Ribeiro, I. W. J., Kampits, C., Rösing, C. K., & Haas, A. N. (2018). Periodontal therapy and endothelial function in coronary artery disease: A randomized controlled trial. Oral Diseases, 24(7), 1349–1357.

[22] Saffi, M. A., Furtado, M. V., Montenegro, M. M., Ribeiro, I. W., Kampits, C., Rabelo-Silva, E. R., Polanczyk, C. A., Rösing, C. K., & Haas, A. N. (2013). The effect of periodontal therapy on C-reactive protein, endothelial function, lipids, and proinflammatory biomarkers in patients with stable coronary artery disease: Study protocol for a randomized controlled trial. Trials, 14, 283.

[23] Ismail, A. B., Balcıoğlu, Ö., Özcem, B., & Ergoren, M. Ç. (2024). APOE gene variation's impact on cardiovascular health: A case-control study. Biomedicines, 12(3), 695.

[24] Jyotsna, F., Ahmed, A., Kumar, K., Kaur, P., Chaudhary, M. H., & Kumar, S. et al. (2023). Exploring the complex connection between diabetes and cardiovascular disease: Analyzing approaches to mitigate cardiovascular risk in patients with diabetes. Cureus, 15, e43882.

[25] Siam, N. H., Snigdha, N. N., Tabasumma, N., & Parvin, I. (2024). Diabetes mellitus and cardiovascular disease: Exploring epidemiology, pathophysiology, and treatment strategies. Reviews in Cardiovascular Medicine, 25(12), 436.

[26] Ge, J., Zhu, X., Weng, C., Yuan, D., Zhao, J., Zhao, L., Wang, T., & Wu, Y. (2024). Periodontitis impacts on thrombotic diseases: From clinical aspect to future therapeutic approaches. International Journal of Oral Science, 16(1), 1–15.

[27] Wurschi, L. C., Hölzle, F., Craveiro, R. B., Wolf, M., & Noels, H. (2024). Crosstalk between periodontitis and cardiovascular risk. Frontiers in Immunology, 15, 1469077.

[28] Ranbhise, J. S., Ju, S., Singh, M. K., Han, S., Akter, S., Ha, J., Choe, W., Kim, S. S., & Kang, I. (2025). Chronic inflammation and glycemic control: Exploring the bidirectional link between periodontitis and diabetes. Dentistry Journal, 13(3), 100.

[29] Shen, Y., Lu, H., Cheng, F., Li, J., Kuo, M., Wu, H., Liu, H., Hsieh, C., Tsai, Y., & Yu, L. (2024). Advanced glycation end-products acting as immunomodulators for chronic inflammation, inflammaging, and carcinogenesis in patients with diabetes and immune-related diseases. Biomedicines, 12(8), 1699.

[30] Nonaka, K., Kajiura, Y., & Bando, M. et al. (2018). Advanced glycation end-products increase IL-6 and ICAM-1 expression via RAGE, MAPK, and NF-κB pathways in human gingival fibroblasts. Journal of Periodontal Research, 53(3), 334–344.

[31] Giri, B., Dey, S., Das, T., Sarkar, M., Banerjee, J., & Dash, S. K. (2018). Chronic hyperglycemia-mediated physiological alteration and metabolic distortion leads to organ dysfunction, infection, cancer progression, and other pathophysiological consequences: An update on glucose toxicity. Biomedicine and Pharmacotherapy, 107, 306–328.

[32] Thimmappa, P. Y., Vasishta, S., Ganesh, K., Nair, A. S., & Joshi, M. B. (2023). Neutrophil (dys)function due to altered immuno-metabolic axis in type 2 diabetes: Implications in combating infections. Human Cell, 36(4), 1265–1278.

[33] Wu, Y., Xiao, E., & Graves, D. T. (2015). Diabetes mellitus-related bone metabolism and periodontal disease. International Journal of Oral Science, 7(2), 63–72.

[34] Qu, Y., Zeng, H., Wang, L., Ge, Z., Liu, B., & Fan, Z. (2025). Microenvironment-regulated dual-layer microneedle patch for promoting periodontal soft and hard tissue regeneration in diabetic periodontitis. Advanced Functional Materials, 35(19), 2418076.

[35] Taylor, J. J., Preshaw, P. M., & Lalla, E. (2013). A review of the evidence for pathogenic mechanisms that may link periodontitis and diabetes. Journal of Clinical Periodontology, 40(Suppl 14), S113–S134.

[36] Preshaw, P. M., Alba, A. L., & Herrera, D. et al. (2012). Periodontitis and diabetes: A two-way relationship. Diabetologia, 55(1), 21–31.

[37] Jia, L., Han, N., Du, J., Guo, L., Luo, Z., & Liu, Y. (2019). Pathogenesis of important virulence factors of *Porphyromonas gingivalis* via Toll-like receptors. Frontiers in Cellular Infection and Microbiology. 9, 262.

[38] Muñoz-Medel, M., Pinto, M. P., Goralsky, L., Cáceres, M., Villarroel-Espíndola, F., Manque, P., Pinto, A., Garcia-Bloj, B., Godoy, J. A., Garrido, M., & Retamal, I. N. (2024). *Porphyromonas gingivalis*, a bridge between oral health and immune evasion in gastric cancer. Frontiers in Oncology. 14, 1403089.

[39] Cao, P., Chen, Q., & Shi, C. et al. (2022). *Fusobacterium nucleatum* promotes the development of acute liver failure by inhibiting the NAD+ salvage metabolic pathway. Gut Pathogens, 14, 29.

[40] Muske, J., & Knoop, K. (2023). Contributions of the microbiota to the systemic inflammatory response. Microbiota Host, 1(1), e230018.

[41] Checa-Ros, A., Hsueh, C., Merck, B., González-Torres, H., & Bermúdez, V. (2024). Obesity and oral health: The link between adipokines and periodontitis. TouchREV Endocrinol, 20(1), 25.

[42] Guo, Z., Peng, Y., Hu, Q., Liu, N., & Liu, Q. (2023). The relationship between leptin and periodontitis: A literature review. PeerJ. 11, e16633.

[43] Naseralavi, F., Nikkhah, M., Etemadi, N., & Salari, A. (2019). Effect of non-surgical periodontal treatment on HbA1c levels in non-diabetic patients with chronic periodontitis in an Iranian population. Journal of Advanced Periodontology & Implant Dentistry, 11(2), 77.

[44] Umeizudike, K. A., Nwhator, S. O., Olaoye, O. I., Ogundana, A. C., Räisänen, I. T., Fasanmade, O. A., Ogundana, O., Ajie, O., & Sorsa, T. (2025). Effects of non-surgical periodontal therapy on glycemic control in prediabetes and diabetes patients with stage II–IV periodontitis as monitored by active-matrix metalloproteinase-8 levels. Biomedicines, 13(4), 969.

[45] Umezaki, Y., Yamashita, A., Nishimura, F., & Naito, T. (2025). The role of periodontal treatment on the reduction of hemoglobin A1c, comparing with existing medication therapy: A systematic review and meta-analysis. Front Clin Diabetes Healthc. 6, 1541145.

[46] Sachelarie, L., Scrobota, I., Romanul, I., Iurcov, R., Potra Cicalau, G. I., & Todor, L. (2024). Probiotic therapy as an adjuvant in the treatment of periodontal disease: An innovative approach. Medicina, 61(1), 126.

[47] Gu, Y., Golub, L. M., Lee, H. M., & Walker, S. G. (2025). Diabetes, periodontal disease, and novel therapeutic approaches: Host modulation therapy. Front Clin Diabetes Healthc. 6, 1529086.

[48] Masi, S., Orlandi, M., Parkar, M., Bhowruth, D., Kingston, I., O'Rourke, C., Virdis, A., Hingorani, A., Hurel, S. J., Donos, N., D'Aiuto, F., & Deanfield, J. (2018). Mitochondrial oxidative stress, endothelial function and metabolic control in patients with type II diabetes and periodontitis: A randomised controlled clinical trial. International Journal of Cardiology Research. 271, 263–268.

[49] Kumar, A., Basra, M., Begum, N., Rani, V., Prasad, S., Lamba, A. K., Verma, M., Agarwal, S., & Sharma, S. (2012). Association of maternal periodontal health with adverse pregnancy outcome. Journal of Obstetrics and Gynaecology Research, 39(1), 40–45.

[50] Fischer, L. A., Demerath, E., Bittner-Eddy, P., & Costalonga, M. (2019). Placental colonization with periodontal pathogens: The potential missing link. The American Journal of Obstetrics & Gynecology, 221(5), 383.

[51] Hashim, N. T., Babiker, R., Padmanabhan, V., Ahmed, A. T., CS, K. C., Mohammed, R., Priya, S. P., Ahmed, A., Bahra, S. E., Islam, M. S., Gismalla, B. G., & Rahman, M. M. (2025). The global burden of periodontal disease: A narrative review on unveiling socioeconomic and health challenges. International Journal of Environmental Research and Public Health, 22(4), 624.

[52] AlSharief, M., & Alabdurubalnabi, E. (2023). Periodontal pathogens and adverse pregnancy outcomes: A narrative review. Life, 13(7), 1559.

[53] Figuero, E., Carrillo-de-albornoz, A., Herrera, D., & Bascones-Martínez, A. (2010). Gingival changes during pregnancy: i. Influence of hormonal variations on clinical and immunological parameters. Journal of Clinical Periodontology, 37(3), 220–229.

[54] Wu, M., Chen, W., & Jiang, Y. (2015). Relationship between gingival inflammation and pregnancy. Inflammatory Mediators, 1–11, 623427.

[55] Vander Haar, E. L., So, J., Gyamfi-Bannerman, C., & Han, Y. W. (2018). *Fusobacterium nucleatum* and adverse pregnancy outcomes: Epidemiological and mechanistic evidence. Anaerobe. 50, 55–59.

[56] Barak, S., Oettinger-Barak, O., Machtei, E. E., Sprecher, H., & Ohel, G. (2007). Evidence of periopathogenic microorganisms in placentas of women with preeclampsia. Journal of Periodontology, 78(4), 670–676.

[57] Fardini, Y., Wang, X., Témoin, S., Nithianantham, S., Lee, D., Shoham, M., & Han, Y. W. (2011). *Fusobacterium nucleatum* adhesin FadA binds vascular endothelial cadherin and alters endothelial integrity. Mol. Microbiol., 82(6), 1468–1480.

[58] Jia, Y. P., Wang, K., Zhang, Z. J., Tong, Y. N., Han, D., & Hu, C. Y. et al. (2017). TLR2/TLR4 activation induces Tregs and suppresses intestinal inflammation caused by *Fusobacterium nucleatum* in vivo. PLoS One, 12(10), e0186179.

[59] Tsikouras, P., Oikonomou, E., Nikolettos, K., Andreou, S., Kyriakou, D., & Damaskos, C. et al. (2024). The impact of periodontal disease on preterm birth and preeclampsia. Journal of Personalized Medicine, 14(4), 345.

[60] Bhuyan, R., SK, B., Mohanty, J. N., Das, S., Juliana, N., & Abu, I. F. (2022). Periodontitis and its inflammatory changes linked to various systemic diseases: A review of its underlying mechanisms. Biomedicines, 10(10), 2659.

[61] Nannan, M., Xiaoping, L., & Ying, J. (2022). Periodontal disease in pregnancy and adverse pregnancy outcomes: Progress in related mechanisms and management strategies. Frontier Medicine. 9, 963956.

[62] Ruffaner-Hanson, C., Noor, S., Sun, M. S., Solomon, E., Marquez, L. E., & Rodriguez, D. E. et al. (2022). The maternal-placental-fetal interface: Adaptations of the HPA axis and immune mediators following maternal stress and prenatal alcohol exposure. ExperimentalNeurology, 355, 114121.

[63] Wen, X., Fu, X., Zhao, C., Yang, L., & Huang, R. (2023). The bidirectional relationship between periodontal disease and pregnancy via the interaction of oral microorganisms, hormone and immune response. Frontiers in Microbiology. 14, 1070917.

[64] Lavu, V., Venkatesan, V., & Rao, S. R. (2015). The epigenetic paradigm in periodontitis pathogenesis. Journal of Indian Society of Periodontology, 19(2), 142–149.

[65] Basak, S., Mallick, R., Navya Sree, B., & Duttaroy, A. K. (2023). Placental epigenome impacts fetal development: Effects of maternal nutrients and gut microbiota. Nutrients, 16(12), 1860.

[66] Jurdziński, K. T., Potempa, J., & Grabiec, A. M. (2020). Epigenetic regulation of inflammation in periodontitis: Cellular mechanisms and therapeutic potential. Clinical Epigenet. 12, 186.

[67] López, N. J., Da Silva, I., Ipinza, J., & Gutiérrez, J. (2005). Periodontal therapy reduces the rate of preterm low birth weight in women with pregnancy-associated gingivitis. Journal of Periodontology. 76, 2144–2153.

[68] López, N. J., Smith, P. C., & Gutiérrez, J. (2002). Periodontal therapy may reduce the risk of preterm low birth weight in women with periodontal disease: A randomized controlled trial. Journal of Periodontology. 73, 911–924.

[69] Tonetti, M. S., D'Aiuto, F., Nibali, L., Donald, A., Storry, C., & Parkar, M. et al. (2007). Treatment of periodontitis and endothelial function. New England Journal of Medicine, 356, 911–920.

[70] Np, P., IP, P., Mauri, D., Tzioras, S., Tsappi, M., & Cortinovis, I. et al. (2009). Effect of periodontal disease treatment during pregnancy on preterm birth incidence: a meta-analysis of randomized trials. The American Journal of Obstetrics & Gynecology, 200, 225–232.

[71] Wu, J., Wu, J., Tang, B., Zhang, Z., Wei, F., & Yu, D. et al. (2024). Effects of different periodontal interventions on the risk of adverse pregnancy outcomes in pregnant women: A systematic review and network meta-analysis of randomized controlled trials. Front Public Health, 12, 1373691.

[72] Gharaibeh, S., Alsabbah, A., Alloubani, A., & Gharaibeh, A. (2025). Reciprocal interactions between periodontal disease and Alzheimer's disease: Implications for mutual triggering, exacerbation, and treatment interventions – a comprehensive review of the literature. Neurology International, 17(6), 81.

[73] Tao, K., Yuan, Y., Xie, Q., & Dong, Z. (2024). Relationship between human oral microbiome dysbiosis and neuropsychiatric diseases: An updated overview. Behavioural Brain Research. 471, 115111.

[74] Kamer, A. R., Craig, R. G., Niederman, R., & Fortea, J. (2020). Periodontal disease as a possible cause for Alzheimer's disease. Periodontol 2000, 83(1), 242–271.

[75] Li, R., Wang, J., Xiong, W., Luo, Y., Feng, H., & Zhou, H. et al. (2024). The oral-brain axis: Can periodontal pathogens trigger the onset and progression of Alzheimer's disease?. Frontiers in Microbiology, 15, 1358179.

[76] Lei, S., Li, J., Yu, J., Li, F., Pan, Y., & Chen, X. et al. (2023). *Porphyromonas gingivalis* bacteremia increases the permeability of the blood-brain barrier via the Mfsd2a/Caveolin-1 mediated transcytosis pathway. International Journal of Oral Science, 15(1), 1–12.

[77] Olsen, I. (2021). *Porphyromonas gingivalis*-induced neuroinflammation in Alzheimer's disease. Frontiers in Neuroscience. 15, 691016.

[78] Liu, D. S., Pan, X. D., & Zhang, J. et al. (2015). APOE4 enhances age-dependent decline in cognitive function by down-regulating an NMDA receptor pathway in EFAD-Tg mice. Molecular Neurodegeneration, 10, 7.

[79] Olsen, I., & Singhrao, S. K. (2020). Interaction between genetic factors, *Porphyromonas gingivalis* and microglia to promote Alzheimer's disease. Journal of Oral Microbiology, 12(1), 1820834.

[80] Korwek, K. M., Trotter, J. H., & LaDu, M. J. et al. (2009). ApoE isoform-dependent changes in hippocampal synaptic function. Molecular Neurodegeneration, 4, 21.

[81] Li, C., Yu, R., & Ding, Y. (2022). Association between *Porphyromonas gingivalis* and systemic diseases: Focus on T cells-mediated adaptive immunity. Frontiers in Cellular Infection and Microbiology. 12, 1026457.

[82] Huang, Z., Hao, M., Shi, N., Wang, X., Yuan, L., & Yuan, H. et al. (2025). *Porphyromonas gingivalis*: a potential trigger of neurodegenerative disease. Frontiers Immunol, 16, 1482033.

[83] Shawkatova, I., Durmanova, V., & Javor, J. (2024). Alzheimer's disease and *Porphyromonas gingivalis*: Exploring the links. Life, 15(1), 96.

[84] Magnusson, A., Wu, R., & Demirel, I. (2024). *Porphyromonas gingivalis* triggers microglia activation and neurodegenerative processes through NOX4. Frontiers in Cellular Infection and Microbiology. 14, 1451683.

[85] Pink, C., Holtfreter, B., & Völzke, H. et al. (2023). Periodontitis and systemic inflammation as independent and interacting risk factors for mortality: Evidence from a prospective cohort study. BMC Medicine, 21, 430.

[86] Söderlund, J., Olsson, S. K., Samuelsson, M., Walther-Jallow, L., Johansson, C., & Erhardt, S. et al. (2011). Elevation of cerebrospinal fluid interleukin-1β in bipolar disorder. Journal of Psychiatry & Neuroscience: JPN, 36(2), 114–118.

[87] Xi, M., Ruan, Q., Zhong, S., Li, J., Qi, W., & Xie, C. et al. (2024). Periodontal bacteria influence systemic diseases through the gut microbiota. Frontiers in Cellular Infection and Microbiology, 14, 1478362.

[88] Dominy, S. S., Lynch, C., Ermini, F., Benedyk, M., Marczyk, A., & Konradi, A. et al. (2019). *Porphyromonas gingivalis* in Alzheimer's disease brains: Evidence for disease causation and treatment with small-molecule inhibitors. Science Advances, 5(1), eaau3333.

[89] Poole, S., Singhrao, S. K., Chukkapalli, S., Rivera, M., Velsko, I., Kesavalu, L., & Crean, S. (2015). Active invasion of *Porphyromonas gingivalis* and infection-induced complement activation in ApoE-/- mice brains. Journal of Alzheimer's Disease, 43(1), 67–80.

[90] Arastu-Kapur, S., Nguyen, M., Raha, D., Ermini, F., Haditsch, U., Araujo, J., De Lannoy, I. A., Ryder, M. I., Dominy, S. S., Lynch, C., & Holsinger, L. J. (2020). Treatment of *Porphyromonas gulae* infection and downstream pathology in the aged dog by lysine-gingipain inhibitor COR388. Pharmacol Res Perspect, 8(1), e00562.

[91] Visentin, D., Gobin, I., & Maglica, Ž. (2023). Periodontal pathogens and their links to neuroinflammation and neurodegeneration. Microorganisms, 11(7), 1832.

[92] Chen, S., Lei, Q., Zou, X., & Ma, D. (2023). The role and mechanisms of Gram-negative bacterial outer membrane vesicles in inflammatory diseases. Frontiers in Immunology, 14, 1157813.

[93] Cirelli, J. A., Thurlings, R. M., Koenders, M. I., & Jr, C. R. (2019). Linkage of periodontitis and rheumatoid arthritis: Current evidence and potential biological interactions. International Journal of Molecular Sciences, 20(18), 4541.

[94] Gawron, K., Bereta, G., Nowakowska, Z., Łazarz, M., Szmigielski, B., Mizgalska, D., Buda, A., Koziel, J., Oruba, Z., & Potempa, J. (2014). Peptidylarginine deiminase from *Porphyromonas gingivalis* (PPAD) contributes to infection of gingival fibroblasts and induction of PGE2-signaling pathway. Molecular Oral Microbiology, 29(6), 321–332.

[95] Maresz, K. J., Hellvard, A., Sroka, A., Adamowicz, K., Bielecka, E., Koziel, J., Gawron, K., Mizgalska, D., Marcinska, K. A., Benedyk, M., Pyrc, K., Quirke, M., Jonsson, R., Alzabin, S., Venables, P. J., Nguyen, A., Mydel, P., & Potempa, J. (2013). *Porphyromonas gingivalis* facilitates the development and progression of destructive arthritis through its unique bacterial peptidylarginine deiminase (PAD). PLoS Pathog, 9(9), e1003627.

[96] Konig, M. F., Abusleme, L., Reinholdt, J., Palmer, R. J., Teles, R. P., Sampson, K., Rosen, A., Nigrovic, P. A., Sokolove, J., Giles, J. T., Moutsopoulos, N. M., & Andrade, F. (2016). *Aggregatibacter actinomycetemcomitans*-induced hypercitrullination links periodontal infection to autoimmunity in rheumatoid arthritis. Science Translational Medicine, 8(369), 369ra176.

[97] Herbert, B. A., Novince, C. M., & Kirkwood, K. L. (2016). *Aggregatibacter actinomycetemcomitans*, a potent immunoregulator of the periodontal host defense system and alveolar bone homeostasis. Molecular Oral Microbiology, 31(3), 207–227.

[98] Neurath, N., & Kesting, M. (2024). Cytokines in gingivitis and periodontitis: From pathogenesis to therapeutic targets. Frontiers in Immunology, 15, 1435054.

[99] Bonsmann, T., Mochol, M., & Pawlik, A. (2023). The role of interleukin 6 in periodontitis and its complications. International Journal of Molecular Sciences, 25(4), 2146.

[100] Kobayashi, T., & Yoshie, H. (2014). Host responses in the link between periodontitis and rheumatoid arthritis. Current Oral Health Reports, 2(1), 1–8.

[101] Ortiz, P., Bissada, N. F., Palomo, L., Han, Y. W., Al-Zahrani, M. S., Panneerselvam, A., & Askari, A. (2009). Periodontal therapy reduces the severity of active rheumatoid arthritis in patients treated with or without tumor necrosis factor inhibitors. Journal of Periodontology, 80(4), 535–540.

[102] Petit, C., Culshaw, S., Weiger, R., Huck, O., & Sahrmann, P. (2024). Impact of treatment of rheumatoid arthritis on periodontal disease: A review. Molecular Oral Microbiology, 39(4), 199–224.

[103] Disale, P. R., Zope, S. A., Suragimath, G., Varma, A. S., & Pisal, A. (2020). Prevalence and severity of periodontitis in patients with established rheumatoid arthritis and osteoarthritis. Journal of Family Medicine and Primary Care, 9(6), 2919–2925.

[104] Guo, Z., & Wang, Z. (2024). Relationship between periodontitis and chronic obstructive pulmonary disease: A bibliometric analysis from 1945 to 2023. Medicina Oral, Patología Oral Y Cirugía Bucal, 30(1), e1.

[105] Xiong, K., Yang, P., Cui, Y., Li, J., Li, Y., & Tang, B. (2023). Research on the association between periodontitis and COPD. International Journal of Chronic Obstructive Pulmonary Disease, 18, 1937–1948.

[106] Wang, D., Dai, L., Cui, Z., Xing, W., Huang, X., Yang, H., & Shan, Y. (2023). Association between periodontal diseases and chronic obstructive pulmonary disease: Evidence from sequential cross-sectional and prospective cohort studies based on UK Biobank. Journal of Clinical Periodontology, 51(1), 97–107.

[107] Zhou, X., Wang, J., Liu, W., Huang, X., Song, Y., Wang, Z., & Jia, X. (2020). Periodontal status and microbiologic pathogens in patients with chronic obstructive pulmonary disease and periodontitis: A case–control study. International Journal of Chronic Obstructive Pulmonary Disease, 15, 2071–2079.

[108] Hajishengallis, G., Wang, M., Bagby, G. J., & Nelson, S. (2008). Importance of TLR2 in early innate immune response to acute pulmonary infection with *Porphyromonas gingivalis* in mice. Journal of Immunology, 181(6), 4141–4149.

[109] Williams, M. D., Kerber, C. A., & Tergin, H. F. (2003). Unusual presentation of Lemierre's syndrome due to *Fusobacterium nucleatum*. Journal of Clinical Microbiology, 41(8), 3445–3448.

[110] Dong, J., Li, W., Wang, Q., Chen, J., Zu, Y., Zhou, X., & Guo, Q. (2022). Relationships between oral microecosystem and respiratory diseases. Frontiers in Molecular Biosciences, 8, 718222.

[111] Vieira Colombo, A. P., Magalhães, C. B., Hartenbach, F. A., Martins Do Souto, R., & Maciel da Silva-boghossian, C. (2016). Periodontal-disease-associated biofilm: A reservoir for pathogens of medical importance. Microbial Pathogenesis, 94, 27–34.

[112] Pathak, J. L., Yan, Y., Zhang, Q., Wang, L., & Ge, L. (2021). The role of oral microbiome in respiratory health and diseases. Respiratory Medicine, 185, 106475.

[113] Suzuki, R., Kamio, N., Kaneko, T., Yonehara, Y., & Imai, K. (2022). *Fusobacterium nucleatum* exacerbates chronic obstructive pulmonary disease in elastase-induced emphysematous mice. FEBS Open Bio, 12(3), 638–649.

[114] Greene, C. M., & McElvaney, N. G. (2005). Toll-like receptor expression and function in airway epithelial cells. Archivum Immunologiae Et Therapiae Experimentalis, 53(5), 418–427.

[115] Wallet, S. M., & Puri, V. (2018). Linkage of infection to adverse systemic complications: Periodontal disease, Toll-like receptors, and other pattern recognition systems Vaccines, 6(2), 21.

[116] Kayongo, A., Robertson, N. M., Siddharthan, T., Ntayi, M. L., Ndawula, J. C., Sande, O. J., Bagaya, B. S., Kirenga, B., Joloba, M. L., & Forslund, S. K. (2023). Airway microbiome-immune crosstalk in chronic obstructive pulmonary disease. Frontiers in Immunology, 13, 1085551.

[117] Nicu, E. A., & Loos, B. G. (2016). Polymorphonuclear neutrophils in periodontitis and their possible modulation as a therapeutic approach. *Periodontology 2000*, 71(1), 140–163.

[118] Qu, J., Yue, L., Gao, J., & Yao, H. (2019). Perspectives on Wnt signal pathway in the pathogenesis and therapeutics of chronic obstructive pulmonary disease. Journal of Pharmacology & Experimental Therapeutics, 369(3), 473–482.

[119] Usher, A. K., & Stockley, R. A. (2013). The link between chronic periodontitis and COPD: A common role for the neutrophil?. BMC Medicine, 11, 241.

[120] Rahman, I. (2005). The role of oxidative stress in the pathogenesis of COPD: Implications for therapy. Treatments in Respiratory Medicine, 4(3), 175–200.

[121] Boukhenouna, S., Wilson, M. A., Bahmed, K., & Kosmider, B. (2018). Reactive oxygen species in chronic obstructive pulmonary disease. Oxidative Medicine and Cellular Longevity, 1–9, 5730395.

[122] Shang, J., Liu, H., Zheng, Y., & Zhang, Z. (2023). Role of oxidative stress in the relationship between periodontitis and systemic diseases. Frontiers in Physiology, 14, 1210449.

[123] Parihar, A. S., Edake, D. N., Nema, S., Laxmipriya, M., Vediya, S. S., Kochar, D., & Laddha, R. (2024). Periodontal inflammation as a modifiable risk factor for COPD exacerbations in the Indian population: A prospective cohort study. Journal of Pharmacy and Bioallied Sciences, 16(Suppl 4), S4006–S4009.

[124] Røsland, A., Bertelsen, R. J., & Heinrich, J. et al. (2025). Effect of periodontal therapy on lung function: A twelve-month follow-up intervention study. Respiratory Research, 26, 172.

[125] Fischer, R. G., Gomes Filho, I. S., Cruz, S. S., Oliveira, V. B., Lira-Junior, R., Scannapieco, F. A., & Rego, R. O. (2021). What is the future of periodontal medicine?. Brazilian Oral Research, 35(suppl 2), e102.

[126] Sachelarie, L., Stefanescu, C. L., Murineanu, R. M., Grigorian, M., Zaharia, A., Scrobota, I., & Hurjui, L. L. (2025). Role of salivary biomarkers IL-1β and MMP-8 in early detection and staging of periodontal disease. Medicina, 61(4), 760.

[127] Slavkin, H. C., Dubois, P. A., Kleinman, D. V., & Fuccillo, R. (2023). Science-informed health policies for oral and systemic health. Journal of Healthcare Leadership, 15, 43–52.

[128] Robertson, S. T., Rosbergen, I. C., Burton-Jones, A., Grimley, R. S., & Brauer, S. G. (2022). The effect of the electronic health record on interprofessional practice: A systematic review. Applied Clinical Informatics, 13(3), 541–558.

[129] Mills, A., Berlin-Broner, Y., & Levin, L. (2023). Improving patient well-being as a broader perspective in dentistry. International Dental Journal, 73(6), 785–791.

[130] Zaman, M. S., Alam, S. M., & Razzaque, M. S. (2025). Oral hygiene and cardiovascular health. Hygiene, 5(2), 14.

[131] Alsalleeh, F., Alhadlaq, A. S., Althumiri, N. A., AlMousa, N., & BinDhim, N. F. (2022). Public awareness of the association between periodontal disease and systemic disease. Healthcare, 11(1), 88.

[132] Martinon, P., Fraticelli, L., Giboreau, A., Dussart, C., Bourgeois, D., & Carrouel, F. (2021). Nutrition as a key modifiable factor for periodontitis and main chronic diseases. Journal of Clinical Medicine, 10(2), 197.

[133] Charchar, F. J., Prestes, P. R., Mills, C., Ching, S. M., Neupane, D., Marques, F. Z., Sharman, J. E., Vogt, L., Burrell, L. M., Korostovtseva, L., Zec, M., Patil, M., Schultz, M. G., Wallen, M. P., Renna, N. F., Islam, S. M. S., Hiremath, S., Gyeltshen, T., Chia, C., & Tomaszewski, M. (2023). Lifestyle management of hypertension: International society of hypertension position paper endorsed by the world hypertension league and European society of hypertension. Journal of Hypertension, 42(1), 23–49.

[134] Dhatariya, K., & Umpierrez, G. E. (2024). Management of diabetes and hyperglycemia in hospitalized patients, In: Feingold, K. R., Ahmed, S. F., & Anawalt, B. et al. (eds) Endotext. MDText.com, Inc: South Dartmouth, MA, 1–40.

[135] Shanmugasundaram, S., & Karmakar, S. (2024). Excess dietary sugar and its impact on periodontal inflammation: A narrative review. BDJ Open, 10, 78.

[136] Surlari, Z., Ciurcanu, O. E., Budala, D. G., Butnaru, O., & Luchian, I. (2023). An update on the interdisciplinary dental care approach for geriatric diabetic patients. Geriatrics, 8(6), 114.

[137] Thyvalikakath, T. P., Padman, R., & Gupta, S. (2013). An integrated risk assessment tool for team-based periodontal disease management. Studies in Health Technology and Informatics, 192, 1150.

[138] Janakiram, C., & Dye, B. A. (2020). A public health approach for prevention of periodontal disease. Periodontology 2000, 84(1), 202–214.

[139] Lyons, K. M., & Darby, I. (2017). Interdisciplinary periodontics: The multidisciplinary approach to the planning and treatment of complex cases. Periodontology 2000, 74(1), 7–10.

Nada Tawfig Hashim, Rasha Babiker, and Riham Mohammed

3 Periodontal-Systemic Links in Rare or Underexplored Diseases

3.1 Introduction

Periodontitis is a well-established inflammatory disease of the tooth-supporting tissues. Nevertheless, it is becoming increasingly apparent that its impact does not remain within the oral cavity [1]. Recurring periodontal inflammation causes systemic effects via the spread of microorganisms, persistent cytokine secretion, and immune response changes [2, 3]. The bidirectional relationships between periodontitis and prevalent systemic diseases, such as diabetes mellitus and cardiovascular disease, have been extensively documented [4–6]. Recent studies, however, indicated that periodontitis can also play a role in influencing or worsening rare or less researched systemic diseases, including psoriasis, inflammatory bowel disease (IBD), autoimmune thyroiditis, and systemic vasculitides [7–10]. The findings highlight the necessity for a broader, interdisciplinary concept in the field of periodontal medicine.

3.2 Pathophysiological Mechanisms Linking Periodontitis to Systemic Conditions

The mechanisms of pathogenesis linking periodontitis to systemic diseases are both multifactorial and intricate. Initially, the periodontal pocket serves as a reservoir for gram-negative bacteria, including *Porphyromonas gingivalis* (*P. gingivalis*), *Treponema denticola* (*T. denticola*), and *Tannerella forsythia* (*T. forsythia*), with a broad array of virulence factors that include lipopolysaccharides (LPS), fimbriae, gingipains, and outer membrane vesicles (OMVs) [2]. These virulence factors are capable of breaching systemic circulation via ulcerated epithelial tissue, thereby inducing bacteremia and endotoxemia [11].

Second, periodontal pathogens trigger toll-like receptor (TLR) signaling in local and secondary tissues that initiate nuclear factor-kappa B (NF-κB) and mitogen-activated protein kinase (MAPK) pathways. This leads to the production of systemic proinflammatory cytokines, such as interleukin-1β (IL-1β), tumor necrosis factor-alpha (TNF-α), and interleukin-6 (IL-6) [12–14] (Figure 3.1). These cytokines disseminate low-grade systemic inflammation and modulate immune responses in distal organ systems. Also, molecular mimicry between microbial antigens and host proteins may trigger autoimmune responses in genetically predisposed individuals [1].

https://doi.org/10.1515/9783112219904-003

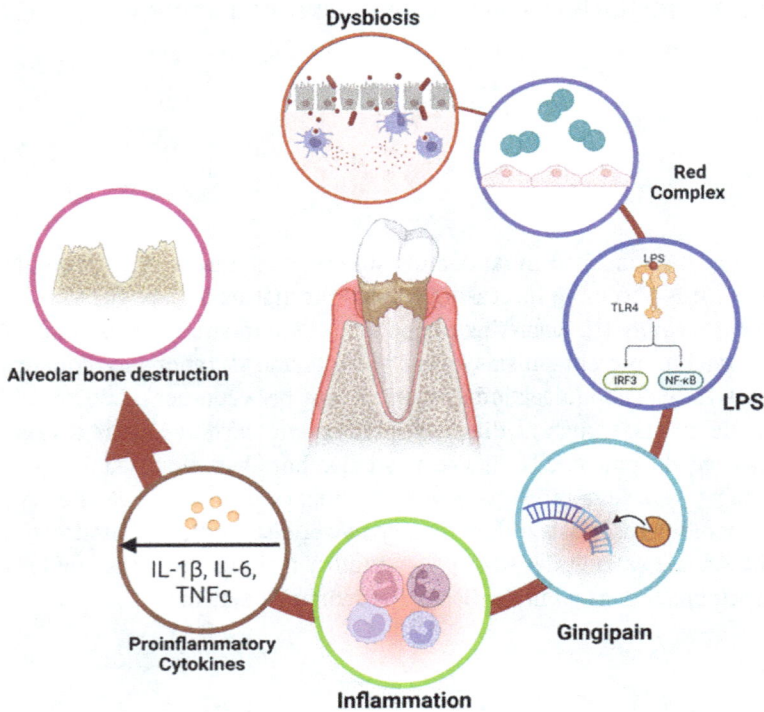

Figure 3.1: Pathogenic cascade in periodontitis. Dysbiosis and red-complex bacteria release LPS/gingipains, provoking inflammation and cytokines that drive alveolar bone loss. Created with Biorender.com.

3.3 Periodontitis and Psoriasis: Shared Inflammatory Landscapes

Psoriasis is a chronic immune-mediated dermatologic disorder affecting 2–3% of the population, marked by erythematous, scaly plaques driven by aberrant activation of T-helper 1 (Th1) and T-helper 17 (Th17) pathways [15]. Similarly, periodontitis involves persistent inflammation of the periodontal tissues initiated by dysbiotic biofilms but perpetuated by an exaggerated host immune response [16]. Beyond the shared elevation of cytokines, such as IL-17, IL-23, TNF-α, and interferon-γ, growing evidence indicates that these diseases are interconnected at both epidemiological and mechanistic levels [17].

Large-scale cohort and case-control studies have consistently shown a higher prevalence and severity of periodontitis among patients with psoriasis, independent of traditional risk factors, such as smoking or diabetes [18, 19]. A meta-analysis by

Qiao et al. [20] reported that psoriasis patients have nearly twice the odds of developing periodontitis compared to healthy controls, suggesting a significant comorbidity burden.

Mechanistically, *P. gingivalis*, a keystone periodontal pathogen, forms a dysbiotic biofilm within periodontal pockets and releases multiple virulence factors, including LPS and gingipains [2]. These microbial components diffuse through ulcerated epithelium and enter the systemic circulation, where they engage TLRs (TLR2 and TLR4) expressed on dendritic cells and macrophages. This interaction activates NF-κB signaling pathways, resulting in the secretion of pro-inflammatory cytokines, such as interleukin-23 (IL-23), IL-1β, and TNF-α [21, 22]. The cytokine milieu drives differentiation and activation of Th17 lymphocytes, which produce interleukin-17 (IL-17), a pivotal effector in sustaining chronic inflammation in both periodontal tissues and psoriatic skin lesions [21, 22]. Simultaneously, infection-induced oxidative stress generates excessive reactive oxygen species, priming neutrophils that not only contribute to local periodontal tissue damage but also circulate systemically [23, 24]. These activated neutrophils migrate to psoriatic plaques, where they release proteases and reactive oxygen intermediates, promoting keratinocyte hyperproliferation and exacerbating cutaneous inflammation [25]. This mechanistic cascade establishes a self-perpetuating inflammatory loop, wherein periodontitis acts as a systemic reservoir of microbial products and cytokines that sustain and amplify psoriatic disease activity, highlighting the intricate immunologic cross-talk between oral infection and chronic autoimmune skin disorders [26] (Figure 3.2).

Clinical studies have also reported that periodontal therapy improves psoriatic symptoms [27, 28]. For example, nonsurgical periodontal treatment in psoriatic patients has been associated with significant reductions in psoriasis area and severity index (PASI) scores, decreased serum C-reactive protein, and improved quality of life measures [29, 30]. This therapeutic effect supports the hypothesis that periodontitis acts as a systemic inflammatory reservoir exacerbating skin disease [31].

These observations underscore the need for integrated care approaches, where dermatologists and dental professionals collaborate to screen and manage both conditions. Further interventional trials are warranted to clarify causality and optimize treatment protocols.

3.4 Inflammatory Bowel Disease (IBD) and Oral-Gut Axis

IBD, which encompasses Crohn's disease and ulcerative colitis, represents chronic relapsing conditions characterized by mucosal immune dysregulation and epithelial barrier dysfunction along the gastrointestinal tract [32]. The oral cavity and gut share extensive microbial and immunological networks, giving rise to a bidirectional "oral-

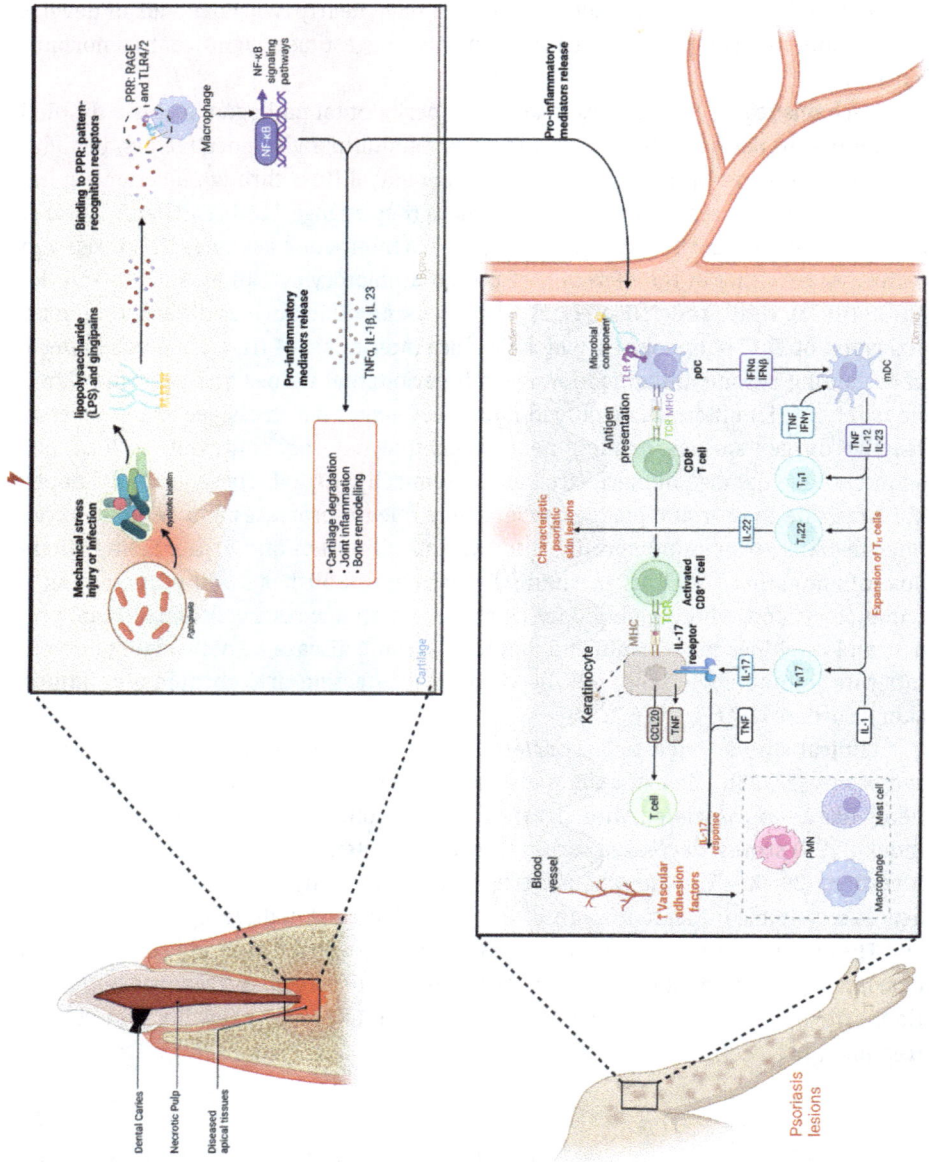

Figure 3.2: Oral-skin axis in psoriasis. Periodontal dysbiosis releases LPS/gingipains that activate PRRs (TLR2/4–NF-κB), elevate cytokines, and prime the IL-23/IL-17 pathway, leading to endothelial activation and psoriatic lesions. Created with Biorender.com.

gut axis" wherein dysbiosis in one site influences inflammation in the other [33]. In periodontitis, overgrowth of pathobionts, such as *Fusobacterium nucleatum* (*F. nucleatum*), *Prevotella* species, and *P. gingivalis* has been shown to contribute to systemic dissemination of bacterial components via saliva swallowing or bacteremia, promoting intestinal colonization and epithelial disruption [34]. *F. nucleatum* in particular is known to adhere to and invade colonic mucosa, exacerbating inflammation and disrupting tight junction proteins critical for gut barrier integrity [35]. Concurrently, TLR (TLR) activation and upregulation of IL-1β, IL-6, and TNF-α in periodontal disease can prime systemic immune responses and lowering the threshold for gut inflammation [1] (Figure 3.3). Experimental models have demonstrated that oral inoculation with *P. gingivalis* increases intestinal permeability, drives Th17 cell polarization, and alters gut microbiota composition, collectively aggravating colitis severity [36, 37].

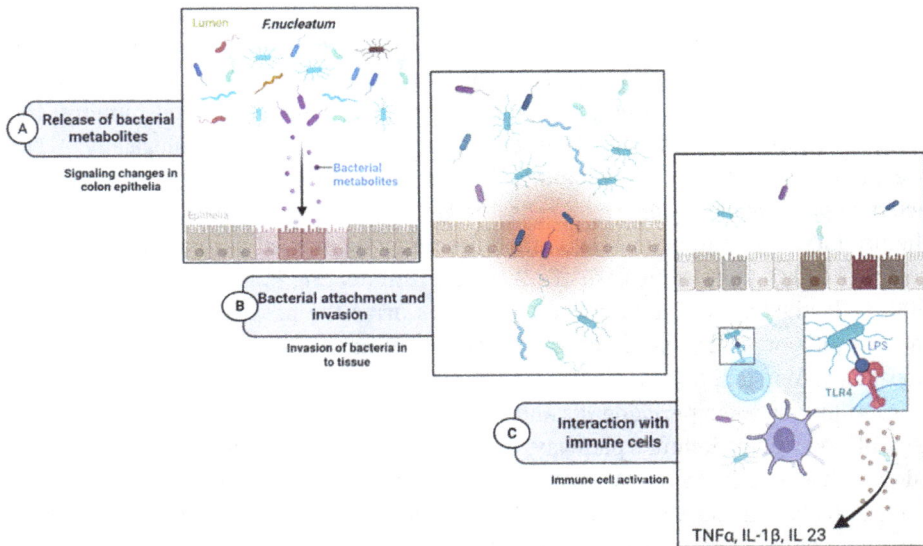

Figure 3.3: Oral-gut axis. Periodontal bacteria and metabolites disrupt intestinal epithelium, enable attachment/invasion, and activate TLR-mediated immune responses (TNF-α, IL-1β, and IL-23). Created with Biorender.com.

Epidemiological studies consistently report a higher prevalence and severity of periodontitis among IBD patients, and there is evidence that periodontal therapy may alleviate gastrointestinal disease activity [38–40]. In parallel, Helicobacter pylori (*H. pylori*), a major etiological agent of gastric ulcers and gastritis, has been frequently identified in dental plaque and periodontal pockets, suggesting that the oral cavity may serve as a reservoir for gastric reinfection [41]. Oral colonization by *H. pylori* can facilitate repeated inoculation of the gastric mucosa, perpetuating chronic gastritis and ulcer recurrence, particularly in individuals with inadequate oral hygiene or untreated periodontal disease [42]. This interconnected pathogenic network underscores the need for integrated management of oral and gastrointestinal health, as addressing periodontal inflammation may contribute to improved outcomes in both IBD and gastric disease.

3.5 Autoimmune Thyroiditis and Periodontitis: A Hypothesized Connection

Autoimmune thyroid diseases (AITDs) represent the most common organ-specific autoimmune disorders, affecting approximately 2–5% of the population, with a marked predominance among women – occurring in 5–15% of females compared to 1–5% of males [43, 44]. The spectrum of AITD primarily includes Hashimoto's thyroiditis (HT) and Graves' disease (GD), which constitute the leading causes of hypothyroidism and hyperthyroidism, respectively [45]. These conditions reflect a fundamental breakdown in immunological tolerance, characterized by both cellular and humoral immune responses directed against thyroid-specific antigens. Histopathologically, AITDs are distinguished by dense lymphocytic infiltration of the thyroid gland, involving reactive populations of T cells and B cells [46, 47]. This immune activation culminates in the production of pathogenic autoantibodies targeting thyroid peroxidase (TPO), thyroglobulin (Tg), and, in the case of GD, thyroid-stimulating hormone (TSH) receptors [48]. Collectively, these immunologic processes drive the progressive destruction or overstimulation of thyroid tissue, ultimately manifesting as the clinical syndromes of thyroid dysfunction.

The link between periodontitis and AITD is still under research; however, the presence of overlapping immune pathways presents an interesting biological rationale. Periodontal disease-associated pathogens have the potential to induce epitope spreading and molecular mimicry. For example, *P. gingivalis* can citrullinate host peptides via its peptidylarginine deiminase enzyme, which in turn may trigger the formation of autoantibodies [26, 49]. Furthermore, systemic inflammation driven by IL-6 and TNF-α in periodontitis may influence thyroid autoimmunity [50]. Studies have reported increased serum levels of these cytokines in AITD patients [51, 52], and periodontal therapy may lower their concentrations [53, 54]. An altered Treg/Th17 balance, characteristic of both diseases, may be a critical immunological intersection [55, 56].

3.6 Systemic Vasculitides

Vasculitides, such as Behçet's disease, granulomatosis with polyangiitis (GPA), and Takayasu arteritis are characterized by inflammation affecting the vascular tissue, resulting in a range of oral manifestations [57, 58]. While periodontitis might not be the most salient issue, it can nevertheless contribute towards the underlying pathophysiologic processes or complicate the progression of these conditions [59].

In GPA, oral ulcers and gingival hyperplasia are common. *P. gingivalis* and *F. nucleatum* have been detected in subgingival biofilms of GPA patients and may contribute to neutrophil priming and ANCA (Anti- neutrophil Cytoplasmic Antibodies) formation [60].

In Behçet's disease, cross-reactivity between streptococcal heat-shock proteins (HSPs) and host antigens suggests a role for oral microbiota in disease flares. In this chronic relapsing multisystem vasculitis, accumulating evidence implicates the oral microbiota as a critical environmental trigger contributing to disease exacerbation [61].

One of the most compelling mechanistic links involves the phenomenon of molecular mimicry between microbial HSPs and host antigens [62]. *Streptococcus sanguinis* (*S. sanguinis*), a commensal bacterium abundant in dental plaque, expresses a 65-kDa HSP (HSP-65) with a high degree of homology to human HSP-60 [63, 64]. This antigenic similarity can provoke cross-reactive immune responses wherein T cells sensitized to streptococcal HSP-65 also recognize and attack host endothelial and epithelial cells expressing homologous HSPs under stress conditions [62] (Figure 3.4).

Immunologically, this cross-reactivity leads to enhanced activation of γδ T cells and CD4+ Th cells producing proinflammatory cytokines, notably interferon-γ (IFN-γ), TNF-α, and IL-17, which are central to the pathogenesis of mucocutaneous ulcers and vasculitis lesions characteristic of Behçet's disease [63, 65, 66]. In parallel, the innate immune system is activated through tollTLRs and nucleotide-binding oligomerization domain-like receptors (NOD-like receptors), further amplifying cytokine release and neutrophil hyper-responsiveness. Neutrophils in Behçet's disease exhibit increased chemotaxis, phagocytic activity, and reactive oxygen species production, contributing to tissue injury and ulcer formation [67, 68].

Clinically, patients with active disease often demonstrate higher colonization levels of *S. sanguinis* and elevated serum antibodies against streptococcal antigens compared to healthy controls [62]. Salivary and mucosal immune responses targeting these bacteria have been proposed as key drivers of the recurrent oral ulcerations that frequently herald systemic flares [62]. The observation that dental plaque control and systemic antibiotic therapy can reduce the frequency and severity of mucosal lesions further underscores the pathogenic role of oral bacteria in Behçet's disease [61].

Overall, these findings support the concept that oral microbiota, through molecular mimicry and innate immune activation, act as a reservoir of antigens capable of perpetuating chronic systemic inflammation in genetically susceptible individuals [69]. The systemic release of proinflammatory mediators from periodontal tissues can exacerbate endothelial dysfunction and immune dysregulation in these disorders. The treatment of oral inflammation in vasculitis patients can potentially reduce systemic disease activity, but interventional studies are still lacking [70].

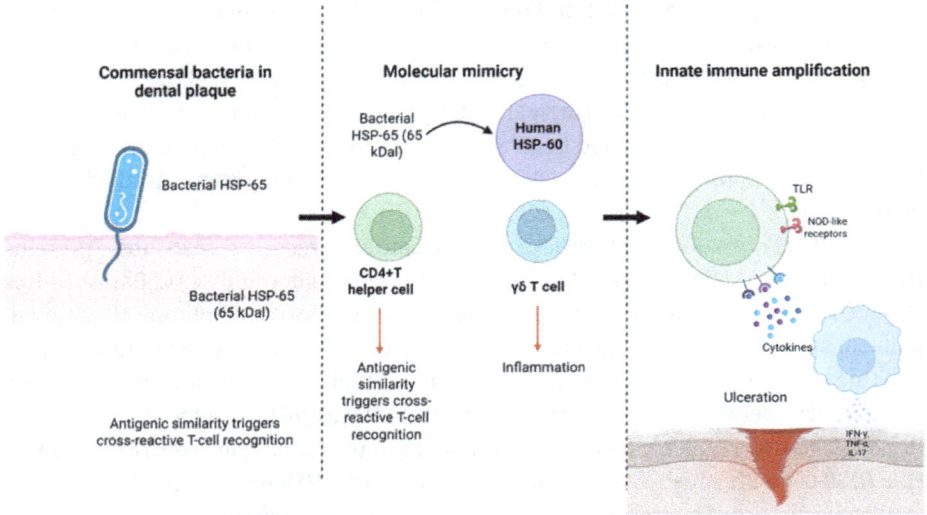

Figure 3.4: Molecular mimicry linking dental plaque to mucosal inflammation. Bacterial HSP60 mimics human HSP60, activating CD4⁺ and γδ T cells; cytokines/ROS amplify innate responses and epithelial injury. Created with Biorender.com.

3.7 Other Rare Conditions: Sarcoidosis and Systemic Sclerosis

Sarcoidosis, characterized by granuloma development and with an unknown etiology, rarely presents as oral lesions and can be worsened by chronic periodontal infections [71, 72].

Systemic sclerosis, characterized by its vascular abnormalities and fibrotic changes, frequently involves the oral mucosa and is associated with increased periodontal attachment loss [73, 74].

In both diseases, chronic inflammation and immune dysregulation intersect with oral health. Salivary cytokine profiles in affected patients often mirror those seen in periodontitis, including elevated IL-6 and MMP-9. Xerostomia and reduced manual dexterity in systemic sclerosis further predispose patients to plaque accumulation and periodontal breakdown [75–77].

3.8 Therapeutic Implications and Future Directions

The identification of the association of periodontitis with comparatively uncommon systemic conditions holds new therapeutic potential for integrated approaches and targeted treatment regimes. Integrated approaches for interdisciplinary screening among rheumatologists, dermatologists, endocrinologists, and gastroenterologists can enhance the timely identification and treatment of periodontitis and immune-mediated states [78].

Biomarker-driven treatment strategies are a promising field of investigation. Salivary IL-1β, MMP-8, and micro-RNA levels, such as miR-146a, can serve as indicators of oral and systemic inflammatory burdens [79, 80]. In addition, new drugs, e.g., monoclonal antibodies (e.g., anti-IL-17 and anti-TNF), used in the management of psoriasis or IBD, can have adjunctive benefits in enhancing periodontal treatment outcomes [81].

Preventive strategies should include enhanced oral hygiene measures, frequent professional dental cleaning, and perhaps additional antimicrobial or host-modulatory treatments tailored according to the individual inflammatory status [82]. Future studies should emphasize longitudinal research designs, mechanistic insights enabled by omics technologies, and randomized clinical trials assessing the effect of periodontal treatment on the progression of systemic diseases.

3.9 Conclusion

Periodontitis is not merely a local oral disease but also a systemic inflammatory condition with far-reaching implications. While its association with prevalent systemic diseases is well recognized, the emerging links with underexplored conditions, such as psoriasis, IBD, autoimmune thyroiditis, and systemic vasculitides deserve focused attention. Through a better understanding of shared immunological and microbial pathways, periodontal care can become a cornerstone of systemic disease management, reinforcing the paradigm of oral-systemic health integration.

References

[1]   Martínez-García, M., & Hernández-Lemus, E. (2021). Periodontal inflammation and systemic diseases: An overview. Frontiers in Physiology, 12, 709438.

[2]   Bui, F. Q., Almeida-da Silva, C. L. C., Huynh, B., Trinh, A., Liu, J., & Woodward, J. et al. (2019). Association between periodontal pathogens and systemic disease. Biomedical Journal, 42, 27–35.

[3]   Ramadan, D. E., Hariyani, N., Indrawati, R., Ridwan, R. D., & Diyatri I. (2020). Cytokines and chemokines in periodontitis. European Journal of Dentistry, 14, 483.

[4]   Nazir, M. A. (2017). Prevalence of periodontal disease, its association with systemic diseases and prevention. International Journal of Health Sciences, 11, 72.

[5]   Păunică, I., Giurgiu, M., Dumitriu, A. S., Păunică, S., Pantea Stoian, A. M., Martu, M. A., & Serafinceanu, C. (2023). The bidirectional relationship between periodontal disease and diabetes mellitus – a review. Diagnostics, 13(4), 681.

[6]   Herrera, D., Sanz, M., Shapira, L., Brotons, C., Chapple, I., Frese, T., Graziani, F., Hobbs, F. D. R., Huck, O., Hummers, E., Jepsen, S., Kravtchenko, O., Madianos, P., Molina, A., Ungan, M., Vilaseca, J., Windak, A., & Vinker, S. (2023). Association between periodontal diseases and cardiovascular diseases, diabetes and respiratory diseases: Consensus report of the joint workshop by the European Federation of Periodontology (EFP) and WONCA Europe. Journal of Clinical Periodontology, 50(6), 819–841.

[7]   Di Spirito, F., Di Palo, M. P., Rupe, A., Piedepalumbo, F., Sessa, A., De Benedetto, G., Russo Barone, S., & Contaldo, M. (2024). Periodontitis in psoriatic patients: Epidemiological insights and putative etiopathogenic links. Epidemiologia, 5(3), 479–498.

[8]   La Rosa, G. R., Ismael, A., Caponio, V. C., & Puci, M. V. (2025). Apical periodontitis in inflammatory bowel disease: A meta-analysis at patient and tooth level. Frontiers in Dental Medicine, 6, 1553914.

[9]   Inchingolo, F., Inchingolo, A. M., Inchingolo, A. D., Fatone, M. C., Ferrante, L., Avantario, P., Fiore, A., Palermo, A., Amenduni, T., Galante, F., & Dipalma, G. (2024). Bidirectional association between periodontitis and thyroid disease: A scoping review. International Journal of Environmental Research and Public Health, 21(7), 860.

[10]   Ge, J., Zhu, X., Weng, C., Yuan, D., Zhao, J., Zhao, L., Wang, T., & Wu, Y. (2024). Periodontitis impacts on thrombotic diseases: From clinical aspect to future therapeutic approaches. International Journal of Oral Science, 16(1), 1–15.

[11]   Abdulkareem, A. A., Al-Taweel, F. B., Al-Sharqi, A. J. B., Gul, S. S., Sha, A., & Chapple, I. L. C. (2023). Current concepts in the pathogenesis of periodontitis: From symbiosis to dysbiosis. Journal of Oral Microbiology, 15(1), 2197779.

[12]   Gu, Y., & Han, X. (2020). Toll-like receptor signaling and immune regulatory lymphocytes in periodontal disease. International Journal of Molecular Sciences, 21(9), 3329.

[13]   Hashim, N. T., Babiker, R., Chaitanya, N. C. S. K., Mohammed, R., Priya, S. P., Padmanabhan, V., Ahmed, A., Dasnadi, S. P., Islam, M. S., Gismalla, B. G., & Rahman, M. M. (2025). New insights in natural bioactive compounds for periodontal disease: Advanced molecular mechanisms and therapeutic potential. Molecules, 30(4), 807.

[14]   Hashim, N. T., Babiker, R., Priya, S. P., Mohammed, R., Chaitanya, N. C., Padmanabhan, V., El Bahra, S., Rahman, M. M., & Gismalla, B. G. (2024). Microbial dynamics in periodontal regeneration: Understanding microbiome shifts and the role of antifouling and bactericidal materials. Current Issues in Molecular Biology, 46(11), 12196–12213.

[15]   Dhabale, A., & Nagpure, S. (2022). Types of psoriasis and their effects on the immune system. Cureus, 14(9), e29536.

[16]   Bunte, K., & Beikler, T. (2019). Th17 cells and the IL-23/IL-17 axis in the pathogenesis of periodontitis and immune-mediated inflammatory diseases. International Journal of Molecular Sciences, 20(14), 3394.

[17]   Meneu, J. J., Fabiana, C., & Silvestre, F. J. (2023). Could periodontitis aggravate psoriasis? An update by systematic review. Oral, 3(1), 57–66.

[18]   Preus, H. R., Khanifam, P., Kolltveit, K., Mørk, C., & Gjermo, P. (2010). Periodontitis in psoriasis patients: A blinded, case-controlled study. Acta Odontologica Scandinavica, 68, 165–170.

[19]   Egeberg, A., Mallbris, L., Gislason, G., Hansen, P. R., & Mrowietz, U. (2017). Risk of periodontitis in patients with psoriasis and psoriatic arthritis. Journal of the European Academy of Dermatology & Venereology, 31, 288–293.

[20] Qiao, P., Shi, Q., Zhang, R., E, L., Wang, P., Wang, J., & Liu, H. (2019). Psoriasis patients suffer from worse periodontal status: A meta-analysis. Frontiers in Medicine, 6, 212.

[21] Li, C., Yu, R., & Ding, Y. (2022). Association between *Porphyromonas gingivalis* and systemic diseases: Focus on T cell-mediated adaptive immunity. Frontiers in Cellular and Infection Microbiology, 12, 1026457.

[22] Lowes, M. A., Russell, C. B., Martin, D. A., Towne, J. E., & Krueger, J. G. (2013). The IL-23/T17 pathogenic axis in psoriasis is amplified by keratinocyte responses. Trends in Immunology, 34(4), 174–181.

[23] Shang, J., Liu, H., Zheng, Y., & Zhang, Z. (2023). Role of oxidative stress in the relationship between periodontitis and systemic diseases. Frontiers in Physiology, 14, 1210449.

[24] Czerwińska, J. (2021). The role of the neutrophilic network in the pathogenesis of psoriasis. International Journal of Molecular Sciences, 23(3), 1840.

[25] Garcia, G., Chen, S. J., Westerland, M. R., Wu, X., Hwang, S. T., & Simon, S. I. (2024). Psoriatic neutrophils are primed in circulation for enhanced β2-integrin-dependent recruitment and effector function on E-selectin and ICAM-1. Journal of Investigative Dermatology, 144(4), 901–905.e4.

[26] Hajishengallis, G. (2015). Periodontitis: From microbial immune subversion to systemic inflammation. Nature Reviews Immunology, 15(1), 30–44.

[27] Ucan Yarkac, F., Ogrum, A., & Gokturk, O. (2020). Effects of non-surgical periodontal therapy on inflammatory markers of psoriasis: A randomized controlled trial. Journal of Clinical Periodontology, 47(2), 193–201.

[28] Marruganti, C., Gaeta, C., Falciani, C., Cinotti, E., Rubegni, P., Alovisi, M., Scotti, N., Baldi, A., Bellan, C., Defraia, C., Bertaggia, E., Fiorino, F., Valensin, S., Bellini, E., De Rosa, A., Graziani, F., D'Aiuto, F., & Grandini, S. (2025). The synergetic effect of periodontal therapy and TNF-α inhibitor for the treatment of comorbid periodontitis and psoriasis. Journal of Clinical Periodontology, 52(6), 907–919.

[29] Keller, J. J., & Lin, H. C. (2012). The effects of chronic periodontitis and its treatment on the subsequent risk of psoriasis. British Journal of Dermatology, 167, 1333–1344.

[30] Marruganti, C., Malvicini, G., Cinotti, E., Fuso, A., Trovato, E., Rubegni, P., Grandini, S., & Gaeta, C. (2025). Association between apical periodontitis and psoriasis vulcaris: A cross-sectional study. International Endodontic Journal, 58(6), 848–861.

[31] Di Spirito, F., Di Palo, M. P., Rupe, A., Piedepalumbo, F., Sessa, A., De Benedetto, G., Russo Barone, S., & Contaldo, M. (2024). Periodontitis in psoriatic patients: Epidemiological insights and putative etiopathogenic links. Epidemiologia, 5(3), 479.

[32] Corridoni, D., Arseneau, K. O., & Cominelli, F. (2014). Inflammatory bowel disease. Immunology Letters, 161(2), 231.

[33] Zhong, Y., Kang, X., Bai, X., Pu, B., Smerin, D., Zhao, L., & Xiong, X. (2024). The oral-gut-brain axis: The influence of microbes as a link of periodontitis with ischemic stroke. CNS Neuroscience and Therapeutics, 30(12), e70152.

[34] Xi, M., Ruan, Q., Zhong, S., Li, J., Qi, W., Xie, C., Wang, X., Abuduxiku, N., & Ni, J. (2024). Periodontal bacteria influence systemic diseases through the gut microbiota. Frontiers in Cellular and Infection Microbiology, 14, 1478362.

[35] Zheng, Z., Jin, W., Guo, W., Jin, Z., & Zuo, Y. (2025). Oral *Fusobacterium nucleatum* exacerbates ulcerative colitis via the oral-gut axis: Mechanisms and therapeutic implications. Frontiers in Cellular and Infection Microbiology, 15, 1564169.

[36] Sun, J., Wang, X., Xiao, J., Yang, Q., Huang, X., Yang, Z., Liu, H., Liu, Y., Wang, H., Huang, Z., Ma, L., & Cao, Z. (2024). Autophagy mediates the impact of *Porphyromonas gingivalis* on short-chain fatty acids metabolism in periodontitis-induced gut dysbiosis. Scientific Reports, 14(1), 26291.

[37] Jia, L., Jiang, Y., Wu, L., Fu, J., Du, J., Luo, Z., Guo, L., Xu, J., & Liu, Y. (2024). *Porphyromonas gingivalis* aggravates colitis via a gut microbiota-linoleic acid metabolism-Th17/Treg cell balance axis. Nature Communications, 15(1), 1617.

[38] Baima, G., Muwalla, M., Testa, G., Mazza, F., Bebars, A., Perotto, S., Vernero, M., Massano, A., Romano, F., Ribaldone, D. G., & Aimetti, M. (2023). Periodontitis prevalence and severity in inflammatory bowel disease: A case-control study. Journal of Periodontology, 94(3), 313–322.

[39] Bertl, K., Burisch, J., Pandis, N., Bruckmann, C., Klinge, B., & Stavropoulos, A. (2022). Periodontitis prevalence in patients with ulcerative colitis and Crohn's disease: A case-control study. Journal of Clinical Periodontology, 49(12), 1262–1274.

[40] Piras, V., Usai, P., Mezzena, S., Susnik, M., Ideo, F., Schirru, E., & Cotti, E. (2017). Prevalence of apical periodontitis in patients with inflammatory bowel diseases: A retrospective clinical study. Journal of Endodontics, 43(3), 389–394.

[41] Marques Payão, S. L., & Rasmussen, L. T. (2016). *Helicobacter pylori* and its reservoirs: a correlation with gastric infection. World Journal of Gastrointestinal Pharmacology and Therapeutics, 7(1), 126.

[42] Sert, S. Y., Ozturk, A., Bektas, A., & Cengiz, M. I. (2020). Periodontal treatment is more effective in gastric *Helicobacter pylori* eradication in those patients who maintain good oral hygiene. International Dental Journal, 69(5), 392.

[43] Simmonds, M. J., & Gough, S. C. (2004). Unravelling the genetic complexity of autoimmune thyroid disease: HLA, CTLA-4 and beyond. Clinical and Experimental Immunology, 136, 1–10.

[44] Dayan, C. M., & Daniels, G. H. (1996). Chronic autoimmune thyroiditis. New England Journal of Medicine, 335, 99–107.

[45] Stathatos, N., & Daniels, G. H. (2012). Autoimmune thyroid disease. Current Opinion in Rheumatology, 24, 70–75.

[46] Tomer, Y., & Davies, T. F. (2003). Searching for the autoimmune thyroid disease susceptibility genes: From gene mapping to gene function. Endocrine Reviews, 24, 694–717.

[47] Anaya, J. M., Castiblanco, J., & Rojas-Villarraga, A. et al. (2012). The multiple autoimmune syndromes: A clue for the autoimmune tautology. Clinical Reviews in Allergy & Immunology, 43, 256–264.

[48] Antonelli, A., Ferrari, S. M., Corrado, A., Di Domenicantonio, A., & Fallahi, P. (2015). Autoimmune thyroid disorders. Autoimmunity Reviews, 14(2), 174–180.

[49] Bonilla, M., & Mesa, F. (2023). Impact of protein citrullination by periodontal pathobionts on oral and systemic health: A systematic review of preclinical and clinical studies. Journal of Clinical Medicine, 13(22), 6831.

[50] Song, E., Park, M. J., Kim, J. A., Roh, E., Yu, J. H., Kim, N. H., Yoo, H. J., Seo, J. A., Kim, S. G., Kim, N. H., Baik, S. H., & Choi, K. M. (2021). Implication of thyroid function in periodontitis: A nationwide population-based study. Scientific Reports, 11(1), 22127.

[51] Mikos, H., Mikos, M., Rabska-Pietrzak, B., & Niedziela, M. (2014). The clinical role of serum concentrations of selected cytokines: IL-1β, TNF-α and IL-6 in diagnosis of autoimmune thyroid disease in children. Autoimmunity, 47(7), 466–472.

[52] Markoš, I. Š., Franceschi, M., Vidranski, V., Markoš, P., Jukić, T., Fröbe, A., & Kes, V. B. (2023). The concentration of interleukin-6 and tumor necrosis factor alpha in saliva and blood of patients with inactive multiple sclerosis and coexisting Hashimoto's thyroiditis. Acta Clinica Croatica, 62(2), 339.

[53] Ren, J., & Li, H. (2022). Effects of periodontal treatment on levels of proinflammatory cytokines in patients with chronic periodontitis: a meta-analysis. Computational and Mathematical Methods in Medicine, 2022, 9349598.

[54] Arregoces, F. M., Roa, N. S., Rodríguez, L. V., Merchan, M. J., Poveda, J. C., Otero, L., Ruiz, Á. J., & Uriza, C. L. (2025). Changes in serum inflammatory markers and clinical periodontal condition after non-surgical periodontal treatment in hypertensive patients. Biomedicines, 13(2), 374.

[55] Li, C., Yuan, J., Zhu, Y. F., Yang, X. J., Wang, Q., Xu, J., He, S. T., & Zhang, J. A. (2016). Imbalance of Th17/Treg in different subtypes of autoimmune thyroid diseases. Cellular Physiology and Biochemistry, 40(1–2), 245–252.

[56] Gaffen, S. L., & Hajishengallis, G. (2008). A new inflammatory cytokine on the block: Re-thinking periodontal disease and the Th1/Th2 paradigm in the context of Th17 cells and IL-17. Journal of Dental Research, 87(9), 817–828.

[57] Watts, R. A., & Scott, D. G. (2009). Recent advances in the classification and assessment of vasculitis. Best Practice and Research Clinical Rheumatology, 23, 429–443.

[58] Waller, R., Ahmed, A., Patel, I., & Luqmani, R. (2013). Update on the classification of vasculitis. Best Practice and Research Clinical Rheumatology, 27, 3–17.

[59] Kiramira, D., Uphaus, T., Othman, A., Heermann, R., Deschner, J., & Müller-Heupt, L. K. (2024). Stroke caused by vasculitis induced by periodontitis-associated oral bacteria after wisdom teeth extraction. Brain Sciences, 14(6), 550.

[60] Szczeklik, K., Włudarczyk, A., Wawrzycka-Adamczyk, K., Górka, J., Fuks-Kulska, M., Darczuk, D., Pytko-Polończyk, J., & Szczeklik, W. (2019). Oral manifestations of granulomatosis with polyangiitis: Clinical and radiological assessment. Journal of Dental Sciences, 14(1), 54–60.

[61] Mumcu, G., & Fortune, F. (2021). Oral health and its aetiological role in Behçet's disease. Frontiers in Medicine, 8, 613419.

[62] Kireçtepe Aydın, A. K., & Hatemi, G. (2023). Heat shock proteins in Behçet syndrome. Balkan Medical Journal, 40(5), 314–323.

[63] Ghasemi, Y., Dabbagh, F., Rasoul-Amini, S., Borhani Haghighi, A., & Morowvat, M. H. (2012). The possible role of HSPs in Behçet's disease: A bioinformatic approach. Computers in Biology and Medicine, 42(11), 1079–1085.

[64] Narikawa, S., Suzuki, Y., Takahashi, M., Furukawa, A., Sakane, T., & Mizushima, Y. (1995). *Streptococcus oralis* previously identified as uncommon *Streptococcus sanguis* in Behçet's disease. Archives of Oral Biology, 40(8), 685–690.

[65] Cunningham, M. W. (2019). Molecular mimicry, autoimmunity, and infection: The cross-reactive antigens of group A streptococci and their sequelae. Microbiology Spectrum, 7(4), gpp3–0045–2018.

[66] Hasan, A., Shinnick, T., Mizushima, Y., Van der Zee, R., & Lehner, T. (2002). Defining a T-cell epitope within HSP65 in recurrent aphthous stomatitis. Clinical and Experimental Immunology, 128(2), 318–325.

[67] Perazzio, S. F., Andrade, L. E. C., & De Souza, A. W. S. (2020). Understanding Behçet's disease in the context of innate immunity activation. Frontiers in Immunology, 11, 586558.

[68] Shimizu, J., Murayama, M. A., Mizukami, Y., Arimitsu, N., Takai, K., & Miyabe, Y. (2023). Innate immune responses in Behçet disease and relapsing polychondritis. Frontiers in Medicine, 10, 105575.

[69] Suárez, L. J., Garzón, H., Arboleda, S., & Rodríguez, A. (2020). Oral dysbiosis and autoimmunity: From local periodontal responses to an imbalanced systemic immunity. Frontiers in Immunology, 11, 591255.

[70] Celik, D., & Kantarci, A. (2021). Vascular changes and hypoxia in periodontal disease as a link to systemic complications. Pathogens, 10(10), 1280.

[71] Radochová, V., Radocha, J., Laco, J., & Slezák, R. (2016). Oral manifestation of sarcoidosis: a case report and review of the literature. Journal of Indian Society of Periodontology, 20(6), 627–629.

[72] Gupta, S., Tripathi, A. K., Kumar, V., & Saimbi, C. S. (2015). Sarcoidosis: Oral and extra-oral manifestation. Journal of Indian Society of Periodontology, 19(5), 582–585.

[73] Jagadish, R., Mehta, D. S., & Jagadish, P. (2012). Oral and periodontal manifestations associated with systemic sclerosis: A case series and review. Journal of Indian Society of Periodontology, 16(2), 271–274.

[74] Sharma, M., Fadl, A., & Leask, A. (2024). Orofacial complications of the connective tissue disease systemic sclerosis. Journal of Dental Research, Advance online publication, 103, 689–696.

[75] Kobak, S., Sever, F., Sivrikoz, O., & Karaarslan, A. (2013). Coexistence of sarcoidosis and systemic sclerosis. Case Reports in Rheumatology, 2013, 684216.

[76] Crincoli, V., Fatone, L., Fanelli, M., Rotolo, R. P., Chialà, A., Favia, G., & Lapadula, G. (2016). Orofacial manifestations and temporomandibular disorders of systemic scleroderma: An observational study. International Journal of Molecular Sciences, 17(7), 1189.

[77] Antonacci, A., Praino, E., Abbinante, A., Favia, G., Rotondo, C., Bartolomeo, N., Giotta, M., Iannone, F., Orrù, G., Agneta, M. T., Capodiferro, S., Barile, G., & Corsalini, M. (2023). Orofacial manifestation of systemic sclerosis: a cross-sectional study and future prospects of oral capillaroscopy. Diagnostics, 14(4), 437.

[78] Mohd Norwir, N. A., Mohd-Said, S., Abdul Aziz, A. F., & Mohd-Dom, T. N. (2025). Leveraging dental visits for systemic health: Diabetes screening and referral compliance in periodontitis patients in Malaysia. Journal of Clinical Medicine, 14(3), 739.

[79] Sachelarie, L., Stefanescu, C. L., Murineanu, R. M., Grigorian, M., Zaharia, A., Scrobota, I., & Hurjui, L. L. (2025). Role of salivary biomarkers IL-1β and MMP-8 in early detection and staging of periodontal disease. Medicina, 61(4), 760.

[80] Bastías, D., Maturana, A., Marín, C., Martínez, R., & Niklander, S. E. (2023). Salivary biomarkers for oral cancer detection: An exploratory systematic review. International Journal of Molecular Sciences, 25(5), 2634.

[81] Jiraskova Zakostelska, Z., Reiss, Z., Tlaskalova-Hogenova, H., & Rob, F. (2023). Paradoxical reactions to anti-TNFα and anti-IL-17 treatment in psoriasis patients: Are skin and/or gut microbiota involved?. Dermatology and Therapy, 13(4), 911–933.

[82] Tonetti, M. S., Bottenberg, P., & Conrads, G. et al. (2017). Dental caries and periodontal diseases in the ageing population: Call to action to protect and enhance oral health and well-being as an essential component of healthy ageing – consensus report of group 4 of the joint EFP/ORCA workshop on the boundaries between caries and periodontal diseases. Journal of Clinical Periodontology, 44(Suppl 18), S135–S144.

Nada Tawfig Hashim, Rasha Babiker, Riham Mohammed, and
Muhammed Mustahsen Rahman

4 Molecular and Genetic Biomarkers in Periodontitis

4.1 Introduction

Periodontitis is described as a chronic and complex inflammatory process that results in the destruction of the supportive structures of the teeth [1]. Although microbial dysbiosis is the main etiological factor, individual predispositions and the regulation of immune responses are important factors that determine the severity, progression, and treatment of the disease [2]. Traditional diagnostic methods – probing and radiographic assessments, are by nature retrospective, detecting the disease only after significant tissue destruction has occurred [3].

Within the framework of this dynamic environment, molecular and genetic biomarkers have become important tools for achieving early diagnosis, the customization of risk assessments, continuous monitoring, and preventive and anticipatory interventions [4]. They are detectable in saliva, gingival crevicular fluid (GCF), and serum and include cytokines, matrix-degrading enzymes, genetic polymorphisms, microRNAs (miRNAs), and various host response mediators [4–6]. The growing importance of these biomarkers puts periodontitis squarely within the domain of personalized medicine – moving toward precision-based prevention and intervention as opposed to reactive approaches.

4.2 The Rationale for Biomarker Use in Periodontology

Traditional diagnostic modalities in periodontology, such as clinical probing, BOP, and radiographic assessment, are retrospective [3]. They provide information about past tissue destruction but offer limited insight into current disease activity, predictive risk, or individual treatment response [7, 8]. This limitation has prompted a growing interest in molecular diagnostics, particularly the use of biomarkers that reflect real-time biological processes occurring within the periodontium [2, 9]. Unlike structural or clinical assessments, biomarkers capture dynamic events at the molecular and cellular levels, offering a functional perspective on disease onset, activity, and resolution [10].

An ideal periodontal biomarker should meet several critical criteria [11]. First, it must be detectable in biological fluids, such as saliva or GCF, ensuring non-invasive,

https://doi.org/10.1515/9783112219904-004

repeatable sampling [12]. Second, it should be highly specific to periodontal pathology, meaning its presence or concentration should correlate with disease severity or activity, and not merely reflect systemic inflammation. Third, the biomarker should mirror the underlying pathophysiology-for instance, indicating tissue breakdown, neutrophil activity, or host-microbiome interactions [13]. Fourth, it must be sensitive enough to detect early-stage disease, ideally before irreversible destruction occurs. Finally, a clinically useful biomarker should be responsive to therapeutic interventions, allowing practitioners to monitor treatment efficacy and adjust care accordingly [13, 14].

The emergence of omics technologies – namely, genomics, transcriptomics, proteomics, and metabolomics – has revolutionized biomarker discovery in periodontology. These high-throughput platforms provide comprehensive profiling of biological molecules, enabling the identification of candidate biomarkers based on their differential expression in health versus disease [15]:

– **Transcriptomics**, for example, assesses gene expression profiles using RNA sequencing or microarrays to reveal upregulated or downregulated transcripts associated with inflammation, immune regulation, or tissue remodeling. Many proinflammatory cytokines, chemokines, and regulatory non-coding RNAs (like microRNAs) have been identified this way [16].

– **Proteomics** focuses on protein expression and post-translational modifications, helping to identify enzymes like matrix metalloproteinases (MMPs) and other signaling proteins in GCF, and saliva that reflect real-time tissue degradation [17].

– **Metabolomics** explores small-molecule metabolites that can serve as functional readouts of microbial metabolism or host response, such as oxidative stress markers or nitric oxide pathways [18].

Together, these omics approaches provide a system-level view of periodontal pathogenesis, bridging the gap between microbial ecology, host genetics, and clinical outcomes. By integrating omics data with clinical and radiographic findings, a new frontier of precision periodontics is emerging one that enables personalized diagnosis, risk prediction, and therapeutic targeting based on each patient's unique molecular profile [19].

4.3 Pro-inflammatory Cytokines as Biomarkers

Pro-inflammatory cytokines are among the earliest and the most extensively studied biomarkers in the domain of periodontology, playing significant roles as mediators and amplifiers of the host inflammatory response [20]. Their production is mainly triggered in resident gingival epithelial cells, fibroblasts, macrophages, dendritic cells, and neutrophils in response to bacterial stimuli, i.e., lipopolysaccharides (LPS) from gram-negative periodontogenic bacteria [21]. The cytokine concentrations in the GCF and saliva are reflective of the magnitude and duration of the inflammatory processes occurring in the periodontal environment and show correlations with clinical parameters like probing depth, loss of clinical attachment, and bleeding upon probing [22].

Interleukin-1 beta (IL-1β) is highly investigated within the context of periodontal disease [22]. This cytokine is mainly produced by activated macrophages and fibroblasts upon exposure to bacterial products and endogenously produced danger signals. IL-1β is implicated in leukocyte recruitment, prostaglandin synthesis, and osteoclast differentiation and is associated with the processes of alveolar bone resorption [23]. Elevated levels of IL-1β in GCF are consistently correlated with active periodontal tissue destruction and represent some of the strongest predictive biomarkers for the progression of periodontitis [22]. Certain polymorphisms in the IL1B gene, including the +3954 C/T polymorphism, have been implicated in the development of a hyperinflammatory phenotype, rendering IL-1β as a diagnostic and prognostic biomarker. Importantly, individuals carrying this polymorphism show increased susceptibility to stages III and IV, grade C periodontitis even with low-level plaque presence, highlighting its possible significance in personalized risk assessment [24, 25] (Figure 4.1).

Tumor necrosis factor-alpha (TNF-α), a critical cytokine, is secreted predominantly by T-cells and monocytes/macrophages in response to stimulation with bacterial endotoxins [26]. The biological activities of TNF-α are multifaceted and include the induction of adhesion molecule expression on endothelial cells, promotion of neutrophil transmigration, apoptosis of structural gingival cells, and a notable stimulation of osteoclastogenesis through upregulation of receptor activator of nuclear factor kappa-B ligand (RANKL) [27]. Additionally, TNF-α induces the release of other cytokines, including interleukin-1 (IL-1) and interleukin-6 (IL-6), initiating a pro-inflammatory cascade that contributes to progressive tissue destruction [28].

Genetically, polymorphisms within the TNF gene promoter region have been shown to influence individual variations in TNF-α production and susceptibility to periodontitis. Among these, the TNF-α −308 G/A polymorphism (rs1800629) is the most widely investigated [29]. The presence of the A allele is associated with higher transcriptional activity of the TNF gene, resulting in increased cytokine expression in response to microbial challenge. This polymorphism has been linked to an elevated risk of severe chronic periodontitis, particularly in individuals also harboring polymorphisms in other pro-inflammatory cytokine genes, such as IL-1β. The synergistic effect of these genotypes contributes to a hyperinflammatory phenotype characterized by exaggerated local cytokine production and accelerated alveolar bone resorption [30] (Figure 4.2).

Concentrations of TNF-α are elevated in the GCF and serum of patients with periodontitis and are thought to contribute to the development of associated systemic inflammatory conditions, such as atherosclerosis and insulin resistance. Importantly, levels of TNF-α in saliva and GCF are reduced following successful periodontal therapy, highlighting its potential utility not only as a biomarker for disease activity but also as an indicator of treatment response [31, 32]. Taken together, TNF-α and its gene

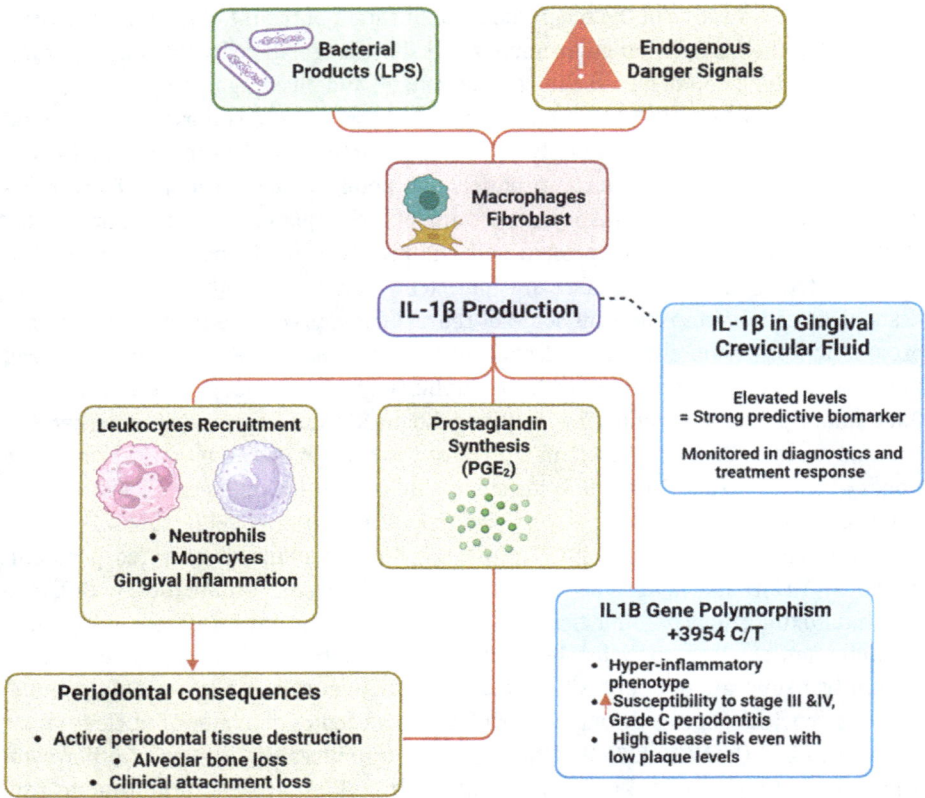

Figure 4.1: IL-1β axis in periodontitis. Bacterial LPS and danger signals activate macrophages/fibroblasts, inducing IL-1β and PGE₂, leukocyte recruitment, and tissue destruction; GCF IL-1β serves as a biomarker, with IL1B +3954 C/T linked to higher risk. Created with Biorender.com.

polymorphisms represent promising molecular biomarkers for both risk assessment and monitoring of periodontal disease progression.

IL-6) plays a dual role, possessing pro-inflammatory as well as anti-inflammatory properties that are context-dependent [33, 34]. As a central mediator in periodontitis, IL-6 is chiefly produced by fibroblasts, monocytes, and endothelial cells as a response to bacterial invasion or IL-1 stimulation [35]. The cytokine is involved in B-cell maturation, affects T-cell differentiation, and is implicated in bone resorption by augmenting the expression of RANKL [22, 36] (Figure 4.3). Elevated levels of IL-6 in GCF and saliva, and their high correlation with disease severity, reflect a strong correlation; additionally, elevated systemic levels have been implicated in oral inflammatory conditions that co-present with systemic diseases like cardiovascular disease, rheumatoid arthritis, and type 2 diabetes. IL-6 levels are generally increased in deep periodontal pockets and inflamed tissues, representing a production gradient, which implicates their site-

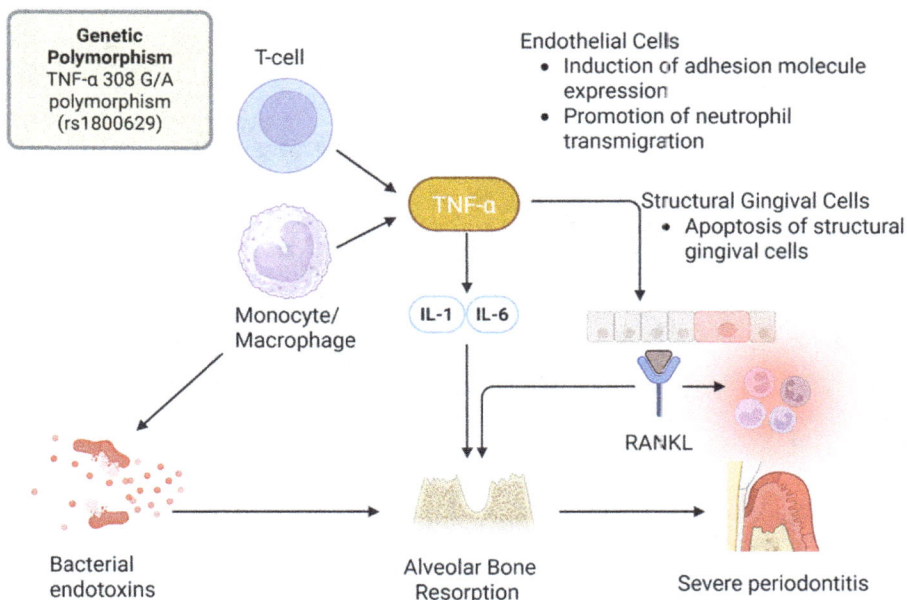

Figure 4.2: TNF-α pathway in periodontitis. The TNF-α −308 G/A (rs1800629) variant and bacterial endotoxins activate T cells/monocytes to elevate TNF-α. Downstream IL-1/IL-6, endothelial adhesion and neutrophil transmigration, apoptosis of structural gingival cells, and RANKL signaling culminate in alveolar bone resorption and severe periodontitis. Created with Biorender.com.

specific diagnostic utility [37–41]. Decreases in IL-6 levels following treatment have been correlated with clinical parameter improvements, thus substantiating its use as a theranostic biomarker [42].

Importantly, the bioavailability and levels of these cytokines are regulated by local factors, such as pocket depth, tissue vascularization, microbial burden, oxidative stress, and the presence of neutrophil extracellular traps (NETs) [43–46]. The diffusion of cytokines into the crevicular fluid is also dependent on tissue permeability and the local inflammatory milieu, which may vary between subjects. Additionally, the methods used for sampling, the amount of fluid sampled, and circadian rhythms may affect the levels of these cytokines detectable, highlighting the need for standardized protocols in biomarker measurement [47–49]. Nevertheless, the inclusion of IL-1β, TNF-α, and IL-6 in multiplex biomarker panels or point-of-care diagnostic tests is already changing risk assessment and therapeutic management within the discipline of periodontology [51–53].

By combining genetic predisposition data (e.g., IL-1 genotype) with real-time cytokine levels, clinicians can now stratify patients based on molecular risk, personalize maintenance protocols, and identify cases at risk of refractory progression, even in

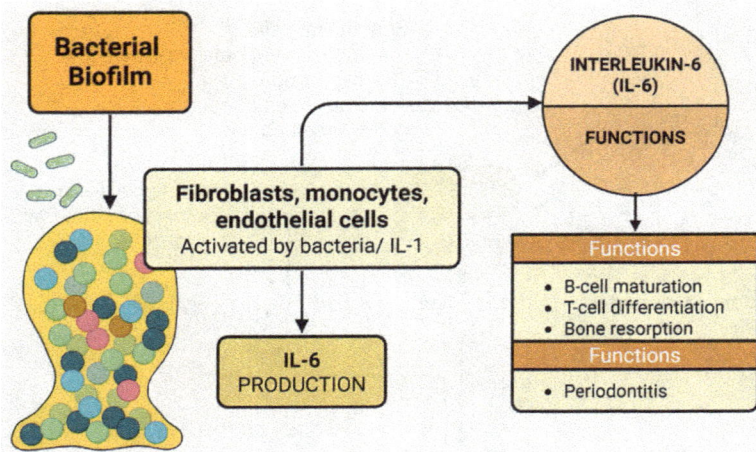

Figure 4.3: IL-6 pathway in periodontitis. Biofilm activates fibroblasts, monocytes, and endothelial cells to produce IL-6, driving B/T-cell responses and bone resorption. Created with Biorender.com.

clinically quiescent states. These insights move periodontics beyond symptom management into the era of predictive and preventive care.

4.4 Matrix Metalloproteinases (MMPs)

MMPs are a family of zinc- and calcium-dependent endopeptidases involved in the turnover of the extracellular matrix (ECM) in both normal physiological conditions and pathological processes [54]. In the context of periodontitis, MMPs are not merely passive bystanders of inflammation but instead play a central role as essential mediators of irreversible connective tissue breakdown, alveolar bone resorption, and periodontal ligament disintegration – hallmark features of disease progression [55]. These enzymes are produced mainly by neutrophils, fibroblasts, macrophages, epithelial cells, and osteoclasts in response to microbial products like LPS, host cytokines (e.g., IL-1β, and TNF-α), and reactive oxygen species (ROS) [56]. Their enzymatic actions are tightly regulated by endogenous inhibitors called tissue inhibitors of metalloproteinases (TIMPs), but in the periodontitis environment, this regulatory balance is tipped in favor of increased matrix breakdown [57].

Among the MMPs, MMP-8, or collagenase-2, has been established as the most sensitive and specific biomarker for the active destruction of periodontal tissues [58, 59]. The enzyme is mainly secreted from activated neutrophils and is highly expressed in inflamed sites, especially in deep periodontal pockets [60]. MMP-8 degrades native type I and III collagens, the chief structural collagenous proteins of periodontal connective tissues, and thus directly causes clinical attachment loss [56, 59]. Several studies have shown that high levels of MMP-8 in GCF, saliva, and peri-implant sulcular fluid strongly correlate with the grade of periodontal disease and agree with clinical measurements of probing pocket depth, BOP, and clinical attachment level [59, 61, 62] (Figure 4.4). Importantly, MMP-8 has the capability to distinguish between active disease sites and inactive locations, and this gives rise to predictive information that goes beyond the information from conventional probing evaluations. Diagnostic kits with point-of-care compatibility, for example, PerioSafe and ImplantSafe, based upon MMP-8 quantification, enable chairside detection of active destruction and the initiation of immediate remedial action [63–65].

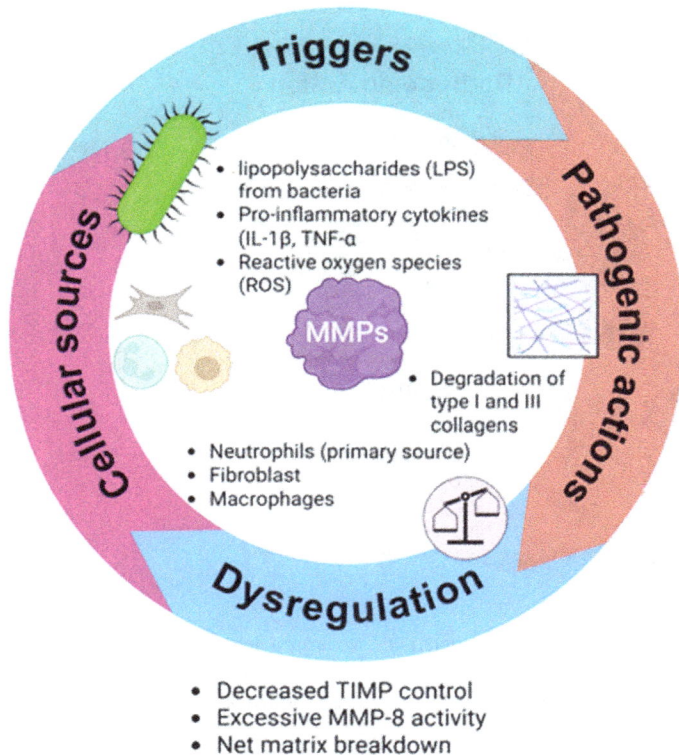

Figure 4.4: Matrix metalloproteinases (MMPs) in periodontitis. Bacterial/PAMP triggers and host cells drive MMP release; inadequate TIMP control causes ECM and collagen breakdown. Created with Biorender.com.

MMP-9 (gelatinase B), the neutrophil-secreted enzyme, is a critical mediator of the process of tissue destruction. MMP-9 targets substrates of denatured collagen (gelatins), elastin, and various basement membrane constituents and thereby contributes to bacterial invasion and immune cell recruitment [66]. Saliva and GCF concentrations of MMP-9 are invariably elevated in periodontitis and gingivitis and are extremely high in stage III and IV periodontitis, hitherto called aggressive periodontitis [67]. Salivary MMP-9 has shown promise of use for population-based screenings because it is highly useful in discriminating among healthy individuals, individuals with gingivitis, and patients with moderate and advanced periodontal disease [67, 68]. The release of MMP-9 is triggered through the process of neutrophil degranulation and stimulation of epithelial cells, and its systemic dissemination could contribute to comorbid disease development, especially cardiovascular and metabolic diseases [69, 70] (Figure 4.5).

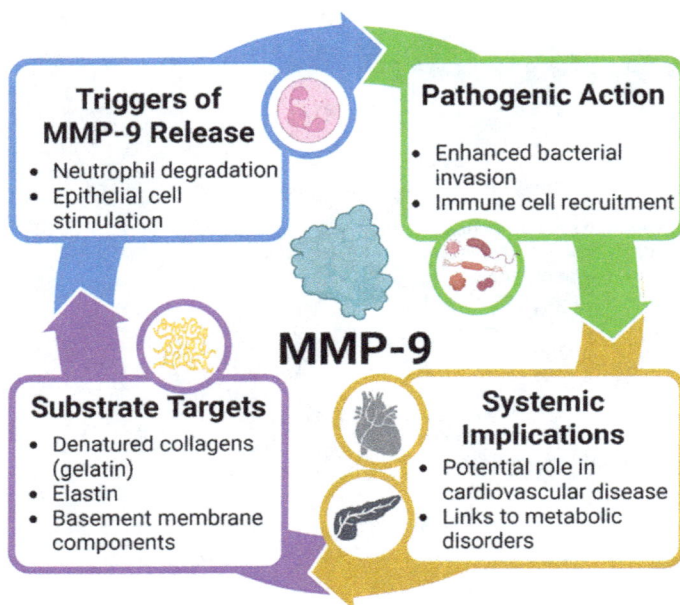

Figure 4.5: Matrix metalloproteinase-9 (MMP-9) in periodontitis. Neutrophil degranulation and epithelial stimulation trigger MMP-9, which degrades gelatin/elastin and basement membranes, facilitating bacterial invasion and immune-cell recruitment; activity is linked to cardiovascular and metabolic comorbidities. Created with Biorender.com.

MMP-13, or collagenase-3, occurs in smaller amounts; nonetheless, it has attracted significant attention due to its exceptional catalytic efficiency against interstitial collagens and its upregulation in later stages of periodontitis, notably in cases of rapid progression [71]. This fibroblast, macrophage, and osteoblast-derived enzyme, induced by inflammatory stimuli, is often increased in severe periodontal disease, especially in stage IV periodontitis or peri-implantitis, where it can cooperate with MMP-8 and MMP-9 to enhance tissue breakdown [56]. More recent evidence also suggests that MMP-13 is involved in alveolar bone remodeling through interaction with RANKL/

OPG (Osteoprotegerin) signaling pathways, thus providing a link between ECM degradation and osteoclastogenesis [72] (Figure 4.6).

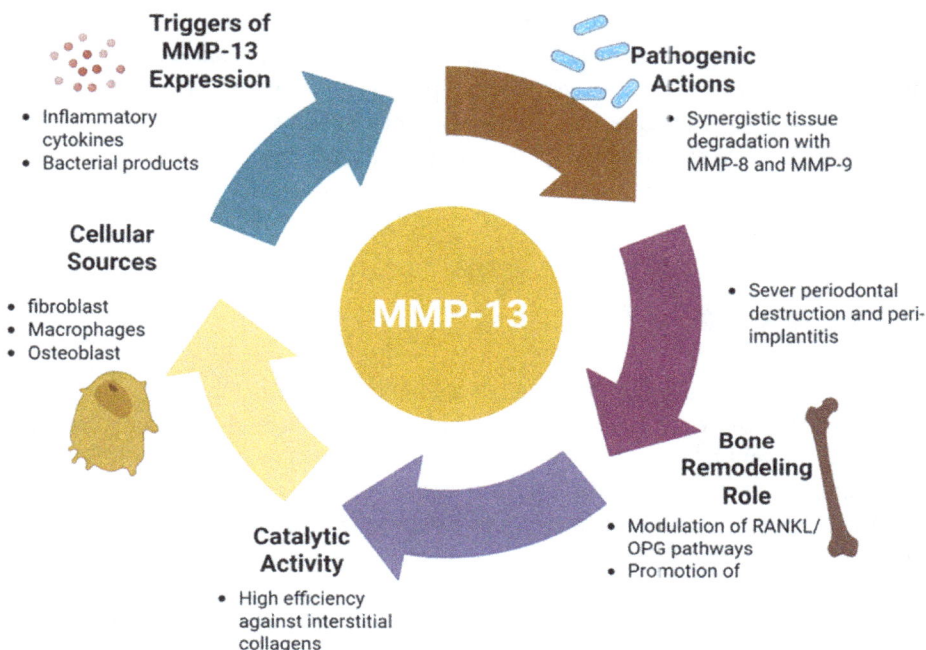

Figure 4.6: Matrix metalloproteinase-13 (MMP-13) in periodontitis. Cytokines and bacterial products induce MMP-13 in fibroblasts, macrophages, and osteoclasts. Its high collagenase activity degrades interstitial collagens and, with RANKL/OPG imbalance, drives bone remodeling and severe periodontal destruction. Created with Biorender.com.

An important counterbalance to MMP activity is provided by TIMPs, particularly TIMP1–4, with TIMP-1 being the most extensively studied in periodontal tissues [73]. Under homeostatic conditions, MMPs and TIMPs maintain equilibrium, but in disease, MMP/TIMP ratios are skewed, favoring degradation [74]. A high MMP-8/TIMP-1 or MMP-9/TIMP-1 ratio is often observed in patients with progressive disease, and these ratios may outperform absolute MMP concentrations in predicting disease activity and progression [75].

From a diagnostic standpoint, MMP profiling is highly beneficial for clinical purposes [60]. It allows for the early detection of tissue damage, the differentiation of active and inactive lesions, and the assessment of the outcome of treatment, as MMP levels tend to decline with the success of nonsurgical and surgical treatments [76]. Additionally, combining MMP levels with cytokines (e.g., IL-1β and TNF-α) and host-derived enzymes (e.g., myeloperoxidase and cathepsin G) in multiplex assays increases diagnostic power considerably and provides the basis for personalized periodontal therapies [77].

MMPs – particularly MMP-8, MMP-9, and MMP-13, serve not only as biochemical markers of periodontal breakdown but also as mechanistic drivers of disease progression [61, 67, 71]. Their dynamic interplay with TIMPs, cytokines, and osteolytic signals underscores their central role in periodontal pathogenesis. As such, MMPs are critical components of any biomarker-based strategy aimed at early diagnosis, risk stratification, and individualized treatment planning in periodontology.

4.5 Genetic Polymorphisms and Periodontal Susceptibility

Periodontitis is increasingly recognized as a complex polygenic disorder wherein the clinical phenotype arises from dynamic interactions between environmental triggers (e.g., oral microbiome, smoking, and diabetes) and host genetic susceptibility [78]. While no single genetic variant is solely responsible for disease onset or progression, a growing body of literature-spanning candidate gene studies, genome-wide association studies, and epigenomic analyses has identified several single nucleotide polymorphisms (SNPs) that modulate individual susceptibility to periodontal tissue destruction, immune response dysregulation, and therapeutic responsiveness [79].

Among the earliest and most validated associations are polymorphisms in the IL-1 gene cluster (IL1A and IL1B) [80]. Specifically, the IL-1β +3954 C/T (rs1143634) and IL-1 α-889 C/T (rs1800587) variants have been strongly linked to enhanced IL-1 production, a cytokine that orchestrates neutrophil recruitment, osteoclast activation, and matrix degradation. Individuals harboring the composite IL-1 genotype (carrying both risk alleles) exhibit a hyperinflammatory phenotype and are more prone to early-onset and severe periodontitis, especially when combined with smoking or systemic risk factors [24]. These polymorphisms have been included in commercial tests, such as PerioPredict®, supporting their potential utility in clinical risk assessment [81].

Another class of important SNPs involves the Fc (Fragement crystallizable region) gamma receptor (FcγR) genes, notably FcγRIIIa (CD16) and FcγRIIa (CD32) [82].These receptors mediate antibody-dependent phagocytosis and clearance of opsonized bacteria. Polymorphisms, such as FcγRIIIa V158F (rs396991) and FcγRIIa H131R (rs1801274) affect binding affinity to IgG (Immnoglobulin G) subclasses and have been associated with impaired neutrophil function and periodontitis, particularly in Asian and African populations [82, 83].

Toll-like receptor (TLR) polymorphisms, particularly TLR4 (rs4986790 and rs4986791) and TLR2 (rs5743708), have garnered significant attention due to their role in pattern recognition and pathogen-associated molecular pattern (PAMP) sensing [84]. These variants lead to altered recognition of bacterial LPS, notably from *Porphyromonas gingivalis* and *Fusobacterium nucleatum*, resulting in delayed or blunted innate immune responses

[85]. Notably, TLR4 Asp299Gly and Thr399Ile variants are linked to hyporesponsiveness to gram-negative LPS, facilitating microbial persistence and chronic inflammation [86].

Another emerging player is glycosyltransferase 6 domain containing 1 (GLT6D1), a gene identified through GWAS to be associated with aggressive periodontitis (stage III and IV grade C periodontitis) [87, 88]. Variants in GLT6D1 are believed to influence B-cell and monocyte function and affect antigen presentation pathways [88]. rs1537415, an SNP in the 5q13 locus, was associated with early-onset periodontitis, indicating a trans-ethnic relevance of this gene in disease pathogenesis [89, 90].

Furthermore, vitamin D receptor (VDR) polymorphisms, such as FokI (rs2228570), BsmI (rs1544410), and TaqI (rs731236), modulate host defense by altering vitamin D-mediated transcription of antimicrobial peptides like cathelicidin and β-defensins [91]. These SNPs have been linked to increased susceptibility, particularly in patients with low vitamin D levels, type 2 diabetes, or smoking habits [92–94].

In the MMP-1 gene, alterations are observed at allele 1607 on the chromosome [95]. Four cohort studies have examined this polymorphism: one involving mixed ethnicities, one conducted in China focusing primarily on Asian populations, one in a Turkish cohort, and one in a Brazilian population. Among these, two studies demonstrated an association with chronic periodontitis, one reported a probable link to either chronic or aggressive periodontitis, and one identified only a limited role. Regarding MMP-2, the polymorphism occurs at the 753C/T locus. Its relationship with periodontal disease has been evaluated in studies among Caucasian, Chinese, and Turkish groups, all of which reported a limited contribution. Notably, in an Asian cohort, an association was identified between aggressive periodontitis and the TIMP-2 −418GC gene polymorphism, assessed using oral swabs [96–100].

For MMP-3, the most common genetic variation is located at 1171 A5/A6. Four investigations have assessed its impact on periodontal disease, including two in Brazil, one in China, and one in Japan. All studies demonstrated an association with disease development except the Japanese study, which did not confirm this link. In the MMP-8 gene, polymorphisms are noted at −17C/G (rs2155052) and −799C/T. Four studies evaluated their role in periodontitis progression: three using peripheral blood samples and one based on gingival fluid. Three of these studies identified a significant association with periodontal disease, while one reported that both SNPs (−799C/T and +17C/G) were not related to periodontitis susceptibility [97, 98, 101–103].

The MMP-9 gene polymorphism at 1562 C/T is among the most extensively investigated. Ten studies have explored MMP-9 alone or in combination with other MMPs in the context of periodontal disease. These included four studies in Caucasian populations, two involving mixed ethnic groups, three conducted in Asian cohorts, and one in India. Most investigations applied polymerase chain reaction methods to analyze DNA extracted from blood or oral samples. Six studies identified either a strong or probable association between MMP-9 variants and periodontitis, whereas four studies did not detect any significant relationship [98–100, 104, 105].

Identifying these diverse polymorphisms contributing to periodontitis may ultimately support the development of novel therapeutic approaches and diagnostic tools.

Other genetic contributors include:
- CD14 (rs2569190): Modulates monocyte response to bacterial LPS [106].
- IL-6 −174 G/C (rs1800795): Alters systemic inflammatory tone and has implications in comorbid diabetes and cardiovascular disease [50].
- TNF-α −308 G/A (rs1800629): Linked to elevated TNF-α levels and enhanced risk of tissue destruction [29].
- CXCL8 (interleukin-8 (IL-8)) −251 A/T (rs4073): Influences neutrophil chemotaxis and biofilm-induced inflammation [107].
- DEFB1 (defensin Œ ≤ 1) polymorphisms: Impact mucosal defense and have been correlated with early-onset periodontitis [108].

Taken together, these polymorphisms represent only the tip of the genetic iceberg. Polygenic risk scores, which integrate multiple SNPs, are being developed to enhance risk prediction accuracy and stratify patients into distinct susceptibility clusters. These approaches promise to transform periodontitis from a reactive, diagnosis-based field into a predictive, precision-guided discipline, where personalized recall intervals, prophylaxis intensity, and host modulation therapy are tailored to individual genetic makeup [109].

As sequencing costs decline and bioinformatic tools improve, integration of genetic biomarkers into routine periodontal care is becoming increasingly feasible. Future models combining host genetics, microbiome profiling, and inflammatory biomarkers may enable deep phenotyping of periodontitis and usher in the era of genotype-guided periodontics [110].

4.6 Epigenetic and miRNA Signatures in Periodontitis

The classical static perspective for the role of genetic predisposition has evolved with the inclusion of a broader emphasis on the role of epigenetic regulation and noncoding RNA mechanisms to allow for adaptive changes in gene expression influenced by the environment and the microbiota [111]. In the context of periodontitis, where immune and inflammatory responses are contextually and temporally regulated, epigenetic changes and microRNA (miRNA) signatures emerged as pivotal disease progression modulators, activity markers, and possible precision medicine targets [112].

4.7 MicroRNAs (miRNAs): Fine-Tuning the Periodontal Inflammatory Network

MicroRNAs (miRNAs) are short, non-coding RNA molecules, roughly 22 nucleotides long, that bind to complementary sequences found in the 3' untranslated regions of target messenger RNAs (mRNAs), inducing post-transcriptional inhibition or degradation [113]. When considering periodontal disease, miRNAs are responsible for orchestrating a multifaceted regulatory framework that modulates the innate and adaptive immune responses, osteoclastogenesis, matrix degradation, and tissue repair mechanisms [114].miR-146a and miR-155 are the most extensively studied microRNAs in periodontal inflammation [115, 116]. miR-146a is a negative feedback modulator induced through nuclear factor kappa B (NF-κB) signaling, which then suppresses the expression of interleukin-1 receptor-associated kinase 1 (IRAK1) and TNF receptor-associated factor 6 (TRAF6), key upstream mediators of the TLR/NF-κB pathway [117]. Overexpression of miR-146a in gingiva and GCF reflects an effort to dampen hyperinflammation, but in chronic disease, this regulatory process could be disrupted or insufficient [118]. In contrast, miR-155, induced through toll-like receptors (TLRs) and cytokines, mainly plays a pro-inflammatory role by promoting Th1/Th17 polarization, macrophage activation, and the production of cytokines like IL-6 and TNF-α, culminating in alveolar bone loss [119] (Figure 4.7).

MicroRNA Regulation of Inflammation in Periodontitis

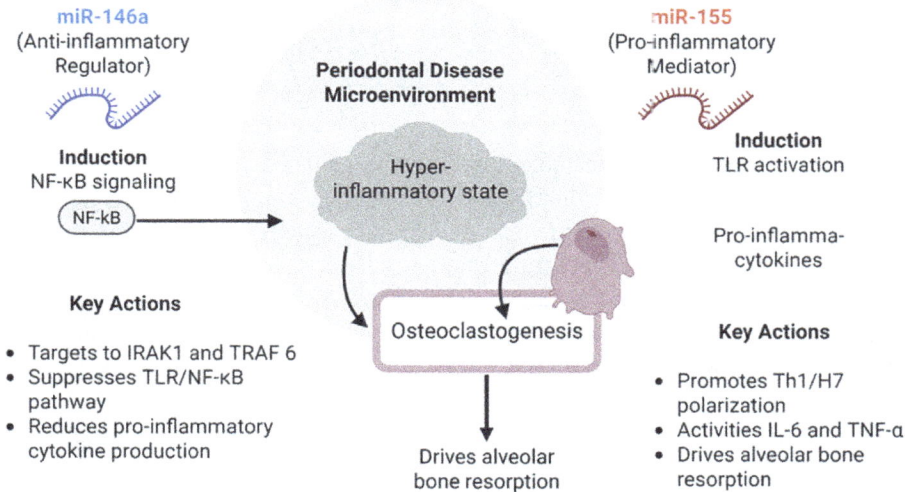

Figure 4.7: MicroRNA regulation of periodontal inflammation. **miR-146a** targets IRAK1/TRAF6 to suppress TLR/NF-κB signaling and cytokines; **miR-155** promotes TLR activation, Th1/Th17 polarization, IL-6/TNF-α release, and **osteoclastogenesis**, accelerating alveolar bone resorption. Created with Biorender.com.

Other microRNAs with important functions are:
- miR-21: Plays a role in osteoclast differentiation, remodeling of tissues, and apoptosis of fibroblasts. It is dual in function, where it is protective during acute inflammation but pro-resorptive during chronic disease [120].
- miR-203: Shows enhanced expression in periodontitis; regulates epithelial integrity, and inflammatory mediators [121].
- miR-146b: shares functional similarity with miR-146a and possesses the capability to modulate immune tolerance in immune and epithelial lineages [122].
- miR-223: Recognized to regulate neutrophil recruitment and resolution processes, particularly critical for balancing destructive versus reparative inflammation [123].
- miR-200 family: Implicated in epithelial-mesenchymal transition, significant in late periodontitis and wound healing [112, 124].

They are disease stage-specific, clearly discriminating between periodontal health, gingivitis, and periodontitis; in addition, they show promise as oral biomarkers that may be quantified using Reverse Transcription Qunatative Polymerase Chain Reaction (RT-qPCR) or miRNA microarrays [112]. Notably, their levels are reversible following periodontal therapy and therefore are valuable for the monitoring of response to treatment or the diagnosis of early recurrence [125, 126].

4.8 Epigenetic Modifications: DNA Methylation, Histone Modifications, and Chromatin Remodeling

Epigenetic changes refer to heritable differences in gene expression that take place without changes to the underlying DNA sequence [127]. Among such changes, DNA methylation particularly at CpG (Cytosine Phosphate Guanine) islands in gene promoters has been most extensively studied in periodontitis [128–130]. The methylation state of genes involved in inflammation or regulation affects the transcriptional responses of host tissues to bacterial biofilms and plays a key part in susceptibility to and chronicity of the disease [131].

The key findings include:
- Suppressor of cytokine signaling 1 (SOCS1): Hypomethylation of its promoter results in overexpression, which dampens STAT signaling and may impair effective immune clearance [132].
- IL-6 and TNF-α: In early periodontal lesions, hypermethylation in the promoter regions of the IL-6 and TNF-α genes can reduce their expression. However, as the disease becomes chronic, these promoter regions often undergo demethylation.

This loss of methylation increases gene activity, leading to persistent overproduction of these cytokines [133, 134].
– TLR2 and TLR4: Changes in methylation status affect receptor sensitivity to LPS and bacterial products, influencing the inflammatory threshold [135].
– CDKN2A and CDH1: Methylation-driven silencing may influence epithelial barrier integrity and cellular senescence, contributing to tissue degradation [136, 137].

Histone modifications, including H3K4me3 and H3K27ac, and nucleosome remodeling events are poorly characterized but are receiving increasing research attention due to their key functions in controlling gene clusters involved in inflammation, angiogenesis, and tissue repair [138]. The growing body of research in this area is not only expanding our knowledge but also sparking new questions and avenues for exploration. Recent studies using chromatin immunoprecipitation sequencing (ChIP-seq) have begun to map these epigenetic landscapes in both gingival fibroblasts and other epithelial cell types, further fueling this exciting area of study [139, 140].

4.9 Translational and Clinical Relevance

The interplay of epigenetics and miRNAs offers exciting translational potential:
– Diagnostic biomarkers: Panels of miRNAs (e.g., miR-146a/miR-155/miR-203) and methylation markers can serve as non-invasive diagnostic tools using GCF or salivary samples [141].
– Prognostic indicators: Aberrant epigenetic patterns may predict rapid progression or poor therapeutic response in otherwise clinically similar patients [142].
– Therapeutic targets: Epigenetic drugs, such as DNA methyltransferase inhibitors (e.g., decitabine) and HDAC (Histone Deacetylase) inhibitors are being explored in systemic inflammatory diseases and may find application in host modulation for periodontitis [143].
– Adjuncts to regenerative therapy: Epigenetic modulation of PDLSCs or gingival MSCs could improve their regenerative efficacy by enhancing osteogenic or anti-inflammatory phenotypes [144].

4.10 Biomarkers in Treatment Monitoring and Prognosis

One useful application of molecular biomarkers in the clinic is that they can predict, assess, and individualize the prognosis of periodontitis [145]. In comparison to conventional clinical parameters, including probing depth, CAL, or BOP, which yield static or retrospective measurements, biomarkers render a dynamic perspective at the molecular level regarding the active inflammatory, immune-modulatory, and re-modeling events. As periodontal therapy moves toward a biologically oriented regimen, biomarker utilization becomes essential to the real-time evaluation of results [146].

An extensive body of evidence has demonstrated that nonsurgical periodontal treatment, specifically scaling and root planning (SRP), leads to a predictable decrease of some inflammatory and tissue-destructive mediators in GCF and saliva [147]. Among such mediators, IL-1β has been the subject of much debate, the concentrations of which consistently decrease within 4–6 weeks following successful SRP. This decrease reflects the resolution of the initial inflammatory cascade. Sustained increases in IL-1β concentrations, however, may reflect ongoing microbial insult or an exaggerated host immune response, requiring ongoing therapeutic measures [148]. MMP-8, integral to type I collagen degradation in periodontal connective tissues, has been recognized as a useful biomarker for active periodontal tissue destruction. Its concentrations significantly decrease after periodontal treatment, and rapid diagnostic point-of-care tests like the PerioSafe test employ monoclonal antibodies to detect the enzymatically active form (aMMP-8), facilitating immediate clinical decision-making [59, 149].

Within the non-coding RNA realm, miR-146a is a well-established regulatory biomarker with sensitivity [117]. The microRNA plays a role in the negative feedback mechanisms governing NF-κB pathway signaling and becomes upregulated in active inflammatory stages [117]. The noted reductions in its levels upon therapeutic interventions, quantified by RT-qPCR assays conducted either on GCF or on saliva samples; signify a return to immunological homeostasis [118, 150]. Similarly, systemic biomarkers, such as C-reactive protein (CRP) and TNF-α exhibit a quantifiable decrease in the saliva and serum after successful periodontal therapies, particularly in patients with concomitant systemic inflammatory conditions, such as diabetes mellitus and cardio disease [151, 152].

To enable the translation of molecular information to clinical practice, several diagnostic platforms have been engineered and validated rigorously for testing. Enzyme-linked immunosorbent assays /continue to be the gold standard for quantifying cytokines, proteases, and chemokines in body fluids. In parallel, lateral flow immunoassays (LFIAs) provide a means for rapid, semi-quantitative point-of-care testing, such as products available for detection of MMP-8 in the time frame of 10–15 min [153, 154]. The application of molecular techniques, such as real-time PCR (qPCR) and RT-qPCR, has enabled the quantitative assessment of microbial burdens and miRNA expression profiles, thus allowing microbial diagnostics and monitoring of host responses [155]. Furthermore, more recent platforms, namely multiplex bead arrays (Luminex®), allow the parallel analysis of several biomarkers with minimal sample consumption, and thus monitor efficiently the complex kinetics of host-microbe interaction under a high-throughput regimen [156].

Novel biosensor technologies have the potential to transform periodontal disease diagnosis. CRISPR (Clustered Regularly Interspaced Short Palindromic Repeats) – Cas-based methods, i.e., SHERLOCK and DETECTR, based on collateral cleavage activities of the reporter molecules on detection of the target RNA or DNA, are being developed for application in diagnostics in saliva for periodontitis [157]. Electrochemical and microfluidic biosensors likewise offer the benefits of portability, improved sensitivity and the potential to be incorporated into smartphone-enabled health monitoring systems [158]. Proteomics and mass spectrometry methodologies are being applied in research to discover novel protein biomarkers and isoforms of diagnostic or prognostic value and thus chart the path for future clinical application [159].

The application of biomarker-based monitoring to clinical practice enables the delivery of customized periodontal therapies by novel and effective means. Patients with persistent biomarker increases following therapeutic treatment – particularly sustained MMP-8 or IL-1β levels – may necessitate reductions in SPT (Supportive Periodontal Therapy) intervals, the introduction of host modulation strategies, or the application of targeted antimicrobial treatment [160]. Biomarker remission, on the other hand, may warrant longer recall intervals, minimizing the potential for unjustified intervention. It should be mentioned that molecular changes within biomarkers typically precede clinically detectable signs of recurrence, thus enabling timely diagnosis and preemptive intervention [161]. Lastly, biomarkers are of invaluable utility in assessing the success of regenerative treatments. Minimization of catabolic markers like MMPs following surgery, together with increases in anabolic markers like VEGF (Vascular Endothelial Growth Factor), BMP-2 (Bone Morphogenetic Protein-2), or OPN (Osteopontin), is a precursor to successful periodontal regeneration [162]. In patients being treated with GTR or EMD therapies, such molecular changes can aid in assessing healing and inform decision-making for subsequent intervention [163]. In addition, in instances where therapeutic outcomes are adverse, sustained increases in cytokines like TNF-α or IL-6 may indicate the necessity for systemic immunomodulation, adjunctive laser therapy, or the re-assessment of risk factors like glycemic control and tobacco use [164].

Tracking molecular biomarkers significantly brings periodontology into the predictive, preventive, and personalized era of medical practice. Integration of the above methods with traditional clinical examinations enables the following of tailored treatment regimens based on the individual's unique biologic characteristics, with resultant enhancement of patient outcomes, elimination of unnecessary interventions, and long-term stability. As validated diagnostic kits and point-of-care devices become more widely available, biomarker-based periodontics is now an integral component of contemporary dental practice.

4.11 Clinical Implementation and Future Perspectives

Despite the potential functions of molecular biomarkers in the improvement of periodontal diagnosis and the tailoring of treatments, routine use for day-to-day clinical periodontics is limited [160]. The gap between concepts and reality is mainly attributed to various technical, logistical, and biological hurdles. Among the foremost challenges is the absence of standardized protocols for sample collection, especially with respect to the preference between saliva and GCF [165, 166]. Although sampling from saliva is convenient and noninvasive, sampling from GCF is more specific and better mirrors the local periodontal condition, but is technically challenging and operator-dependent [167]. Moreover, the expense and availability of advanced molecular test platforms like qPCR, multiplex arrays, and proteomics create access barriers, especially in general dental practices or in resource-challenged environments [168, 169]. Another significant hurdle is the high variability between individuals in the expression of biomarkers, as the expression is dependent upon the genetic profile, overall systemic health, smoking, stress, and even circadian rhythms. The variability makes the standardization of diagnostic thresholds and guidelines impossible [170, 171]. Thus, the clinical use of biomarkers requires population-related validation and patient-specific reference ranges [172]. Nonetheless, new advances in the past several years are rapidly mitigating the obstacles. The elucidation of point-of-care test devices like LFIAs, electrochemical sensors, and CRISPR platforms has made chairside, real-time biomarker analysis realistically possible [173, 174]. Concurrently, advances in the area of lab-on-a-chip diagnostics are providing the ability to detect multiple analytes from tiny sample amounts with in-built processing and readout modules. Furthermore, the integration of biomarker science with machine intelligence has enormous transformative power [175]. Machine-based learning programs can combine heterogeneous biomarker profiles like cytokines, MMPs, microRNAs, and genetic polymorphisms with clinical parameters to build potent prediction models. These tools promise to enable timely diagnosis, classify patients according to disease activity or risk of progression, and guide individualized treatment strategies with significant accuracy [176, 177]. Future applications can be expected to include biosensor devices coupled with smartphones, cloud-based biomarker monitoring platforms, and artificial intelligence-powered decision-support systems, all of which together move us closer to the future of precision periodontics [178]. In summary, while challenges remain, the development of biomarker use within the scope of clinical periodontics represents an era of unprecedented change. Through continued interdisciplinary collaboration, validation studies, and technological innovation, the vision for biologically informed, predictive, and personalized periodontal care is quickly becoming an achievable standard.

4.12 Conclusion

Genetic and molecular biomarkers offer a transformative approach to diagnosing periodontitis, assessing risk, and managing the condition. Their integration into clinical workflows signals a new era of precision periodontics, where disease can be detected before irreversible damage occurs, treatment can be tailored to individual needs, and outcomes can be monitored in real time. As research continues to refine and validate these tools, their role in personalized oral healthcare will only grow more prominent.

References

[1] Trieger, N. (2003). The surgical treatment of periodontal infections. Oral and Maxillofacial Surgery Clinics of North America, 15(1), 123–128.

[2] Łasica, A., Golec, P., Laskus, A., Zalewska, M., Gędaj, M., & Popowska, M. (2024). Periodontitis: Etiology, conventional treatments, and emerging bacteriophage and predatory bacteria therapies. Frontiers in Microbiology, 15, 1469414.

[3] Jacobs, R., Fontenele, R. C., Lahoud, P., Shujaat, S., & Bornstein, M. M. (2024). Radiographic diagnosis of periodontal diseases – current evidence versus innovations. Periodontology 2000, 95(1), 51–69.

[4] M., T. Jr, Kinney, J., Kim, A. S., & W.v, G. (2005). Diagnostic biomarkers for oral and periodontal diseases. Dental Clinics of North America, 49(3), 551–571.

[5] Dolińska, E., Wiśniewski, P., & Pietruska, M. (2023). Periodontal molecular diagnostics: State of knowledge and future prospects for clinical application. International Journal of Molecular Sciences, 25(23), 12624.

[6] Barros, S. P., Williams, R., Offenbacher, S., & Morelli, T. (2016). Gingival crevicular fluid as a source of biomarkers for periodontitis. Periodontology 2000, 70(1), 53–64.

[7] Checherita, L. E., Antohe, M. E., Stamatin, O., Rudnic, I., Lupu, I. C., Croitoru, I., Surdu, A., Cioloca, D., Gradinaru, I., Francu, L., Foia, I., Vascu, B. M., & A.m, F. (2021). Periodontal disease diagnosis in the context of oral rehabilitation approaches. Applied Sciences, 12(18), 9067.

[8] Ramseier, C. A. (2024). Diagnostic measures for monitoring and follow-up in periodontology and implant dentistry. Periodontology 2000, 95(1), 129–155.

[9] Miller, C. S., Foley, J. D., Bailey, A. L., Campell, C. L., Humphries, R. L., Christodoulides, N., Floriano, P. N., Simmons, G., Bhagwandin, B., Jacobson, J. W., Redding, S. W., Ebersole, J. L., & McDevitt, J. T. (2010). Current developments in salivary diagnostics. Biomarkers in Medicine, 4(1), 171–189.

[10] Qasim, S. S., Gul, S. S., & Zafar, M. S. (2019). An evidence-based update on the molecular mechanisms underlying periodontal diseases. International Journal of Molecular Sciences, 21(11), 3829.

[11] Khiste, S. V., Ranganath, V., Nichani, A. S., & Rajani, V. (2011). Critical analysis of biomarkers in the current periodontal practice. Journal of Indian Society of Periodontology, 15(2), 104–110.

[12] Griffith, A., Chande, C., Kulkarni, S., Morel, J., Cheng, H., Shimizu, E., Cugini, C., Basuray, S., & Kumar, V. (2024). Point-of-care diagnostic devices for periodontitis – current trends and urgent need. Sensors & Diagnostics, 3(7), 1119–1131.

[13] Grant, M. M., Taylor, J. J., Jaedicke, K., Creese, A., Gowland, C., Burke, B., Doudin, K., Patel, U., Weston, P., Milward, M., Bissett, S. M., Cooper, H. J., Kooijman, G., Rmaile, A., Preshaw, P. M., & Chapple, I. L. C. (2022). Discovery, validation, and diagnostic ability of multiple protein-based biomarkers in saliva and gingival crevicular fluid to distinguish between health and periodontal diseases. Journal of Clinical Periodontology, 49(7), 622–634.

[14] Gul, S. S., Abdulkareem, A. A., Sha, A. M., & Rawlinson, A. (2020). Diagnostic accuracy of oral fluids biomarker profile to determine the current and future status of periodontal and peri-implant diseases. Diagnostics, 10(10), 838.

[15] Magro, D., Venezia, M., & Balistreri, C. R. (2024). The omics technologies and liquid biopsies: Advantages, limitations, applications. Medicine in Omics, 11, 100039.

[16] Gatsounia, A., Schinas, G., Danielides, G., Grafanaki, K., Mastronikolis, N., Stathopoulos, C., & Lygeros, S. (2025). Epigenetic mechanisms in CRSwNP: The role of microRNAs as potential biomarkers and therapeutic targets. Current Issues in Molecular Biology, 47(2), 114.

[17] Radzki, D., Negri, A., Kusiak, A., & Obuchowski, M. (2024). Matrix metalloproteinases in the periodontium – vital in tissue turnover and unfortunate in periodontitis. International Journal of Molecular Sciences, 25(5), 2763.

[18] Aya, V., Vega, L. C., Cala, M. P., & J.d, R. (2025). Integrating metagenomics and metabolomics to study the gut microbiome and host relationships in sports across different energy systems. Scientific Reports, 15(1), 1–19.

[19] Kabbashi, S., Roomaney, I., & Chetty, M. (2024). Bridging the gap between omics research and dental practice. BDJ Open, 10, 16.

[20] Taylor, J. J. (2014). Protein biomarkers of periodontitis in saliva. ISRN Inflammation, 2014, 593151.

[21] Pan, W., Wang, Q., & Chen, Q. (2019). The cytokine network involved in the host immune response to periodontitis. International Journal of Oral Science, 11(3), 30.

[22] Relvas, M., Gonçalves, M., Salazar, F., & Silvestre, R. (2023). Salivary IL-1β, IL-6, and IL-10 are key biomarkers of periodontitis severity. International Journal of Molecular Sciences, 25(15), 8401.

[23] Cheng, R., Wu, Z., Li, M., Shao, M., & Hu, T. (2020). Interleukin-1β is a potential therapeutic target for periodontitis: A narrative review. International Journal of Oral Science, 12, 2.

[24] Pani, P., Tsilioni, I., McGlennen, R., Brown, C. A., Hawley, C. E., Theoharides, T. C., & Papathanasiou, E. (2021). IL-1B(3954) polymorphism and red complex bacteria increase IL-1β (GCF) levels in periodontitis. Journal of Periodontal Research, 56(3), 501–511.

[25] Resende, R. G., Abreu, M. H., de Souza, L. N., Silva, M. E., Gomez, R. S., & Correia-Silva, J. F. (2013). Association between IL1B (+3954) polymorphisms and IL-1β levels in blood and saliva, together with acute graft-versus-host disease. Journal of Interferon and Cytokine Research, 33(7), 392–397.

[26] Parameswaran, N., & Patial, S. (2010). Tumor necrosis factor-α signaling in macrophages. Critical Reviews in Eukaryotic Gene Expression, 20(2), 87–103.

[27] Kitaura, H., Marahleh, A., Ohori, F., Noguchi, T., Nara, Y., Pramusita, A., Kinjo, R., Ma, J., Kanou, K., & Mizoguchi, I. (2021). Role of the interaction of tumor necrosis factor-α and tumor necrosis factor receptors 1 and 2 in bone-related cells. International Journal of Molecular Sciences, 23(3), 1481.

[28] Bhol, N. K., Bhanjadeo, M. M., Singh, A. K., Dash, U. C., Ojha, R. R., Majhi, S., Duttaroy, A. K., & Jena, A. B. (2024). The interplay between cytokines, inflammation, and antioxidants: Mechanistic insights and therapeutic potentials of various antioxidants and anti-cytokine compounds. Biomedicine & Pharmacotherapy, 178, 117177.

[29] Azab, E., & Elfasakhany, F. M. (2022). Effect of tumor necrosis factor alpha (TNF-α) −308 and −1031 gene polymorphisms on periodontitis among Saudi subjects. Saudi Dental Journal, 34(3), 226–232.

[30] Zhang, X., Zhu, X., & Sun, W. (2021). Association between tumor necrosis factor-α (G-308A) polymorphism and chronic periodontitis, aggressive periodontitis, and peri-implantis: A meta-analysis. Journal of Evidence Based Dental Practice, 21(3), 101528.

[31] Romero-Castro, N. S., Vázquez-Villamar, M., Muñoz-Valle, J. F., Reyes-Fernández, S., Serna-Radilla, V. O., García-Arellano, S., & Castro-Alarcón, N. (2020). Relationship between TNF-α, MMP-8, and MMP-9 levels in gingival crevicular fluid and the subgingival microbiota in periodontal disease. Odontology, 108(1), 25–33.

[32] Kadayıf, A., Ö.e., T., & Karaduman, B. (2025). Effects of non-surgical periodontal therapy on gingival crevicular fluid CTRP-1, TNF-α, and IL-10 levels. Clinical Oral Investigations, 29, 345.

[33]   Tanaka, T., Narazaki, M., & Kishimoto, T. (2014). IL-6 in inflammation, immunity, and disease. Cold
       Spring Harbor Perspectives in Biology, 6(10), a016295.
[34]   Hunter, C. A., & Jones, S. A. (2015). IL-6 as a keystone cytokine in health and disease. Nature
       Immunology, 16(5), 448–457.
[35]   Mazurek-Mochol, M., Bonsmann, T., Mochol, M., Poniewierska-Baran, A., & Pawlik, A. (2024). The
       role of interleukin 6 in periodontitis and its complications. International Journal of Molecular
       Sciences, 25(4), 2146.
[36]   Neurath, N., & Kesting, M. (2024). Cytokines in gingivitis and periodontitis: From pathogenesis to
       therapeutic targets. Frontiers in Immunology, 15, 1435054.
[37]   Majeed, Z. N., Jassim, S. D., & Kamil, Z. H. (2023). Assessment of salivary and gingival crevicular
       fluids IL-6, IL-8, IL-12, and IL-17 levels in healthy subjects and patients with periodontal disease.
       Journal of Oral and Maxillofacial Pathology, 27(3), 494.
[38]   Ali, H. M., Mustafa, M., Suliman, S., Elshazali, O. H., Ali, R. W., & Berggreen, E. (2020). Inflammatory
       mediators in saliva and gingival fluid of children with congenital heart defect. Oral Diseases, 26(5),
       1053–1061.
[39]   Bibi, T., Khurshid, Z., Rehman, A., Imran, E., Srivastava, K. C., & Shrivastava, D. (2020). Gingival
       crevicular fluid (GCF): A diagnostic tool for the detection of periodontal health and diseases.
       Molecules, 26(5), 1208.
[40]   Sanz, M., Jepsen, S., Gonzalez-Juanatey, J. R., Bouchard, P., Chapple, I., Dietrich, T., Gotsman, I.,
       Graziani, F., Herrera, D., Loos, B., Madianos, P., Michel, J. B., Perel, P., Pieske, B., Shapira, L.,
       Shechter, M., Tonetti, M., Vlachopoulos, C., & Wimmer, G. (2020). Periodontitis and cardiovascular
       diseases. Consensus Report. Global Heart, 15(1), 1.
[41]   Kalaivani, V., Kumar, Y. P., & Rajapandian, K. et al. (2023). Association of elevated IL-6 with poor
       glycemic control in periodontitis patients. F1000Research, 12, 595.
[42]   Reis, C., Da Costa, A. V., Guimarães, J. T., Tuna, D., Braga, A. C., Pacheco, J. J., Arosa, F. A., Salazar, F.,
       & Cardoso, E. M. (2014). Clinical improvement following therapy for periodontitis: Association with a
       decrease in IL-1 and IL-6. Experimental and Therapeutic Medicine, 8(1), 323–327.
[43]   Balu, P., Balakrishna Pillai, A. K., Mariappan, V., & Ramalingam, S. (2024). Cytokine levels in gingival
       tissues as an indicator to understand periodontal disease severity. Current Research in
       Immunology, 5, 100080.
[44]   Celik, D., & Kantarci, A. (2021). Vascular changes and hypoxia in periodontal disease as a link to
       systemic complications. Pathogens, 10(10), 1280.
[45]   Liu, W., & Guo, D. (2025). Oxidative stress in periodontitis and the application of antioxidants in
       treatment: A narrative review. Frontiers in Physiology, 16, 1485367.
[46]   Kolaparthy, L. K., Sanivarapu, S., Swarna, C., & Devulapalli, N. S. (2014). Neutrophil extracellular
       traps: Their role in periodontal disease. Journal of Indian Society of Periodontology, 18(6), 693–697.
[47]   Gündoğar, H., Üstün, K., Şenyurt, S. Z., E.ç, Ö., Sezer, U., & Erciyas, K. (2021). Gingival crevicular fluid
       levels of cytokine, chemokine, and growth factors in patients with periodontitis or gingivitis and
       periodontally healthy subjects: A cross-sectional multiplex study. Central European Journal of
       Immunology, 46(4), 474–480.
[48]   Sakai, A., Ohshima, M., Sugano, N., Otsuka, K., & Ito, K. (2006). Profiling the cytokines in gingival
       crevicular fluid using a cytokine antibody array. Journal of Periodontology, 77(5), 856–864.
[49]   Mazurek-Mochol, M., Dembowska, E., Malinowski, D., Safranow, K., & Pawlik, A. (2019). IL-1β
       rs1143634 and rs16944 polymorphisms in patients with periodontal disease. Archives of Oral
       Biology, 98, 47–51.
[50]   Mazurek-Mochol, M., Bonsmann, T., Malinowski, D., Serwin, K., Czerewaty, M., Safranow, K., &
       Pawlik, A. (2024). Interleukin-6 receptor gene rs1800795 polymorphism and expression of
       interleukin-6 in gingival tissue in patients with periodontitis. Microorganisms, 12(10), 1954.

[51] Holla, L. I., Fassmann, A., Stejskalová, A., Znojil, V., Vaněk, J., & Vacha, J. (2003). Analysis of the interleukin-6 gene promoter polymorphisms in Czech patients with chronic periodontitis. Journal of Periodontology, 75(1), 30–36.

[52] Majumder, P., Thou, K., Bhattacharya, M., Nair, V., Ghosh, S., & Dey, S. K. (2018). Association of tumor necrosis factor-α gene promoter polymorphisms with aggressive and chronic periodontitis in the eastern Indian population. Bioscience Reports, 38(4), 1–14. BSR20171212.

[53] Li, Y., Yang, J., Wu, X., & Sun, W. (2020). TNF-α polymorphisms might influence predisposition to periodontitis: A meta-analysis. Microbial Pathogenesis, 143, 104113.

[54] Cabral-Pacheco, G. A., Garza-Veloz, I., Ramirez-Acuña, J. M., Perez-Romero, B. A., Guerrero-Rodriguez, J. F., Martinez-Avila, N., & M.l, M.-F. (2020). The roles of matrix metalloproteinases and their inhibitors in human diseases. International Journal of Molecular Sciences, 21(24), 9739.

[55] Natarajan, P. M., Ganesan, A., Varma, S. R., & Shetty, N. Y. (2024). Delving into matrix metalloproteinase-1 (MMP-1) and its significance in periodontal diseases. Journal of Pharmacy and Bioallied Sciences, 16(Suppl 2), S1080.

[56] Luchian, I., Goriuc, A., Sandu, D., & Covasa, M. (2022). The role of matrix metalloproteinases (MMP-8, MMP-9, MMP-13) in periodontal and peri-implant pathological processes. International Journal of Molecular Sciences, 23(3), 1806.

[57] Andrian, E., Mostefaoui, Y., Rouabhia, M., & Grenier, D. (2007). Regulation of matrix metalloproteinases and tissue inhibitors of matrix metalloproteinases by *Porphyromonas gingivalis* in an engineered human oral mucosa model. Journal of Cellular Physiology, 211(1), 56–62.

[58] Sorsa, T., Hernández, M., Leppilahti, J., Munjal, S., Netuschil, L., & Mäntylä, P. (2010). Detection of gingival crevicular fluid MMP-8 levels with different laboratory and chair-side methods. Oral Diseases, 16(1), 39–45.

[59] Domokos, Z., Simon, F., Uhrin, E., Szabó, B., Váncsa, S., Varga, G., Hegyi, P., Kerémi, B., & Németh, O. (2024). Evaluating salivary MMP-8 as a biomarker for periodontal diseases: A systematic review and meta-analysis. Heliyon, 10(22), e40402.

[60] Al-Majid, A., Alassiri, S., Rathnayake, N., Tervahartiala, T., Gieselmann, R., & Sorsa, T. (2018). Matrix metalloproteinase-8 as an inflammatory and prevention biomarker in periodontal and peri-implant diseases. International Journal of Dentistry, 7891323.

[61] Ramenzoni, L. L., Hofer, D., Solderer, A., Wiedemeier, D., Attin, T., & Schmidlin, P. R. (2021). Origin of MMP-8 and lactoferrin levels from gingival crevicular fluid, salivary glands and whole saliva. BMC Oral Health, 21, 385.

[62] Katsiki, P., Nazmi, K., Loos, B. G., Laine, M. L., Schaap, K., Hepdenizli, E., Bikker, F. J., Brand, H. S., Veerman, C. I., & Nicu, E. A. (2021). Comparing periodontitis biomarkers in saliva, oral rinse and gingival crevicular fluid: A pilot study. Journal of Clinical Periodontology, 48(9), 1250–1259.

[63] Fragkioudakis, I., Batas, L., Vouros, I., & Sakellari, D. (2025). Diagnostic accuracy of active MMP-8 point-of-care test in peri-implantitis. European Journal of Dentistry, 19(3), 743–748.

[64] Lähteenmäki, H., Tervahartiala, T., Räisänen, I. T., Pärnänen, P., Mauramo, M., Gupta, S., Sampson, V., Rathnayake, N., Heikkinen, A. M., Alassiri, S., Gieselmann, D. R., Frankenberger, R., & Sorsa, T. (2022). Active MMP-8 point-of-care/chairside enzyme test as an adjunctive tool for early and real-time diagnosis of peri-implantitis. Clinical and Experimental Dental Research, 8(2), 485–496.

[65] Aji, N. R., Sahni, V., Penttala, M. T., Sakellari, D., Grigoriadis, A., Pätilä, T., Pärnänen, P., Neefs, D., Pfützner, A., Gupta, S., Sorsa, T., & I.t, R. (2025). Oral medicine and oral clinical chemistry game changers for future plaque control and maintenance: PerioSafe® aMMP-8 POCT, Lumoral® 2× PDT, and Lingora® fermented lingonberry oral rinse treatments. Dentistry Journal, 13(3), 127.

[66] Klein, T., & Bischoff, R. (2010). Physiology and pathophysiology of matrix metalloproteases. Amino Acids, 41(2), 271–290.

[67] Arshad, R., Ismail, W. A., Zara, B., Naseer, R., Minhas, S., Ansari, M., Akhter, F., Khokhar, S. A., Alqahtani, A. A., Abutayyem, H., Alswairki, H. J., & Alam, M. K. (2022). Salivary MMP-9 levels in chronic periodontitis patients with type-II diabetes mellitus. Molecules, 27(7), 2174.

[68] Romano, F., Iaderosa, G., Corana, M., Perotto, S., Baima, G., Di Scipio, F., Abbadessa, G., Mariani, G. M., Aimetti, M., & Berta, G. N. (2022). Comparing ionic profile of gingival crevicular fluid and saliva as distinctive signature of severe periodontitis. Biomedicines, 10(3), 687.

[69] Yabluchanskiy, A., Ma, Y., Iyer, R. P., Hall, M. E., & Lindsey, M. L. (2013). Matrix metalloproteinase-9: Many shades of function in cardiovascular disease. Physiology, 28(6), 391–403.

[70] Kowluru, R. A., Zhong, Q., & Santos, J. M. (2012). Matrix metalloproteinases in diabetic retinopathy: Potential role of MMP-9. Expert Opinion on Investigational Drugs, 21(6), 797–805.

[71] Hernandez, M., Valenzuela, M. A., Lopez-Otin, C., Alvarez, J., Lopez, J. M., Vernal, R., & Gamonal, J. (2006). Matrix metalloproteinase-13 is highly expressed in destructive periodontal disease activity. Journal of Periodontology, 77, 1863–1870.

[72] Khoswanto, C. (2023). Role of matrix metalloproteinases in bone regeneration: Narrative review. Journal of Oral Biology and Craniofacial Research, 13(5), 539–545.

[73] Brew, K., Dinakarpandian, D., & Nagase, H. (2000). Tissue inhibitors of metalloproteinases: Evolution, structure and function. Biochimica et Biophysica Acta, 1477(1–2), 267–283.

[74] Muller, M., Trocme, C., Lardy, B., Morel, F., Halimi, S., & Benhamou, P. Y. (2008). Matrix metalloproteinases and diabetic foot ulcers: The ratio of MMP-1 to TIMP-1 is a predictor of wound healing. Diabetic Medicine, 25(4), 419–426.

[75] Bikker, F. J., Brand, H. S., & Kaman, W. E. (2022). Is TIMP-1 a biomarker for periodontal disease? A systematic review and meta-analysis. Journal of Periodontal Research, 57(2), 235–245.

[76] Sopi, M., Koçani, F., Bardhoshi, M., & Meqa, K. (2022). The effect of periodontal therapy on the level of MMP-8 in patients with chronic periodontitis. European Journal of Dentistry, 17(1), 70–75.

[77] Zhang, Q., Wang, Z., Shen, S., Wang, J., Cao, J., Deng, Y., Meng, H., & Ma, L. (2024). Integrating enzyme–nanoparticles bring new prospects for the diagnosis and treatment of immune dysregulation in periodontitis. Frontiers in Cellular and Infection Microbiology, 14, 1494651.

[78] Loos, B. G., & Van Dyke, T. E. (2020). The role of inflammation and genetics in periodontal disease. Periodontology 2000, 83(1), 26–39.

[79] Schaefer, A. S. (2018). Genetics of periodontitis: Discovery, biology, and clinical impact. Periodontology 2000, 78(1), 162–173.

[80] Li, L., Shi, B., Zheng, W., Xing, W., Zhao, Y., Li, F., Xin, D., Jin, T., Zhu, Y., & Yang, X. (2017). Association of IL-1A and IL-1B polymorphisms with ankylosing spondylitis among the Chinese Han population: A case–control study. Oncotarget, 8(17), 28278.

[81] Ko, T. J., Byrd, K. M., & Kim, S. A. (2021). The chairside periodontal diagnostic toolkit: Past, present, and future. Diagnostics, 11, 932.

[82] Chai, L., Song, Y. Q., Zee, K. Y., & Leung, W. K. (2010). SNPs of Fc-gamma receptor genes and chronic periodontitis. Journal of Dental Research, 89(7), 705–710.

[83] Hans, V. M., Mehta, D. S., & Hans, M. (2015). Association of Fc gamma-receptors IIa, IIIa, and IIIb genetic polymorphism with susceptibility to chronic periodontitis in South Indian population. Contemporary Clinical Dentistry, 6(Suppl 1), S141.

[84] Banescu, C., Tripon, F., Bojan, A. S., Trifa, A. P., Muntean, C., & Crauciuc, G. A. et al. (2022). Association of TLR4 rs4986791 polymorphism and TLR9 haplotypes with acute myeloid leukemia susceptibility: A case-control study of adult patients. Journal of Personalized Medicine, 12(3), 409.

[85] Coutinho-Silva, R. (2019). Immunological pathways triggered by *Porphyromonas gingivalis* and *Fusobacterium nucleatum*: Therapeutic possibilities?. Mediators of Inflammation, 2019, 7241312.

[86] Guo, N., Tian, H., Song, T., & Peng, Y. (2024). Association of TLR4 gene rs4986790 and rs4986791 polymorphisms with asthma susceptibility: Meta-analysis and trial sequential analysis. Annals of Saudi Medicine, 44(3), 183.

[87] Schaefer, A. S., Richter, G. M., Nothnagel, M., Manke, T., Dommisch, H., & Jacobs, G. et al. (2010). A genome-wide association study identifies GLT6D1 as a susceptibility locus for periodontitis. Human Molecular Genetics, 19(3), 553–562.

[88] Hashim, N. T., Linden, G. J., Ibrahim, M. E., Gismalla, B. G., Lundy, F. T., Hughes, F. J., & El Karim, I. A. (2015). Replication of the association of GLT6D1 with aggressive periodontitis in a Sudanese population. Journal of Clinical Periodontology, 42(4), 319–324.

[89] Richter, G. M., Wagner, G., Reichenmiller, K., Staufenbiel, I., Martins, O., & Löscher, B. S. et al. (2022). Exome sequencing of 5 families with severe early-onset periodontitis. Journal of Dental Research, 101(2), 151–157.

[90] Rodrigues, R. S., Rêgo, R., Scarel Caminaga, R. M., Goveia, J. M., & Silveira, V. R. S. (2022). Analysis of GLT6D1 and CDKN2BAS gene polymorphisms in Brazilian patients with advanced periodontitis. Brazilian Oral Research, 36, e077.

[91] Mashhadiabbas, F., Neamatzadeh, H., Nasiri, R., Foroughi, E., Farahnak, S., & Piroozmand, P. et al. (2018). Association of vitamin D receptor BsmI, TaqI, FokI, and ApaI polymorphisms with susceptibility of chronic periodontitis: A systematic review and meta-analysis. Dental Research Journal, 15(3), 155.

[92] Deng, H., Liu, F., Pan, Y., Jin, X., Wang, H., & Cao, J. (2011). BsmI, TaqI, ApaI, and FokI polymorphisms in the vitamin D receptor gene and periodontitis: A meta-analysis. Journal of Clinical Periodontology, 38(3), 199–207.

[93] Nibali, L., Parkar, M., Suvan, J. E., Brett, P. M., Griffiths, G. S., Rosin, M., Schwahn, C., & Tonetti, M. S. (2008). Vitamin D receptor polymorphism (−1056 Taq-I) interacts with smoking for the presence and progression of periodontitis. Journal of Clinical Periodontology, 35(7), 561–567.

[94] Zakaria, W. N. A., Yunus, N. M., Yaacob, N. M., Omar, J., Wan Mohamed, W. M. I., Sirajudeen, K. N. S., & Tuan Ismail, T. S. (2021). Association between vitamin D receptor polymorphisms (BsmI and FokI) and glycemic control among patients with type 2 diabetes. International Journal of Environmental Research and Public Health, 18(4), 1595.

[95] Alotaibi, D. H., Altalhi, A. M., Sambawa, Z. M., Koppolu, P., Alsinaidi, A. A., & Krishnan, P. (2020). The association of matrix metalloproteinase gene polymorphisms and periodontitis: An overview. Journal of Pharmacy and Bioallied Sciences, 12(Suppl 1), S37.

[96] Izakovicova Holla, L., Hrdlickova, B., Vokurka, J., & Fassmann, A. (2012). Matrix metalloproteinase-8 (MMP8) gene polymorphisms in chronic periodontitis. Archives of Oral Biology, 57, 188–196.

[97] Emingil, G., Han, B., Gürkan, A., Berdeli, A., Tervahartiala, T., & Salo, T. et al. (2014). MMP-8 and TIMP-1 gene polymorphisms in generalized aggressive periodontitis: GCF MMP-8 and TIMP-1 levels and outcome of periodontal therapy. Journal of Periodontology, 85, 1070–1080.

[98] Keles, G. C., Gunes, S., Sumer, A. P., Sumer, M., Kara, N., & Bagci, H. et al. (2006). Association of MMP-9 promoter polymorphism with chronic periodontitis. Journal of Periodontology, 77, 1510–1514.

[99] Saza-Guzmán, D. M., Arias-Osorio, C., Martínez-Pabón, M. C., & S.i, T.-A. (2011). Salivary MMP-9 and TIMP-1 levels: relationship with periodontal status and MMP-9 (−1562C/T) polymorphism. Archives of Oral Biology, 56, 401–411.

[100] Li, G., Yue, Y., Tian, Y., Wang, M., Liang, H., Liao, P., & Chow, L. W. (2012). Association of MMP-1, -3, -9, IL-2, IL-8 and COX-2 gene polymorphisms with chronic periodontitis in a Chinese population. Cytokine, 60, 552–560.

[101] de Souza, A. P., Trevilatto, P. C., Scarel-Caminaga, R. M., De Brito, R. B. Jr, Barros, S. P., & Line, S. R. (2005). Analysis of MMP-9 (C-1562T) and TIMP-2 (G-418C) promoter polymorphisms in chronic periodontitis. Journal of Clinical Periodontology, 32, 207–211.

[102] Letra, A., Silva, R. M., Motta, L. G., Blanton, S. H., Hecht, J. T., & Granjeiro, J. M. et al. (2012). Association of MMP3 and TIMP2 promoter polymorphisms with nonsyndromic oral clefts. Birth Defects Research Part A: Clinical and Molecular Teratology, 94, 540–548.

[103] Chou, Y. H., Ho, Y. P., Lin, Y. C., Hu, K. F., Yang, Y. H., Ho, K. Y. & et al. (2011). MMP-8 −799 C>T polymorphism and susceptibility to chronic and aggressive periodontitis in Taiwanese. Journal of Clinical Periodontology, 38, 1078–1084.

[104] Hadi, C. A., Suhartono, W., Sulijaya, B., Sarwono, A. T., Yuniastuti, M., & Auerkari, E. I. (2017). Distribution of MMP-9 (−1562 C/T) polymorphism in Indonesian males with periodontitis. Journal of International Dental and Medical Research, 10, 778–781.

[105] Rai, B., Kaur, J., Jain, R., & Anand, S. C. (2010). Levels of GCF metalloproteinases-8 and −9 in periodontitis. Saudi Dental Journal, 22, 129–131.

[106] Zhang, H., Zhou, L., & Han, Y. et al. (2013). Associations between CD14 −159 C>T polymorphism and chronic/aggressive periodontitis susceptibility. Oral Diseases, 19(8), 805–811.

[107] Finoti, L. S., Nepomuceno, R., Pigossi, S. C., Corbi, S. C. T., Secolin, R., & Scarel-Caminaga, R. (2017). Association between interleukin-8 levels and chronic periodontal disease: a PRISMA-compliant systematic review and meta-analysis. Medicine (Baltimore), 96(22), e6932.

[108] Venkata Subbiah, H., Ramesh Babu, P., & Subbiah, U. (2023). Genetic polymorphism and gene expression of β-defensin-1 in periodontitis associated with type 2 diabetes mellitus. Cureus, 15(12), e49814.

[109] Truong, B., Hull, L. E., Ruan, Y., Huang, Q. Q., Hornsby, W., & Martin, H. et al. (2024). Integrative polygenic risk score improves the prediction accuracy of complex traits and diseases. Cell Genomics, 4(4), 100523.

[110] Kikuchi, T., & Mitani, A. (2022). Next-generation examination, diagnosis, and personalized medicine in periodontal disease. Journal of Personalized Medicine, 12(10), 1743.

[111] Kaikkonen, M. U., Lam, M. T., & Glass, C. K. (2011). Non-coding RNAs as regulators of gene expression and epigenetics. Cardiovascular Research, 90(3), 430–440.

[112] Santonocito, S., Polizzi, A., Palazzo, G., & Isola, G. (2021). The emerging role of microRNA in periodontitis: Pathophysiology, clinical potential and future perspectives. International Journal of Molecular Sciences, 22(11), 5456.

[113] Hayder, H., Zayed, Y., & Peng, C. (2018). Overview of microRNA biogenesis, mechanisms of actions, and circulation. Frontiers in Endocrinology, 9, 402.

[114] Luan, X., Zhou, X., Naqvi, A., Francis, M., Foyle, D., Nares, S., & Diekwisch, T. G. H. (2018). MicroRNAs and immunity in periodontal health and disease. International Journal of Oral Science, 10(3), 24.

[115] Wu, P., Feng, J., & Wang, W. (2021). Expression of miR-155 and miR-146a in saliva of patients with periodontitis and its clinical value. American Journal of Translational Research, 13(6), 6670.

[116] Micó-Martínez, P., Almiñana-Pastor, P. J., Alpiste-Illueca, F., & López-Roldán, A. (2021). microRNAs and periodontal disease: A qualitative systematic review of human studies. Journal of Periodontal & Implant Science, 51(6), 386.

[117] Han, R., Gao, J., Wang, L., Hao, P., Chen, X., & Wang, Y. et al. (2023). MicroRNA-146a negatively regulates inflammation via IRAK1/TRAF6/NF-κB in dry eye. Scientific Reports, 13, 11192.

[118] Almiñana-Pastor, P. J., Alpiste-Illueca, F. M., Micó-Martinez, P., García-Giménez, J. L., García-López, E., & López-Roldán, A. (2023). MicroRNAs in gingival crevicular fluid: Differential expression in periodontitis. Non-Coding RNA, 9(6), 73.

[119] Kurowska-Stolarska, M., Alivernini, S., Ballantine, L. E., Asquith, D. L., Millar, N. L., & Gilchrist, D. S. et al. (2011). MicroRNA-155 as a proinflammatory regulator in clinical and experimental arthritis. Proceedings of the National Academy of Sciences USA, 108(27), 11193.

[120] Subramaniam, R., Vijakumaran, U., Shanmuganantha, L., Law, X., Al as, E., & Ng, H. (2023). The role and mechanism of microRNA-21 in osteogenesis: An update. International Journal of Molecular Sciences, 24(14), 11330.

[121] Yang, Y., Ren, D., Zhao, D., Zhang, B., & Ye, R. (2023). MicroRNA-203 mediates *Porphyromonas gingivalis* LPS-induced inflammation and differentiation of periodontal ligament cells. Oral Diseases, 29(4), 1715–1725.

[122] Paterson, M., & Kriegel, A. (2017). MiR-146a/b: a family with shared seeds and different roots. Physiological Genomics, 49, 243–252.

[123] Houshmandfar, S., Saeedi-Boroujeni, A., Rashno, M., Khodadadi, A., & Mahmoudian-Sani, R. (2021). MiRNA-223 as a regulator of inflammation and NLRP3 inflammasome. Naunyn-Schmiedeberg's Archives of Pharmacology, 394(11), 2187.

[124] Hsieh, L., Huang, C., & Yu, C. (2021). Emerging role of microRNA-200 family in dentistry. Non-Coding RNA, 7(2), 35.

[125] Daily, Z. A., Al-Ghurabi, B. H., Al-Qarakhli, A. M. A., & Moseley, R. (2023). MicroRNA-155 as a biomarker of periodontal status and coronary heart disease severity: A case-control study. BMC Oral Health, 23(1), 868.

[126] P., J., & Luis, J. (2023). Study of microRNAs in gingival crevicular fluid as periodontal disease biomarkers: Systematic review. International Journal of Molecular Sciences, 25(15), 8274.

[127] Miska, E. A., & Ferguson-Smith, A. C. (2016). Transgenerational inheritance: Models and mechanisms of non-DNA sequence-based inheritance. Science, 354(6308), 59–63.

[128] Hernandez Martinez, C. D., Glessner, J., Finoti, L. S., Silva, P. F., Messora, M., Coletta, R. D., Hakonarson, H., & Palioto, D. B. (2024). Methylome-wide analysis in systemic microbial-induced experimental periodontal disease in mice with different susceptibility. Frontiers in Cellular and Infection Microbiology, 14, 1369226.

[129] Long, H. K., King, H. W., Patient, R. K., Odom, D. T., & Klose, R. J. (2016). Protection of CpG islands from DNA methylation is DNA-encoded and conserved. Nucleic Acids Research, 44(14), 6693.

[130] Viana, M. B., Cardoso, F. P., Diniz, M. G., Costa, F. O., Da Costa, J. E., Gomez, R. S., & Moreira, P. R. (2011). Methylation pattern of IFN-γ and IL-10 genes in periodontal tissues. Immunobiology, 216(8), 936–941.

[131] Qin, W., & Scicluna, B. P. (2021). The role of host cell DNA methylation in the immune response to bacterial infection. Frontiers in Immunology, 12, 696280.

[132] Tukek, T., Pehlivan, S., Medetalibeyoglu, A., Serin, I., Oyacı, Y., & Arıcı, H. et al. (2022). SOCS1 gene polymorphism and promoter methylation correlate with the course of COVID-19. Pathogens and Global Health, 117(4), 392–400.

[133] Zhang, S., Barros, S. P., Moretti, A. J., Yu, N., Zhou, J., Preisser, J. S., & Offenbacher, S. (2013). Epigenetic regulation of TNFA expression in periodontal disease. Journal of Periodontology, 84(11), 1606.

[134] Chiang, C. Y., Hsu, C. C., Chen, Y. W., & Fu, E. (2025). Hypomethylation of the interleukin-6 promoter in gingival tissue of patients with periodontitis. Journal of Periodontology, Epub ahead of print.

[135] De Oliveira, N. F., Andia, D. C., Planello, A. C., Pasetto, S., Marques, M. R., F.h., N. Jr, Line, S. R., & A.p, D. S. (2011). TLR2 and TLR4 promoter methylation status during chronic periodontitis. Journal of Clinical Periodontology, 38(11), 975–983.

[136] Pawlowska, E., Szczepanska, J., Derwich, M., Sobczuk, P., Düzgüneş, N., & Blasiak, J. (2024). DNA methylation in periodontal disease: A focus on folate, folic acid, mitochondria, and dietary intervention. International Journal of Molecular Sciences, 26(7), 3225.

[137] Chen, S., Zhou, D., Liu, O., Chen, H., Wang, Y., & Zhou, Y. (2022). Cellular senescence and periodontitis: mechanisms and therapeutics. Biology, 11(10), 1419.

[138] Chi, P., Allis, C. D., & Wang, G. G. (2010). Covalent histone modifications: Miswritten, misinterpreted, and miserased in human cancers. Nature Reviews Cancer, 10(7), 457–469.

[139] Larsson, L. (2017). Current concepts of epigenetics and its role in periodontitis. Current Oral Health Reports, 4, 286–293.

[140] Patten, D. K., Corleone, G., & Magnani, L. (2018). ChIP-seq: Tips and tricks for protocol and initial analysis. Methods in Molecular Biology, 1767, 271–288.

[141] Schmalz, G., Li, S., Burkhardt, R., Rinke, S., Krause, F., Haak, R., & Ziebolz, D. (2016). MicroRNAs as salivary markers for periodontal diseases: A new diagnostic approach?. BioMed Research International, 2016, 1027525.

[142] Al-Rawi, N. H., Al-Marzooq, F., Al-Nuaimi, A. S., Hachim, M. Y., & Hamoudi, R. (2020). Salivary microRNA-155, −146a/b and −203 as potential non-invasive biomarkers of periodontitis and diabetes mellitus. PLoS One, 15(8), e0237004.

[143] Dai, W., Qiao, X., Fang, Y., Guo, R., Bai, P., & Liu, S. et al. (2024). Epigenetics-targeted drugs: Current paradigms and future challenges. Signal Transduction and Targeted Therapy, 9, 332.

[144] Rashed, F., Taher, E. S., Abdeen, A., Taymour, N., Soliman, M. M., & Shalaby, H. K. et al. (2024). Prospective and challenges of locally applied repurposed pharmaceuticals for periodontal tissue regeneration. Frontiers in Bioengineering and Biotechnology, 12, 1400472.

[145] Blanco-Pintos, T., Regueira-Iglesias, A., Seijo-Porto, I., Balsa-Castro, C., Castelo-Baz, P., Nibali, L., & Tomás, I. (2023). Accuracy of periodontitis diagnosis using multiple molecular biomarkers in oral fluids: Systematic review and meta-analysis. Journal of Clinical Periodontology, 50(11), 1420–1443.

[146] Sunila, B. S., Shivakumar, G. C., Abdul, N. S., Sudhakar, N., Franco, R., Ronsivalle, V., Cicciù, M., & Minervini, G. (2025). Conventional periodontal probing versus salivary biomarkers in type 2 diabetes with chronic periodontitis. Minerva Dental and Oral Science, 74(3), 187–194.

[147] Kadayıf, A., Taşçi, Ö.E., & Karaduman, B. (2025). Effects of non-surgical periodontal therapy on GCF CTRP-1, TNF-α, and IL-10 levels. Clinical Oral Investigations, 29(7), 345.

[148] Chaudhari, A. U., Byakod, G. N., Waghmare, P. F., & Karhadkar, V. M. (2011). Correlation of IL-1β in GCF to clinical parameters of chronic periodontitis. Journal of Contemporary Dental Practice, 12, 52–59.

[149] Reinhardt, R. A., Stoner, J. A., Golub, L. M., Lee, H. M., Nummikoski, P. V., Sorsa, T., & Payne, J. B. (2010). Association of GCF biomarkers during periodontal maintenance with subsequent progressive periodontitis. Journal of Periodontology, 81, 251–259.

[150] Saba, R., Sorensen, D. L., & Booth, S. A. (2014). MicroRNA-146a: A dominant, negative regulator of the innate immune response. Frontiers in Immunology, 5, 578.

[151] Koppolu, P., Durvasula, S., Palaparthy, R., Rao, M., Sagar, V., Reddy, S. K., & Lingam, S. (2013). CRP and TNF-α before and after periodontal therapy in cardiovascular disease patients. Pan African Medical Journal, 15, 92.

[152] Mouliou, D. S. (2023). C-reactive protein: Pathophysiology, diagnosis, false results and a diagnostic algorithm. Diseases, 11(4), 132.

[153] Liu, C., Chu, D., George, J., Young, H. A., & Liu, G. (2021). Cytokines: From clinical significance to quantification. Advanced Science, 8(15), 2004433.

[154] Fojtíková, L., Šuláková, A., Blažková, M., Holubová, B., Kuchař, M., Mikšátková, P., Lapčík, O., & Fukal, L. (2017). LFIA and ELISA as immunomethods for detecting synthetic cannabinoid JWH-200. Toxicology Reports, 5, 65–72.

[155] Nolan, T., Hands, R. E., & Bustin, S. A. (2006). Quantification of mRNA using real-time RT-PCR. Nature Protocols, 1(3), 1559–1582.

[156] Tighe, P. J., Ryder, R. R., Todd, I., & Fairclough, L. C. (2015). ELISA in the multiplex era: Potentials and pitfalls. Proteomics: Clinical Applications, 9(3–4), 406–422.

[157] Mustafa, M. I., & Makhawi, A. M. (2021). SHERLOCK and DETECTR: CRISPR-Cas systems as rapid diagnostics. Journal of Clinical Microbiology, 59(3), e00745–20.

[158] Xing, E., Chen, H., Xin, X., Cui, H., Dou, Y., & Song, S. (2025). Recent advances in smartphone-based biosensors. Chemosensors, 13(7), 221.

[159] Al-Amrani, S., Al-Jabri, Z., Al-Zaabi, A., Alshekaili, J., & Al-Khabori, M. (2021). Proteomics: Concepts and applications in human medicine. World Journal of Biological Chemistry, 12(5), 57.

[160] Sachelarie, L., Stefanescu, C. L., Murineanu, R. M., Grigorian, M., Zaharia, A., Scrobota, I., & Hurjui, L. L. (2025). Role of salivary biomarkers IL-1β and MMP-8 in early detection and staging of periodontal disease. Medicina (Kaunas), 61(4), 760.

[161] Said, K. N., Al-Momani, A. M., Almaseeh, J. A., Marouf, N., Shatta, A., & Al-Abdulla, J. et al. (2022). Association of periodontal therapy with inflammatory biomarkers and complications in COVID-19 patients. Clinical Oral Investigations, 26(11), 6721.

[162] Gürsoy, U. K., Gürsoy, M., & Könönen, E. (2022). Biomarkers and periodontal regenerative approaches. Dental Clinics of North America, 66(1), 157–167.

[163] Ramseier, C. A., Rasperini, G., Batia, S., & Giannobile, W. V. (2012). Advanced regenerative technologies for periodontal tissue repair. Periodontology 2000, 59(1), 185–202.

[164] Ni, Z., Zhang, P., & Zhang, Y. (2025). Effectiveness of antimicrobial photodynamic therapy for peri-implant diseases in type 2 diabetes: Systematic review and meta-analysis. Photodiagnosis and Photodynamic Therapy, 54, 104684.

[165] Gürsoy, U. K., & Kantarci, A. (2022). Molecular biomarker research in periodontology: Roadmap for translation to clinical assay validation. Journal of Clinical Periodontology, 49(6), 556–567.

[166] McLeod, C., Norman, R., Litton, E., Saville, B. R., Webb, S., & Snelling, T. L. (2019). Choosing primary endpoints for clinical trials of health care interventions. Contemporary Clinical Trials Communications, 12, 100486.

[167] Romano, F., Iaderosa, G., Corana, M., Perotto, S., Baima, G., & Di Scipio, F. et al. (2022). Comparing ionic profile of GCF and saliva as signature of severe periodontitis. Biomedicines, 10(3), 687.

[168] Li, Y., Ou, Y., Fan, K., & Liu, G. (2024). Salivary diagnostics: Opportunities and challenges. Theranostics, 14(18), 6969.

[169] Kreitmann, L., Miglietta, L., Xu, K., Malpartida-Cardenas, K., D'Souza, G., & Kaforou, M. et al. (2023). Next-generation molecular diagnostics: Digital technologies to enhance multiplexing in real-time PCR. Trends in Analytical Chemistry, 160, 116963.

[170] Skubic, C., Zevnik, U., Nahtigal, K., Dolenc Grošelj, L., & Rozman, D. (2025). Circadian biomarkers in humans: Detecting melatonin and cortisol. Biomolecules, 15(7), 1006.

[171] Rijo-Ferreira, F., & Takahashi, J. S. (2019). Genomics of circadian rhythms in health and disease. Genome Medicine, 11, 82.

[172] Drabovich, A. P., Martínez-Morillo, E., & Diamandis, E. P. (2015). Toward an integrated pipeline for protein biomarker development. Biochimica Et Biophysica Acta: Proteins and Proteomics, 1854(6), 677–686.

[173] Macovei, G., Irimes, B., Hosu, O., Cristea, C., & Tertis, M. (2022). Point-of-care electrochemical testing of inflammatory biomarkers. Analytical and Bioanalytical Chemistry, 415(6), 1033–1046.

[174] Gowri, A., Kumar, N. A., & Anand, B. S. (2021). Advances in nanomaterials-based PoC diagnosis of COVID-19: Minireview. Trends in Analytical Chemistry, 137, 116205.

[175] Wang, S., Guan, X., & Sun, S. (2024). Microfluidic biosensors: Enabling advanced disease detection. Sensors, 25(6), 1936.

[176] Quazi, S. (2022). Artificial intelligence and machine learning in precision and genomic medicine. Medical Oncology, 39(8), 120.

[177] Felekkis, K., & Papaneophytou, C. (2024). The circulating biomarkers league: Combining miRNAs with cell-free DNAs and proteins. International Journal of Molecular Sciences, 25(6), 3403.

[178] Vo, K., & Trinh, K. L. (2025). Advances in wearable biosensors for wound healing and infection monitoring. Biosensors, 15(3), 139.

Nada Tawfig Hashim, Md Sofiqul Islam, and Rasha Babiker

5 Periodontitis as a Model of Inflammaging and Immunosenescence

5.1 Aging, Inflammation, and the Oral Cavity

Aging is an inevitable biological process marked by a gradual decline in physiological function and an increased susceptibility to chronic diseases [1]. Among the hallmarks of aging is a state of chronic, low-grade systemic inflammation, commonly referred to as inflammaging [2]. This condition is characterized by elevated levels of circulating pro-inflammatory cytokines, such as interleukin-6 (IL-6), tumor necrosis factor-alpha (TNF-α), and C-reactive protein (CRP), even in the absence of overt infection [3]. Alongside inflammaging, aging is also associated with immunosenescence, a term that encapsulates the age-related deterioration of both innate and adaptive immune responses [4]. These systemic alterations profoundly impact the host's ability to mount effective immune responses, increasing vulnerability to infections, impaired wound healing, autoimmune dysregulation, and cancer [5, 6].

Periodontitis, a chronic inflammatory disease that affects the supporting structures of teeth, is increasingly recognized as both a consequence and a contributor to systemic aging processes [7]. In elderly individuals, the prevalence and severity of periodontitis are markedly higher, with tooth loss, alveolar bone resorption, and systemic inflammatory burden becoming dominant concerns [8]. Periodontitis may thus serve as a localized model of inflammaging and a reflection of immune aging, offering a unique and accessible system for studying the complex interface between microbial stimuli, host response, and systemic health in older adults [8, 9].

5.2 The Oral Microbiome and Aging-Related Dysbiosis

Aging alters the composition and function of the oral microbiome, a dynamic microbial ecosystem intricately involved in maintaining periodontal health [10]. In young, healthy individuals, the oral microbiome is characterized by a predominance of symbiotic species that contribute to mucosal immunity, nitric oxide metabolism, and epithelial integrity [11]. With advancing age, shifts in dietary habits, salivary flow, medication use, and immune surveillance create a permissive environment for dysbiosis [10, 12] (Figure 5.1).

Periodontal dysbiosis in elderly individuals is marked by increased colonization by anaerobic, proteolytic, and pathogenic bacteria, such as *Porphyromonas gingivalis*

https://doi.org/10.1515/9783112219904-005

(*P. gingivalis*), *Tannerella forsythia* (*T. forsythia*), and *Treponema denticola* (*T. denticola*) [13, 14]. These organisms not only disrupt local tissue homeostasis but also amplify systemic inflammation through the release of lipopolysaccharides, gingipains, and other virulence factors [15, 16]. The heightened microbial load and reduced microbial diversity observed in aged individuals further complicate the host-microbiome equilibrium, establishing a chronic feed-forward loop of tissue damage and immune stimulation. As a result, the oral cavity becomes a persistent source of systemic inflammatory burden [17, 18].

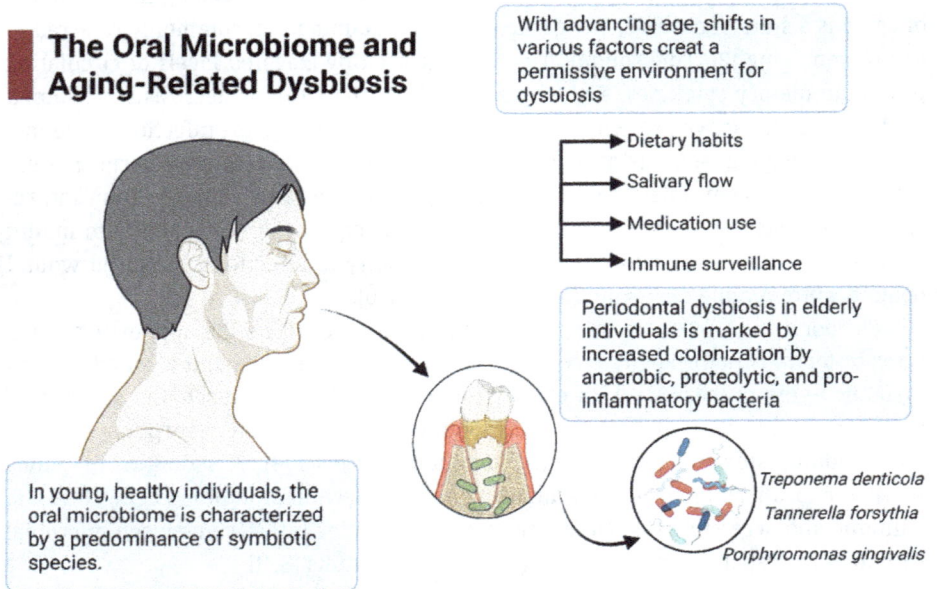

The Oral Microbiome and Aging-Related Dysbiosis

With advancing age, shifts in various factors creat a permissive environment for dysbiosis

Dietary habits

Salivary flow

Medication use

Immune surveillance

Periodontal dysbiosis in elderly individuals is marked by increased colonization by anaerobic, proteolytic, and pro-inflammatory bacteria

In young, healthy individuals, the oral microbiome is characterized by a predominance of symbiotic species.

Treponema denticola

Tannerella forsythia

Porphyromonas gingivalis

Figure 5.1: The oral microbiome and aging-related dysbiosis. With aging, changes in diet, salivary flow, medication use, and immune surveillance create a permissive environment for dysbiosis, leading to increased colonization by anaerobic, proteolytic, and pro-inflammatory bacteria, such as *Treponema denticola*, *Tannerella forsythia*, and *Porphyromonas gingivalis*. Created with Biorender.com.

5.3 Immune Dysregulation in Aging and Its Reflection in Periodontitis

Immunosenescence profoundly modifies the host defense system, exerting distinct effects on both innate and adaptive immunity [19]. Within the periodontium, the innate immune response undergoes significant phenotypic and functional alterations [20]. Neutrophils, which act as the primary responders to periodontal bacterial invasion, display impaired chemotaxis, delayed apoptosis, and heightened production of reactive oxygen species (ROS) [21]. This results in a hyper-inflammatory yet ineffective response. Additionally, monocytes and macrophages in aged individuals often acquire a senescence-associated secretory phenotype (SASP), characterized by persistent secretion of pro-inflammatory mediators, such as interleukin-1 beta (IL-1β), TNF-α, and matrix metalloproteinases (MMPs), thereby driving connective tissue degradation and alveolar bone resorption [22, 23].

In terms of adaptive immunity, aging leads to a shift toward memory and senescent T cell populations with compromised effector functions. Regulatory T cells (Tregs) frequently exhibit impaired suppressive activity, while Th17 responses become exaggerated, amplifying periodontal tissue damage [24, 25]. B cell diversity and repertoire decline with age, diminishing the quality and specificity of antibody-mediated defense mechanisms [26] (Figure 5.2). These age-driven immune alterations not only shape the local periodontal microenvironment but also exacerbate the progression and chronicity of periodontitis, reinforcing a systemic pro-inflammatory loop [27].

IMMUNOSENESCENCE

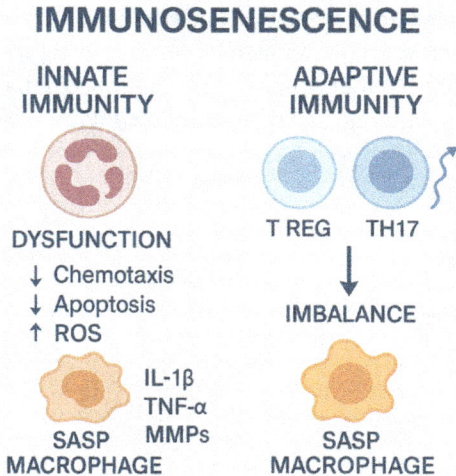

INNATE IMMUNITY

DYSFUNCTION
↓ Chemotaxis
↓ Apoptosis
↑ ROS

IL-1β
TNF-α
MMPs

SASP MACROPHAGE

ADAPTIVE IMMUNITY

T REG   TH17

IMBALANCE

SASP MACROPHAGE

Figure 5.2: Immunosenescence and its impact on innate and adaptive immunity. Aging is associated with impaired innate immune responses, including reduced chemotaxis, increased apoptosis, and elevated ROS production, leading to dysfunctional macrophages with a senescence-associated secretory phenotype (SASP). On the adaptive side, an imbalance between T regulatory (Treg) and TH17 cells contributes to chronic inflammation, further promoting SASP macrophage activity. Created with Biorender.com.

5.4 Molecular Markers of Inflammaging in the Periodontium

Aging-associated periodontal tissues and gingival crevicular fluid exhibit a distinctive biomarker profile that parallels systemic signatures of inflammaging [28]. Notably, elevated concentrations of pro-inflammatory mediators, such as interleukin-6 (IL-6), CRP, TNF-α, MMP-8, and cathepsin B have been detected, correlating strongly with clinical attachment loss and alveolar bone resorption [29, 30] (Figure 5.3). Additionally, the accumulation of advanced glycation end products (AGEs) – a hallmark of aging – is prominent in aged periodontal tissues. Engagement of AGEs with their receptor (RAGEs) triggers sustained nuclear factor kappa B (NF-κB) signaling, leading to enhanced cytokine release, oxidative stress, and further amplification of the inflammatory cascade [31, 32].

Emerging evidence also highlights the upregulation of senescence-associated markers, such as p16INK4a, p21, and β-galactosidase in gingival tissues from older individuals with periodontitis [33–35]. These biomarkers reflect cellular senescence and the activation of the SASP, which perpetuates a pro-inflammatory, non-resolving microenvironment. Collectively, these molecular signatures underscore the concept that the aging periodontium functions as a sentinel tissue, mirroring and amplifying systemic inflammatory aging [36, 37].

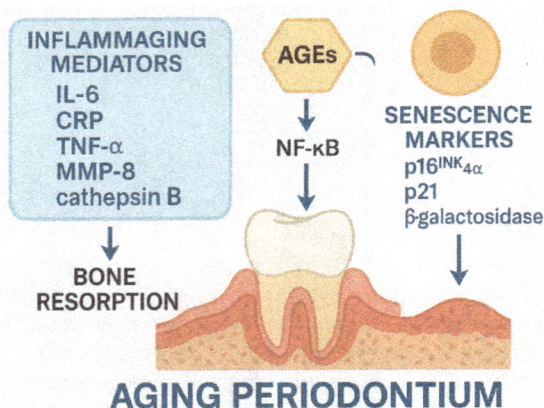

Figure 5.3: Mechanisms of aging in the periodontium. Inflammaging mediators (IL-6, CRP, TNF-α, MMP-8, cathepsin B) promote bone resorption, while advanced glycation end products (AGEs) activate NF-κB signaling. These processes, together with cellular senescence markers, such as p16^INK4a, p21, and β-galactosidase, contribute to periodontal tissue breakdown and age-related susceptibility to disease. Created with Biorender.com.

5.5 Impact of Chronic Periodontal Inflammation on Systemic Aging Phenotypes

Periodontitis has been implicated in a number of age-associated systemic conditions, including cardiovascular disease, type 2 diabetes, rheumatoid arthritis, Alzheimer's disease, frailty, and osteoporosis [38, 39]. In each of these conditions, chronic low-grade inflammation acts as a shared pathogenic mechanism, and periodontitis serves as a peripheral amplifier [9, 38] (Figure 5.4).

In cardiovascular disease, for example, periodontal pathogens and their products can enter the bloodstream, induce endothelial dysfunction, and contribute to athero-genesis [40]. In neurodegenerative disorders, such as Alzheimer's disease, *P. gingivalis* DNA and gingipains have been detected in brain tissue, where they may activate microglia and accelerate neuroinflammation [41, 42]. In osteoporosis, inflammatory cytokines from periodontal sites enhance osteoclast activity systemically, leading to increased bone resorption [43].These findings reinforce the role of periodontitis as a model of inflammaging, where a chronic localized infection promotes systemic immune activation and accelerates age-related decline in other tissues.

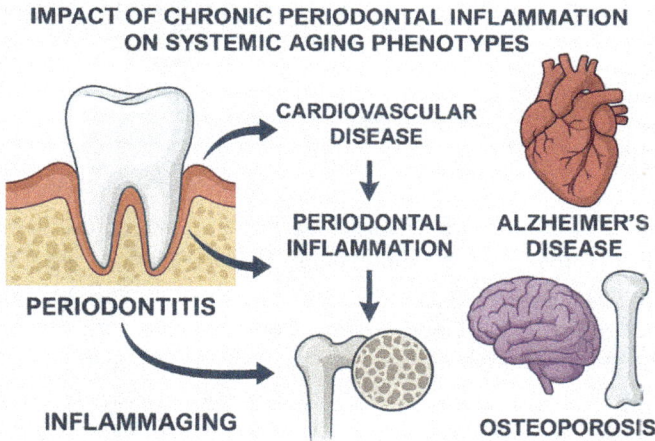

IMPACT OF CHRONIC PERIODONTAL INFLAMMATION ON SYSTEMIC AGING PHENOTYPES

PERIODONTITIS

CARDIOVASCULAR DISEASE

PERIODONTAL INFLAMMATION

ALZHEIMER'S DISEASE

INFLAMMAGING

OSTEOPOROSIS

Figure 5.4: Impact of chronic periodontal inflammation on systemic aging phenotypes. Periodontitis-driven inflammaging contributes to systemic diseases, including cardiovascular disease, Alzheimer's disease, and osteoporosis, linking oral inflammation with age-related conditions. Created with Biorender.com.

5.6 Therapeutic Implications: Targeting the Inflammatory-Aging Interface

Understanding the bidirectional relationship between periodontitis and systemic inflammaging opens new avenues for integrated therapy [44–46]. Traditional periodontal treatments, such as scaling and root planing and antimicrobial therapy may transiently reduce local inflammation, but addressing the immunosenescent component may require more targeted approaches [46–48].

Host modulation therapies, including sub-antimicrobial-dose doxycycline, resolvins, and omega-3 fatty acids, have shown promise in downregulating chronic inflammation [49, 50]. Immunonutrition, antioxidant therapy (e.g., curcumin, resveratrol), and senolytic agents targeting senescent cells in periodontal tissues are emerging as adjunctive strategies [51]. Moreover, the use of systemic anti-inflammatory agents, such as IL-6 or TNF-α blockers, though still under investigation, could offer dual benefits in managing periodontitis and comorbid inflammatory conditions [52].

Importantly, geriatric periodontal care should be personalized, accounting for biological age, systemic health, immunological profile, and medication interactions. Biomarker-driven approaches that monitor systemic inflammatory burden and periodontal disease activity may aid in stratifying patients for more precise therapeutic interventions [53, 54].

5.7 Conclusion

Periodontitis in the elderly is more than a localized oral disease; it is a clinical manifestation of the broader immunological and inflammatory changes that characterize aging. By examining the interplay between dysbiotic microbial communities and immunosenescent host responses, periodontitis serves as a valuable model for studying inflammaging. The insights gained from this model may not only improve periodontal care but also inform strategies for managing chronic inflammatory diseases in aging populations. As research deepens, the integration of periodontal health into geriatric medicine will become increasingly essential, reaffirming the mouth as a mirror and mediator of systemic health.

References

[1]   Tenchov, R., Sasso, J. M., Wang, X., & Zhou, Q. A. (2023). Aging hallmarks and progression and age-related diseases: A landscape view of research advancement. ACS Chemical Neuroscience, 15(1), 1.
[2]   Ferrucci, L., & Fabbri, E. (2018). Inflammageing: Chronic inflammation in ageing, cardiovascular disease, and frailty. Nature Reviews Cardiology, 15(9), 505.

[3] Baechle, J. J., Chen, N., Makhijani, P., Winer, S., Furman, D., & Winer, D A. (2023). Chronic inflammation and the hallmarks of aging. Molecular Metabolism, 74, 101755.

[4] Theodorakis, N., Feretzakis, G., Hitas, C., Kreouzi, M., Kalantzi, S., Spyridaki, A., Kollia, Z., Verykios, V. S., & Nikolaou, M. (2024). Immunosenescence: How aging increases susceptibility to bacterial infections and virulence factors. Microorganisms, 12(10), 2052.

[5] Yu, W., Yu, Y., Sun, S., Lu, C., Zhai, J., Lei, Y., Bai, F., Wang, R., & Chen, J (2023). Immune alterations with aging: Mechanisms and intervention strategies. Nutrients, 16(22), 3830.

[6] Wrona, M. V., Ghosh, R., Coll, K., Chun, C., & Yousefzadeh, M. J. (2024) The 3 I's of immunity and aging: immunosenescence, inflammaging, and immune resilience. Frontiers in Aging, 5, 1490302.

[7] Bhuyan, R., Bhuyan, S. K., Mohanty, J. N., Das, S., Juliana, N., & Abu, I. F. (2022). Periodontitis and its inflammatory changes linked to various systemic diseases: A review of its underlying mechanisms. Biomedicines, 10(10), 2659.

[8] Zhu, L., Tang, Z., Hu, R., Gu, M., & Yang, Y. (2023). Ageing and inflammation: What happens in periodontium?. Bioengineering, 10(11), 1274.

[9] Bertolini, M., & Clark, D. (2023). Periodontal disease as a model to study chronic inflammation in aging. GeroScience, 46(4), 3695.

[10] Pei, M., Zhou, X., Tsang, W., Tai, W. C. S., & Wong, C. C. (2024). The oral microbial ecosystem in age-related Xerostomia: A critical review. International Journal of Molecular Sciences, 25(23), 12815.

[11] Sedghi, L., DiMassa, V., Harrington, A., Lynch, S. V., & Kapila, Y. L. (2021). The oral microbiome: Role of key organisms and complex networks in oral health and disease. Periodontology 2000, 87(1), 107.

[12] Shintani, T., Obayashi, N., Yoshimoto, T., Ando, T., Morihara, N., Kataoka, N., Miyata, R., Yoshino, M., Yoshii, H., Morimoto, S., Hayashi, Y., Suzuki, M., Tanimoto, K., & Kajiya, M. (2025). Effect of stimulated salivary volume on dysbiosis of the salivary microbiome in children and young adults. International Dental Journal, 75(3), 1759.

[13] Tan, K. H., Seers, C. A., Dashper, S. G., Mitchell, H. L., Pyke, J. S., Meuric, V., Slakeski, N., Cleal, S. M., Chambers, J. L., McConville, M. J., & Reynolds, E. C. (2014). Porphyromonas gingivalis and Treponema denticola exhibit metabolic symbioses. PLoS Pathogens, 10(3), e1003955.

[14] Kamer, A. R., Pushalkar, S., Gulivindala, D., Butler, T., Li, Y., Annam, K. R. C., Glodzik, L., Ballman, K. V., Corby, P. M., Blennow, K., Zetterberg, H., & Saxena, D. (2021). Periodontal dysbiosis associates with reduced CSF Aβ42 in cognitively normal elderly. Alzheimer's & Dementia: Diagnosis, Assessment & Disease Monitoring, 13(1), e12172.

[15] Tamai, R., Deng, X., & Kiyoura, Y. (2009). Porphyromonas gingivalis with either Tannerella forsythia or Treponema denticola induces synergistic IL-6 production by murine macrophage-like J774.1 cells. Anaerobe, 15(3), 87–90.

[16] Rosenfeld, Y., & Shai, Y. (2006). Lipopolysaccharide (Endotoxin)-host defense antibacterial peptides interactions: Role in bacterial resistance and prevention of sepsis. Biochimica Et Biophysica Acta (BBA) – Biomembranes, 1758(9), 1513–1522.

[17] Lamont, R. J., Koo, H., & Hajishengallis, G. (2018). The oral microbiota: Dynamic communities and host interactions. Nature Reviews Microbiology, 16(12), 745.

[18] Hu, W., Chen, S., Zou, X., Chen, Y., Luo, J., Zhong, P., & Ma, D. (2025). Oral microbiome, periodontal disease and systemic bone-related diseases in the era of homeostatic medicine. Journal of Advanced Research, 73, 443–458.

[19] Liu, Z., Liang, Q., Ren, Y., Guo, C., Ge, X., Wang, L., Cheng, Q., Luo, P., Zhang, Y., & Han, X. (2023). Immunosenescence: Molecular mechanisms and diseases. Signal Transduction and Targeted Therapy, 8(1), 1–16.

[20] Hajishengallis, G. (2014). Aging and its impact on innate immunity and inflammation: Implications for periodontitis. Journal of Oral Biosciences, 56(1), 30.

[21] Wang, Z., Saxena, A., Yan, W., Uriarte, S. M., Siqueira, R., & Li, X. (2025). The impact of aging on neutrophil functions and the contribution to periodontitis. International Journal of Oral Science, 17, 10.

[22] Rattanaprukskul, K., Xia, X. J., Jiang, M., Albuquerque-Souza, E., Bandyopadhyay, D., & Sahingur, S. E. (2024). Molecular signatures of senescence in periodontitis: Clinical insights. Journal of Dental Research, 103(8), 800–808.

[23] Wang, L., Hong, W., Zhu, H., He, Q., Yang, B., Wang, J., & Weng, Q. (2024). Macrophage senescence in health and diseases. Acta Pharmaceutica Sinica B, 14(4), 1508.

[24] Xu, L., Chen, X., & Cheng, J. (2024). The effect of T cell aging on the change of human tissue structure. Immunity & Ageing, 21, 26.

[25] Afzali, B., Lombardi, G., Lechler, R. I., & Lord, G. M. (2007). The role of T helper 17 (Th17) and regulatory T cells (Treg) in human organ transplantation and autoimmune disease. Clinical and Experimental Immunology, 148(1), 32.

[26] Dunn-Walters, D. K., & Ademokun, A. A. (2010). B cell repertoire and ageing. Current Opinion in Immunology, 22(4), 514–520.

[27] Ebersole, J. L., Dawson, D. A., Huja, P. E., Pandruvada, S., Basu, A., Nguyen, L., Zhang, Y., & Gonzalez, O. A. (2018). Age and periodontal health – immunological view. Current Oral Health Reports, 5(4), 229.

[28] Tsalikis, L. (2010). The effect of age on the gingival crevicular fluid composition during experimental gingivitis: A pilot study. The Open Dentistry Journal, 4, 13.

[29] Taylor, J. J. (2014). Protein biomarkers of periodontitis in saliva. ISRN Inflammation, 2014, 593151.

[30] Jakovljevic, A., Miletic, M., Nikolic, N., Beljic-Ivanovic, K., Andric, M., & Milasin, J. (2019). Notch signaling pathway mediates alveolar bone resorption in apical periodontitis. Medical Hypotheses, 124, 87–90.

[31] Chaudhuri, J., Bains, Y., Guha, S., Kahn, A., Hall, D., Bose, N., Gugliucci, A., & Kapahi, P. (2018). The role of advanced glycation end products in aging and metabolic diseases: Bridging association and causality. Cell Metabolism, 28(3), 337.

[32] Ramasamy, R., Vannucci, S. J., Yan, S. S., Herold, K., Yan, S. F., & Schmidt, A. M. (2005). Advanced glycation end products and RAGE: A common thread in aging, diabetes, neurodegeneration, and inflammation. Glycobiology, 15(7), 16R–28R.

[33] Huang, W., Hickson, L. J., Eirin, A., Kirkland, J. L., & Lerman, L. O. (2022). Cellular senescence: The good, the bad and the unknown. Nature Reviews Nephrology, 18(10), 611.

[34] Wang, S., Mou, J., Jiang, J., He, Q., Qahar, M., Santis, D. D., Qi, F., Xu, G., & Liu, J. (2025). Accelerated senescence animal models and application in dentistry: A scoping review. Journal of Dental Sciences, 20, 2026–2038.

[35] Khosla, S., Farr, J. N., & Monroe, D. G. (2019). Periodontal disease and senescent cells: New players for an old oral health problem?. International Journal of Molecular Sciences, 21(20), 7441.

[36] Rattanaprukskul, K., Xia, J., Jiang, M., Albuquerque-Souza, E., Bandyopadhyay, D., & Sahingur, S. (2024). Molecular signatures of senescence in periodontitis: Clinical insights. Journal of Dental Research, 103(8), 800.

[37] Chu, X., Elashiry, M., Carroll, A., Cornelius, C. J., Cutler, C. W., & Elsayed, R. (2024). The role of senescence in experimental periodontitis at the causal level: An in vivo study. Cells, 14(3), 226.

[38] Clark, D., Kotronia, E., & Ramsay, S. E. (2021). Frailty, aging, and periodontal disease: Basic biological considerations. Periodontology 2000, 87(1), 143.

[39] Holmstrup, P., Damgaard, C., Olsen, I., Klinge, B., Flyvbjerg, A., Nielsen, C. H., & Hansen, P. R. (2017). Comorbidity of periodontal disease: Two sides of the same coin? An introduction for the clinician. Journal of Oral Microbiology, 9(1), 1332710.

[40] Angjelova, A., Jovanova, E., Polizzi, A., Laganà, L., Santonocito, S., Ragusa, R., & Isola, G. (2024). Impact of periodontitis on endothelial risk dysfunction and oxidative stress improvement in patients with cardiovascular disease. Journal of Clinical Medicine, 13(13), 3781.

[41] Magnusson, A., Wu, R., & Demirel, I. (2024). Porphyromonas gingivalis triggers microglia activation and neurodegenerative processes through NOX4. Frontiers in Cellular and Infection Microbiology, 14, 1451683.

[42] Jiang, Y., Xu, L., Zhao, X., Shen, H., Qiu, C., He, Z., Song, Z., & Zhou, W. (2025). Porphyromonas gingivalis-induced periodontitis promotes neuroinflammation and neuronal loss associated with dysfunction of the brain barrier. Frontiers in Cellular and Infection Microbiology, 15, 1559182.

[43] Hienz, S. A., Paliwal, S., & Ivanovski, S. (2015). Mechanisms of bone resorption in periodontitis. Journal of Immunology Research, 2015, 615486.

[44] Tang, Q., Xu, W., Zhang, F., Yuan, G., & Zhou, D. (2025). Interdisciplinary research on periodontitis and depression: a bibliometric analysis of research trends, hotspots and future directions. Frontiers in Oral Health, 6, 1588737.

[45] Seyedmoalemi, M. A., & Saied-Moallemi, Z. (2025). Association between periodontitis and Alzheimer's disease: A narrative review. IBRO Neuroscience Reports, 13, 360–365.

[46] Ranbhise, J. S., Ju, S., Singh, M. K., Han, S., Akter, S., Ha, J., Choe, W., Kim, S. S., & Kang, I. (2025). Chronic Inflammation and Glycemic control: Exploring the bidirectional link between periodontitis and diabetes. Dentistry Journal, 13(3), 100.

[47] Radu, C., Radu, C. C., Arbănaşi, E., Hogea, T., Murvai, V. R., Chiş, I., & Zaha, D. C. (2024). Exploring the efficacy of novel therapeutic strategies for periodontitis: A literature review. Life, 14(4), 468.

[48] Alassy, H., Pizarek, J. A., Kormas, I., Pedercini, A., & Wolff, L. F. (2021). Antimicrobial adjuncts in the management of periodontal and peri-implant diseases and conditions: a narrative review. Frontiers in Oral and Maxillofacial Medicine, 3, 16.

[49] Deore, G. D., Gurav, A. N., Patil, R., Shete, A. R., NaikTari, R. S., & Inamdar, S. P. (2014). Omega 3 fatty acids as a host modulator in chronic periodontitis patients: a randomised, double-blind, placebo-controlled clinical trial. Journal of Periodontal & Implant Science, 44(1), 25.

[50] Sufaru, I., Teslaru, S., Pasarin, L., Iovan, G., Stoleriu, S., & Solomon, S. M. (2022). Host response modulation therapy in the diabetes mellitus – periodontitis conjuncture: A narrative review. Pharmaceutics, 14(8), 1728.

[51] Hashim, N. T., Babiker, R., Chaitanya, C. S. K., Mohammed, R., Priya, S. P., Padmanabhan, V., Ahmed, A., Dasnadi, S. P., Islam, M. S., Gismalla, B. G., & Rahman, M. M. (2025). New insights in natural bioactive compounds for periodontal disease: Advanced molecular mechanisms and therapeutic potential. Molecules, 30(4), 807.

[52] Ancuţa, C., Chirieac, R., Ancuţa, E., Ţănculescu, O., Solomon, S. M., Făţu, A. M., Doloca, A., & Iordache, C. (2021). Exploring the role of Interleukin-6 receptor inhibitor tocilizumab in patients with active rheumatoid arthritis and periodontal disease. Journal of Clinical Medicine, 10(4), 878.

[53] Foroughi, M., Torabinejad, M., & Angelov, N. (2025). Bridging oral and systemic health: exploring pathogenesis, biomarkers, and diagnostic innovations in periodontal disease. Infection. 2025, e1003933.

[54] Laniado, N., Levin, L., & Lamster, I. (2022). Management of periodontal disease in older adults, In: Hogue, C. M., & Ruiz, J. G. (eds), Oral Health and Aging. Springer: Cham.109–129. https://doi.org/10.1007/978-3-030-85993-0_6.

Nada Tawfig Hashim, Rasha Babiker,
and Muhammed Mustahsen Rahman

6 Microbiome Therapeutics and Ecological Periodontal Therapy

6.1 Introduction: A Shift in Periodontal Therapeutic Philosophy

Periodontal diseases, particularly periodontitis, have long been conceptualized through a reductionist model that centers on the elimination of specific pathogenic bacteria [1]. However, emerging evidence from microbial ecology and systems biology has revolutionized this framework [2, 3]. Rather than viewing periodontitis as the result of infection by exogenous pathogens, it is now recognized as a polymicrobial dysbiosis, a disruption of the homeostatic balance of the oral microbiome and host immune interactions [4]. This shift demands therapeutic strategies that do not merely suppress bacteria indiscriminately but rather restore a balanced, health-compatible microbial community. Ecological periodontal therapy (EPT) embraces this paradigm, focusing on modulating the entire microbiome rather than targeting individual pathogens [5].

6.2 Ecological Concept of Periodontal Disease

The oral cavity represents a highly complex and dynamic ecosystem, home to over 700 microbial species, including bacteria, archaea, viruses, and fungi [6]. In a state of health, this community is dominated by symbiotic species such as *Streptococcus sanguinis* (*S. sanguinis*), *Actinomyces naeslundii* (*A. naeslundii*), and Veillonella spp., which contribute to colonization resistance, immune modulation, and metabolic cross-feeding [7–9]. Periodontitis arises when ecological pressures, such as poor oral hygiene, smoking, systemic disease, or immunosenescence, alter the local habitat, favoring the overgrowth of pathobionts like *Porphyromonas gingivalis* (*P. gingivalis*), *Tannerella forsythia* (*T. forsythia*), and *Treponema denticola* (*T. denticola*) [10]. Although often present at low abundance, these organisms can act as keystone pathogens, initiating a cascade of immune dysregulation and microbial synergy that drives the community toward a pathogenic state [11, 12]. Once this dysbiotic shift occurs, the biofilm becomes enriched with virulent species that secrete proteolytic enzymes, lipopolysaccharides (LPS), and other virulence factors capable of degrading extracellular matrix components while manipulating the host immune response [13]. Keystone pathogens such as *P. gingivalis* can subvert neutrophil activity, dysregulate comple-

https://doi.org/10.1515/9783112219904-006

ment pathways, and provoke the excessive release of pro-inflammatory cytokines, including IL-1β, TNF-α, and IL-6 [14, 15]. This chronic, ineffective inflammatory response fails to eliminate the biofilm but instead drives collateral tissue destruction, including connective tissue breakdown and alveolar bone resorption. Additionally, microbial synergy among anaerobic species enhances their evasion of host defenses, resulting in a self-sustaining dysbiotic ecosystem [16, 17].

Crucially, the oral microbiome is not static but highly responsive to changes in environmental and host-related factors [18] (Figure 6.1). As such, modulating the composition and virulence of the oral microbiome – through meticulous oral hygiene, targeted antimicrobial approaches, host-modulating therapies, and lifestyle interventions – remains central to preventing and controlling periodontitis. Ultimately, effective regulation of the oral microbiome translates to effective control of the disease itself [19].

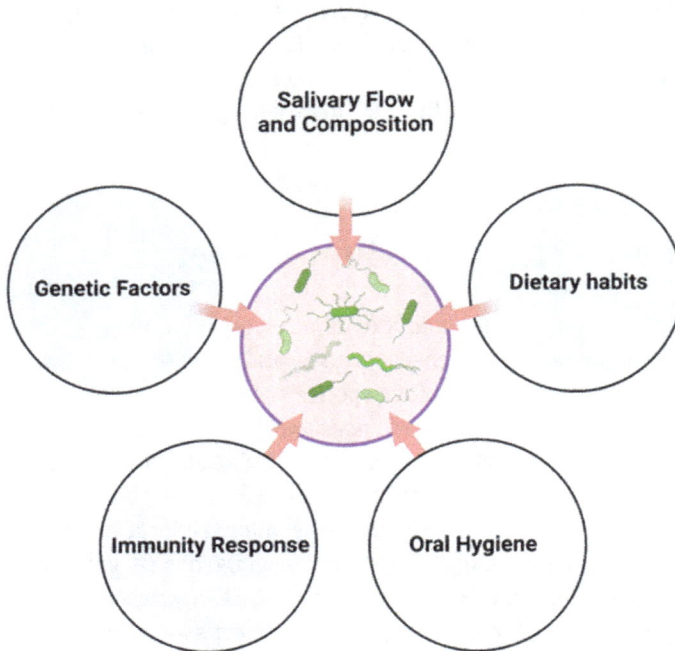

Figure 6.1: Key determinants of the oral microbiome. Factors influencing microbial balance include salivary flow and composition, dietary habits, oral hygiene practices, host immune response, and genetic predisposition. Created with Biorender.com.

6.3 Probiotics in Periodontal Therapy

Probiotics are defined as live microorganisms that, when administered in adequate amounts, confer health benefits to the host [20]. In the context of periodontitis, probiotics have shown promise in suppressing inflammation, inhibiting pathogen adhesion, and promoting recolonization by beneficial bacteria [21]. Commonly studied probiotic strains include *Lactobacillus reuteri* (*L. reuteri*), *Lactobacillus salivarius* (*L. salivarius*), and *Streptococcus salivarius* (*S. salivarius*) [22–24]. These strains exert their effects through competitive exclusion of pathogens, production of antimicrobial peptides such as reuterin and bacteriocins, and modulation of host immune responses [25]. For example, *L. reuteri* has been shown to reduce IL-1β and TNF-α levels in gingival crevicular fluid, enhancing clinical attachment levels when used adjunctively with scaling and root planning [26, 27].

Clinical trials have demonstrated that probiotic lozenges, mouth rinses, or chewing gums can reduce plaque scores, bleeding on probing, and periodontal pocket depths [28–30]. However, colonization resistance in the oral cavity poses a significant challenge for the long-term effectiveness of probiotics, as the indigenous microbiota, organized within complex and highly competitive biofilms, limits the ability of introduced strains to establish stable colonization [31]. Factors such as nutrient competition, lack of appropriate adhesion molecules, and constant mechanical clearance by salivary flow and oral hygiene practices contribute to the transient nature of probiotic presence [32–34] (Figure 6.2). To overcome these limitations, synbiotic approaches, which combine probiotics with selective prebiotics, are being explored [35].

6.4 Prebiotics and Synbiotics: Feeding the Friendly Microbiota

Prebiotics are nondigestible food components that selectively stimulate the growth or activity of beneficial bacteria [36]. In the oral cavity, potential prebiotics include xylitol, arginine, and polyphenol-rich compounds such as those found in green tea or cranberries [37]. Arginine metabolism by commensals like *Streptococcus gordonii* (*S. gordonii*) increases local pH through ammonia production, countering acidogenic pathogens and supporting microbial homeostasis [38]. Xylitol, beyond its anticariogenic effects, inhibits biofilm formation and reduces adhesion of *P. gingivalis* [39] (Figure 6.3).

Synbiotics refer to combinations of probiotics and prebiotics that synergistically enhance microbial balance [40]. For instance, a formulation combining *L. reuteri* with inulin or arginine could enhance probiotic survival and metabolic activity in the gingival sulcus [41].

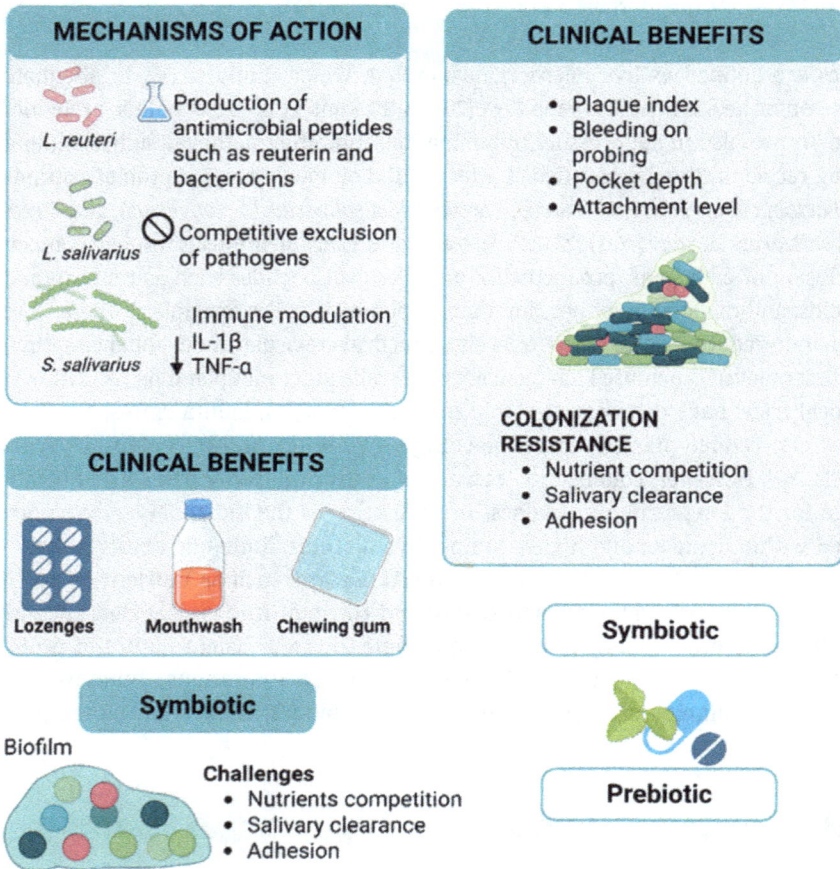

MECHANISMS OF ACTION

L. reuteri
Production of antimicrobial peptides such as reuterin and bacteriocins

L. salivarius
Competitive exclusion of pathogens

S. salivarius
Immune modulation
↓ IL-1β
↓ TNF-α

CLINICAL BENEFITS

Lozenges   Mouthwash   Chewing gum

Biofilm

Symbiotic

Challenges
- Nutrients competition
- Salivary clearance
- Adhesion

CLINICAL BENEFITS

- Plaque index
- Bleeding on probing
- Pocket depth
- Attachment level

COLONIZATION RESISTANCE
- Nutrient competition
- Salivary clearance
- Adhesion

Symbiotic

Prebiotic

Figure 6.2: Mechanisms of action and clinical benefits of probiotics in oral health. Probiotics act by producing antimicrobial peptides, competing with pathogens, and modulating immune responses. Their clinical benefits include plaque reduction, decreased bleeding on probing, improved pocket depth, and enhanced attachment level. Delivery can occur via lozenges, mouth rinses, or chewing gum. Symbiotics and prebiotics provide further ecological support by promoting colonization resistance. Created with Biorender.com.

Emerging delivery technologies, such as biofilm-compatible carriers, slow-release lozenges, and synbiotic-enriched oral gels – are being developed to prolong retention time in the oral cavity and improve colonization efficiency, thereby facilitating microbial balance restoration [42, 43]. Although clinical evidence on synbiotics in periodontology remains limited, early studies report enhanced plaque control and greater modulation of inflammation compared to probiotics alone [44, 45] (Figure 6.3).

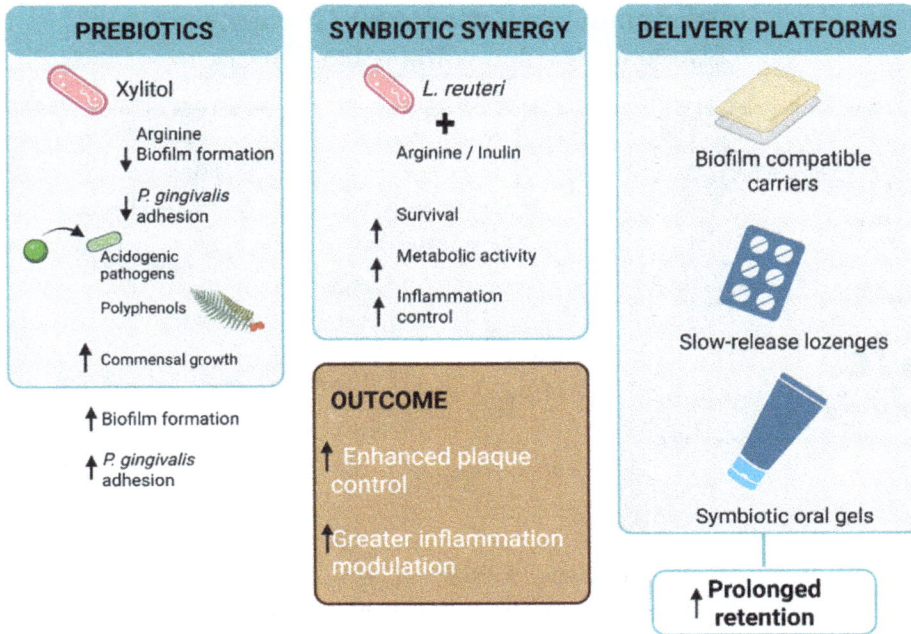

Figure 6.3: Prebiotics, synbiotic synergy, and delivery platforms for oral health. Prebiotics such as xylitol reduce biofilm formation and inhibit pathogens, while synbiotic synergy with *L. reuteri* enhances plaque control and inflammation modulation. Delivery platforms including biofilm-compatible carriers, slow-release lozenges, and symbiotic oral gels provide prolonged retention and therapeutic efficacy. Created with Biorender.com.

6.5 Postbiotics: Microbial Metabolites as Bioactive Agents

Postbiotics encompass the bioactive metabolites, cell wall components, and secreted proteins produced by probiotics that exert health effects without requiring live microorganisms [46]. This category includes short-chain fatty acids (SCFAs), antimicrobial peptides, extracellular vesicles, and exopolysaccharides. SCFAs like butyrate and acetate have demonstrated anti-inflammatory effects by modulating NF-κB signaling and promoting regulatory T-cell activity [47, 48].

In periodontal therapy, postbiotics offer several advantages over live probiotics, including stability, safety, and precise dosing [49]. For example, bacteriocins derived from *L. salivarius* can inhibit *P. gingivalis* growth, while extracellular polysaccharides from Bifidobacteria can block pathogen adhesion to epithelial cells [50]. These molecules can be formulated into oral rinses, hydrogels, or biodegradable delivery systems for targeted application to periodontal pockets [51] (Figure 6.4).

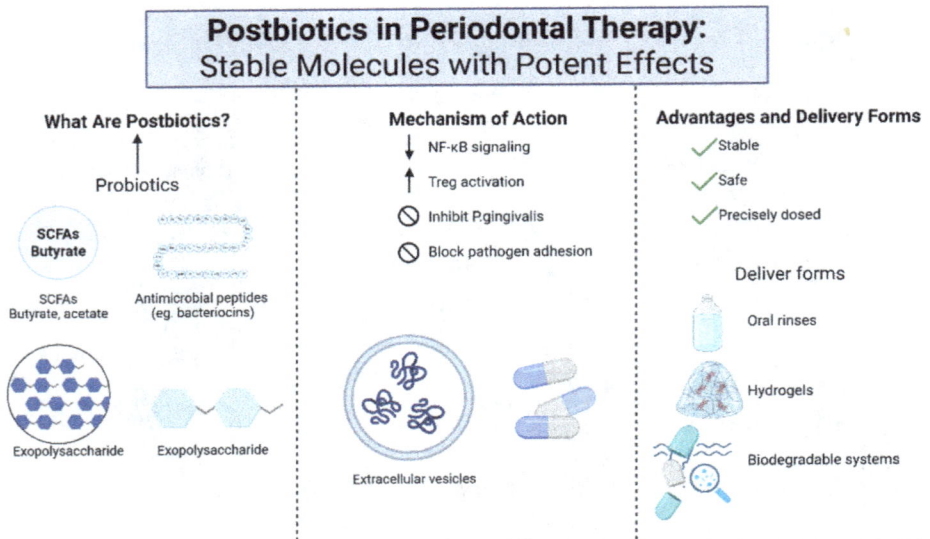

Figure 6.4: Postbiotics in periodontal therapy: Stable microbial-derived molecules with therapeutic effects. Postbiotics, including SCFAs, bacteriocins, and enzymes, act by inhibiting pathogens, modulating immune responses, and blocking pathogenic activation. Their advantages include safety, stability, and clinical efficacy. Delivery forms include oral rinses, hydrogels, and biodegradable systems. Created with Biorender.com.

6.6 Bacteriophage Therapy: Targeted Elimination of Periodontal Pathogens

Bacteriophages (phages) are viruses that specifically infect and lyse bacterial cells [52]. Unlike broad-spectrum antibiotics, phages can be engineered to selectively eliminate pathogenic bacteria while preserving commensal flora [53]. In periodontology, phage therapy has been explored for targeting key pathogens such as *P. gingivalis* and *Aggregatibacter actinomycetemcomitans* (*A. actinomycetemcomitans*) [54, 55]. Phages can be applied locally via gels, films, or rinses and can penetrate biofilms through enzymatic degradation of the extracellular polymeric matrix [56]. Additionally, CRISPR-Cas systems have been integrated into phages to enhance specificity and deliver gene-editing tools to disrupt virulence genes or antibiotic resistance elements (Figure 6.5). While still experimental, phage therapy represents a promising ecological tool to reshape subgingival communities without contributing to dysbiosis [57, 58].

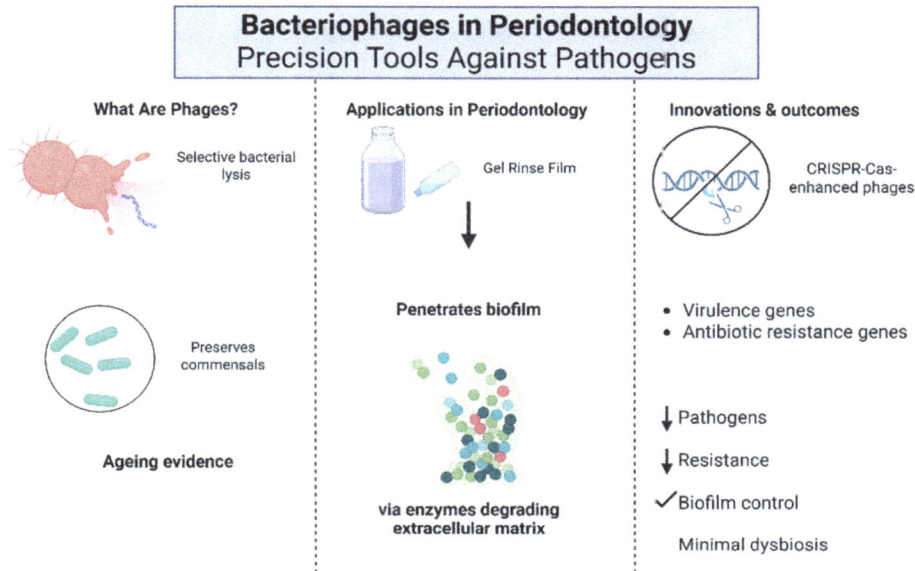

Figure 6.5: Bacteriophages in periodontology as precision tools against pathogens. Phages selectively target bacterial cells, penetrate biofilms, and degrade the extracellular matrix. Their applications include biofilm disruption, bacterial clearance, and CRISPR-Cas–enhanced phage therapies. Outcomes include pathogen reduction, antibiotic resistance control, and preservation of microbial balance. Created with Biorender.com.

6.7 Microbiome Transplants: Conceptualizing Oral Fecal Microbiota Transplantation

Inspired by the success of fecal microbiota transplantation in treating *Clostridioides difficile* infections, oral microbiome transplantation (OMT) have emerged as a theoretical approach to restore microbial balance in refractory periodontitis [59, 60]. The concept involves collecting the oral microbiome from healthy donors and transplanting it to dysbiotic sites via gels, rinses, or scaffold-based delivery systems [61] (Figure 6.6). Although OMT remains in preclinical stages, proof-of-concept studies in animal models have demonstrated the feasibility of recolonizing diseased sites with health-associated microbiota [62]. Key challenges include donor screening, safety regulation, and ensuring stable engraftment of transplanted communities. Advances in microbial culturomics and synthetic community design may facilitate standardized oral microbiota consortia for therapeutic use [63].

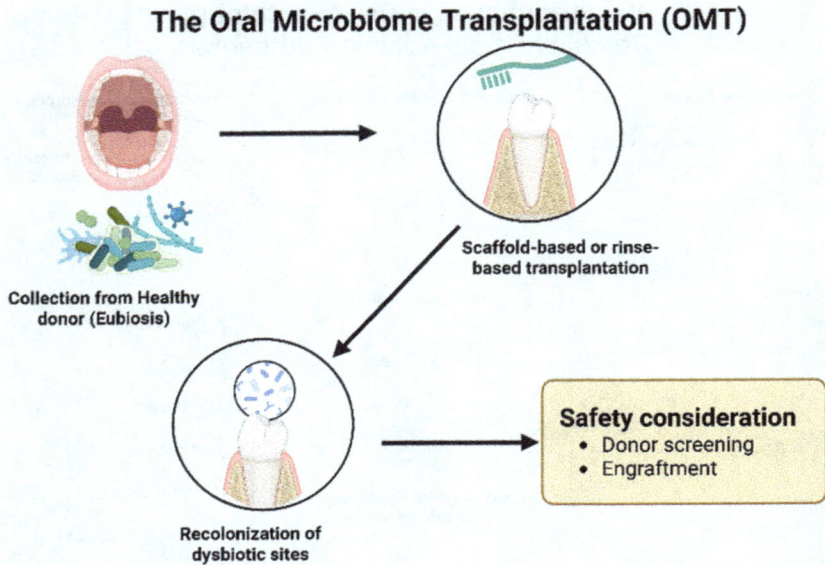

Figure 6.6: Oral microbiome transplantation (OMT) as a therapeutic strategy. Healthy donor microbiota is collected and transplanted via swab-based or scaffold-based methods into dysbiotic sites. Safety considerations include donor screening and successful microbial engraftment. Created with Biorender. com.

6.8 Ecological Periodontal Therapy in Clinical Practice

Integrating microbiome therapeutics into periodontal practice requires a paradigm shift in diagnosis, treatment, and maintenance [64]. Diagnosis should move beyond pathogen detection to microbial community profiling using next-generation sequencing or rapid molecular diagnostics. Treatment planning should consider not just biofilm removal but ecological rehabilitation, selecting adjuvants that promote beneficial taxa and suppress dysbiosis [65, 66]. For example, adjunctive use of a probiotic mouth rinse post-SRP could accelerate the restoration of microbial homeostasis. Incorporating dietary counseling to support prebiotic intake, such as polyphenol-rich foods or arginine-containing products, can further enhance treatment outcomes [67, 68]. Maintenance protocols should include periodic microbiome monitoring and personalized interventions based on microbial and host-inflammatory markers [37].

6.9 Challenges and Future Directions

Despite the promise of microbiome-based therapies, several challenges remain. The resilience and redundancy of the oral microbiome make it difficult to induce long-lasting changes. Interindividual variability, influenced by genetics, diet, hygiene, and systemic health, affects therapeutic outcomes. Moreover, standardized protocols for dosing, duration, and delivery of probiotics or phages are lacking.

Future research must prioritize randomized clinical trials with robust microbiological and immunological endpoints. Advances in synthetic biology, systems microbiology, and AI-driven microbiome modeling will enable the rational design of targeted microbial interventions. Regulatory frameworks must evolve to accommodate live biotherapeutic products and genetically engineered microbiome tools.

6.10 Conclusion: From Pathogen Elimination to Microbial Harmony

The future of periodontal therapy lies not in eradicating microbes, but in restoring ecological balance. Microbiome therapeutics, encompassing probiotics, prebiotics, postbiotics, phage therapy, and potentially microbiome transplants, represent a sophisticated approach that aligns with the principles of precision and personalized dentistry. As our understanding of microbial ecology deepens and technology advances, ecological periodontal therapy may redefine how we treat, monitor, and prevent periodontitis in the era of microbial harmony.

References

[1]   Bartold, P. M., & Van Dyke, T. E. (2013). Periodontitis: A host-mediated disruption of microbial homeostasis. Unlearning learned concepts. Periodontology 2000, 62(1), 203–217.

[2]   Łasica, A., Golec, P., Laskus, A., Zalewska, M., Gędaj, M., & Popowska, M. (2024). Periodontitis: Etiology, conventional treatments, and emerging bacteriophage and predatory bacteria therapies. Frontiers in Microbiology, 15, 1469414.

[3]   Di Spirito, F., Pisano, M., Di Palo, M. P., De Benedetto, G., Rizki, I., Franci, G., & Amato, M. (2025). Periodontal status and *Herpes viridae*, bacteria, and fungi in gingivitis and periodontitis of systemically compromised pediatric subjects: A systematic review. Children, 12(3), 375.

[4]   Hajishengallis, G., & Lamont, R. J. (2021). Polymicrobial communities in periodontal disease: Their quasi-organismal nature and dialogue with the host. Periodontology 2000, 86(1), 210.

[5]   Hasturk, H., Kantarci, A., & Van Dyke, T. E. (2011). Paradigm shift in the pharmacological management of periodontal diseases. Frontiers of Oral Biology, 15, 160.

[6]   Zhang, Y., Wang, X., Li, H., Ni, C., Du, Z., & Yan, F. (2018). Human oral microbiota and its modulation for oral health. Biomedicine & Pharmacotherapy, 99, 883–893.

[7]   Hasan, F., Budi, H. S., Ramasamy, R., Tantiana, T., Ridwan, R. D., Winoto, E. R., Nuraini, P., Handajani, J., Djais, A. A., & Anitasari, S. (2025). A systematic review of *Streptococcus mutans* and *Veillonellae* species interactions in dental caries progression: Positive or negative impact?. F1000Research, 13, 1080.

[8]   Zhu, B., Green, S. P., Ge, X., Puccio, T., Nadhem, H., Ge, H., Bao, L., Kitten, T., & Xu, P. (2021). Genome-wide identification of *Streptococcus sanguinis* fitness genes in human serum and discovery of potential selective drug targets. Molecular Microbiology, 115(4), 658–671.

[9]   Kumar, P. S., & Mason, M. R. (2015). Mouthguards: does the indigenous microbiome play a role in maintaining oral health?. Frontiers in Cellular and Infection Microbiology, 5, 35.

[10] Di Stefano, M., Polizzi, A., Santonocito, S., Romano, A., Lombardi, T., & Isola, G. (2022). Impact of oral microbiome in periodontal health and periodontitis: a critical review on prevention and treatment. International Journal of Molecular Sciences, 23(9), 5142.

[11] Zhu, Y., Dashper, S. G., Chen, Y., Crawford, S., Slakeski, N., & Reynolds, E. C. (2013). *Porphyromonas gingivalis* and *Treponema denticola* synergistic polymicrobial biofilm development. PLoS ONE, 8(8), e71727.

[12] Verma, R. K., Rajapakse, S., Meka, A., Hamrick, C., Pola, S., Bhattacharyya, I., Nair, M., Wallet, S. M., Aukhil, I., & Kesavalu, L. (2010). *Porphyromonas gingivalis* and *Treponema denticola* mixed microbial infection in a rat model of periodontal disease. Interdisciplinary Perspectives on Infectious Diseases, 2010, 605125.

[13] Roy, R., Tiwari, M., Donelli, G., & Tiwari, V. (2017). Strategies for combating bacterial biofilms: A focus on anti-biofilm agents and their mechanisms of action. Virulence, 9(1), 522.

[14] Olsen, I., Lambris, J. D., & Hajishengallis, G. (2017). *Porphyromonas gingivalis* disturbs host–commensal homeostasis by changing complement function. Journal of Oral Microbiology, 9(1), 1340085.

[15] Mei, F., Xie, M., Huang, X., Long, Y., Lu, X., Wang, X., & Chen, L. (2020). *Porphyromonas gingivalis* and its systemic impact: Current status. Pathogens, 9(11), 944.

[16] Messina, B. M., Grippaudo, C., Polizzi, A., Blasi, A., & Isola, G. (2024). The key role of *Porphyromonas gingivalis* in the pathogenesis of periodontitis linked with systemic diseases. Applied Sciences, 15(12), 6847.

[17] Li, C., Yu, R., & Ding, Y. (2022). Association between *Porphyromonas gingivalis* and systemic diseases: Focus on T cells-mediated adaptive immunity. Frontiers in Cellular and Infection Microbiology, 12, 1026457.

[18] Sedghi, L., DiMassa, V., Harrington, A., Lynch, S. V., & Kapila, Y. L. (2021). The oral microbiome: Role of key organisms and complex networks in oral health and disease. Periodontology 2000, 87(1), 107.

[19] Bostanghadiri, N., Kouhzad, M., Taki, E., Elahi, Z., Khoshbayan, A., & Navidifar, T. (2024). Oral microbiota and metabolites: Key players in oral health and disorder, and microbiota-based therapies. Frontiers in Microbiology, 15, 1431785.

[20] Hill, C., Guarner, F., Reid, G., Gibson, G. R., Merenstein, D. J., & Pot, B. et al. (2014). The International scientific association for probiotics and prebiotics consensus statement on the scope and appropriate use of the term probiotic. Nature Reviews Gastroenterology & Hepatology, 11, 506–514.

[21] Nguyen, T., Brody, H., Radaic, A., & Kapila, Y. (2021). Probiotics for periodontal health – current molecular findings. Periodontology 2000, 87(1), 254.

[22] Haukioja, A. (2010). Probiotics and oral health. European Journal of Dentistry, 4(3), 348.

[23] Lee, C., Hsu, J., Ho, H., Hsieh, H., Kuo, W., Sung, C., & Huang, C. (2020). *Lactobacillus salivarius* subsp. *salicinius* SA-03 is a new probiotic capable of enhancing exercise performance and decreasing fatigue. Microorganisms, 8(4), 545.

[24] Jansen, P. M., Abdelbary, M. M. H., & Conrads, G. (2021). A concerted probiotic activity to inhibit periodontitis-associated bacteria. PLoS ONE, 16(3), e0248308.

[25] Liu, Z., Cao, Q., Wang, W., Wang, B., Yang, Y., Xian, C. J., Li, T., & Zhai, Y. (2024). The impact of *Lactobacillus reuteri* on oral and systemic health: A comprehensive review of recent research. Microorganisms, 13(1), 45.

[26] Ochôa, C., Castro, F., Bulhosa, J. F., Manso, C., Hasse Fernandes, J. C., & Oliveira Fernandes, G. V. (2023). Influence of the probiotic *L. reuteri* on periodontal clinical parameters after nonsurgical treatment: A systematic review. Microorganisms, 11(6), 1449.

[27] Alshareef, A., Attia, A., Almalki, M., Alsharif, F., Melibari, A., Mirdad, B., Azab, E., Youssef, R., & Dardir, A. (2020). Effectiveness of probiotic lozenges in periodontal management of chronic periodontitis patients: Clinical and immunological study. European Journal of Dentistry, 14(2), 281.

[28] Deshmukh, M. A., Suresh Dodamani, A., Karibasappa, G., Khairnar, M. R., Naik, R. G., & Jadhav, H. C. (2017). Comparative evaluation of the efficacy of probiotic, herbal and chlorhexidine mouthwash on gingival health: A randomized clinical trial. Journal of Clinical and Diagnostic Research, 11(3).

[29] Manjunathappa, T. H., Jojo, J. J., Kenganora, M., & Kumar, M. N. (2020). Effect of tulsi extract and probiotic mouthrinse on plaque and gingivitis among school children – a randomized controlled trial. Journal of Datta Meghe Institute of Medical Sciences University, 15(1).

[30] Kandaswamy, S. K., Sharath, A., & Priya, P. R. G. (2018). Comparison of the effectiveness of probiotic, chlorhexidine-based mouthwashes, and oil pulling therapy on plaque accumulation and gingival inflammation in 10–12-year-old schoolchildren: a randomized controlled trial. International Journal of Clinical Pediatric Dentistry, 11(2), 66–70.

[31] Caballero-Flores, G., Pickard, J. M., & Núñez, G. (2022). Microbiota-mediated colonization resistance: Mechanisms and regulation. Nature Reviews Microbiology, 21(6), 347.

[32] Akimbekov, N. S., Digel, I., Yerezhepov, A. Y., Shardarbek, R. S., Wu, X., & Zha, J. (2022). Nutritional factors influencing microbiota-mediated colonization resistance of the oral cavity: A literature review. Frontiers in Nutrition, 9, 1029324.

[33] Carpenter, G. (2020). Salivary factors that maintain the normal oral commensal microflora. Journal of Dental Research, 99(6), 644.

[34] Wang, R., Liu, Y., Wen, Y., Chen, S., Zhang, X., Zhang, C., & Liu, X. (2025). Unraveling the secrets of probiotic adhesion: An overview of adhesion-associated cell surface components, adhesion mechanisms, and the effects of food composition. Trends in Food Science & Technology, 159, 104945.

[35] Pandey, K. R., Naik, S. R., & Vakil, B. V. (2015). Probiotics, prebiotics and synbiotics – a review. Journal of Food Science and Technology, 52(12), 7577.

[36] Davani-Davari, D., Negahdaripour, M., Karimzadeh, I., Seifan, M., Mohkam, M., Masoumi, S. J., Berenjian, A., & Ghasemi, Y. (2019). Prebiotics: definition, types, sources, mechanisms, and clinical applications. Foods, 8(3), 92.

[37] Guo, Y., Li, Z., Chen, F., & Chai, Y. (2023). Polyphenols in oral health: Homeostasis maintenance, disease prevention, and therapeutic applications. Nutrients, 15(20), 4384.

[38] Huang, X., Schulte, R. M., Burne, R. A., & Nascimento, M. M. (2015). Characterization of the arginolytic microflora provides insights into pH homeostasis in human oral biofilms. Caries Research, 49(2), 165.

[39] Chen, S. Y., Delacruz, J., Kim, Y., Kingston, R., Purvis, L., & Sharma, D. (2023). Effect of xylitol on *Porphyromonas gingivalis*: a systematic review. Clinical and Experimental Dental Research, 9(2), 265.

[40] Parhi, P., Liu, S. Q., & Choo, W. S. (2024). Synbiotics: Effects of prebiotics on the growth and viability of probiotics in food matrices. Bioactive Carbohydrates and Dietary Fibre, 32, 100462.

[41] Virk, M. S., Virk, M. A., He, Y., Tufail, T., Gul, M., Qayum, A., Rehman, A., Rashid, A., Ekumah, N., Han, X., Wang, J., & Ren, X. (2024). The anti-inflammatory and curative exponent of probiotics: a comprehensive and authentic ingredient for the sustained functioning of major human organs. Nutrients, 16(4), 546.

[42] Govindarajan, D. K., Mohanarangam, M., Kadirvelu, L., Sivaramalingam, S. S., Jothivel, D., Ravichandran, A., Periasamy, S., & Kandaswamy, K. (2025). Biofilms and oral health: Nanotechnology for biofilm control. Discover Nano, 20(1), 114.

[43] Udawatte, N. S., Liu, C., Staples, R., Han, P., Kumar, P. S., Arumugam, T. V., Ivanovski, S., & Seneviratne, C. J. (2024). Short-term probiotic colonization alters molecular dynamics of 3D oral biofilms. International Journal of Molecular Sciences, 26(13), 6403.

[44] Hernández, Y., Medina, B., Mendoza, E., Sánchez-Vargas, L. O., Alvarado, D., & Aranda-Romo, S. (2020). Short-term effect of a synbiotic in salivary viscosity and buffering capacity: A quasi-experimental study. Journal of Oral Research, 9, 96–101.

[45] Ercan, N., Olgun, E., Kisa, Ü., & Yalim, M. (2020). Effect of synbiotics in the treatment of smokers and non-smokers with gingivitis: Randomized controlled trial. Australian Dental Journal, 65, 210–219.

[46] Prajapati, N., Patel, J., Singh, S., Yadav, V. K., Joshi, C., Patani, A., Prajapati, D., Sahoo, D. K., & Patel, A. (2023). Postbiotic production: Harnessing the power of microbial metabolites for health applications. Frontiers in Microbiology, 14, 1306192.

[47] Gurunathan, S., Thangaraj, P., & Kim, H. (2023). Postbiotics: Functional food materials and therapeutic agents for cancer, diabetes, and inflammatory diseases. Foods, 13(1), 89.

[48] Hijová, E. (2023). Postbiotics as metabolites and their biotherapeutic potential. International Journal of Molecular Sciences, 25(10), 5441.

[49] Zdybel, K., Śliwka, A., Polak, P., & Waśko, A. (2024). Postbiotics formulation and therapeutic effect in inflammation: a systematic review. Nutrients, 17(13), 2187.

[50] Mulla, M., Hegde, S., Koshy, A., & Mulla, M. (2021). Effect of probiotic *Lactobacillus salivarius* on peri-implantitis pathogenic bacteria: An in vitro study. Cureus, 13(12), e20808.

[51] Scribante, A., Appendino, P., Maiorani, C., Fontanarosa, P., Pascadopoli, M., Cammisuli, S., Azouz, B., Buttiglieri, S., & Butera, A. (2025). Home efficacy of a postbiotic-based gel compared with a gel without active ingredients for the treatment of gingival inflammation in patients with Down syndrome: a randomized controlled study. Dentistry Journal, 13(2), 62.

[52] Hamdi, M. F., Alsaedi, A. A., & Hayder, A. Q. et al. (2025). Invasive bacteriophages between a bell and a hammer: A comprehensive review of pharmacokinetics and bacterial defense systems. Discover Life, 55, 10.

[53] Jo, S. J., Kwon, J., Kim, S. G., & Lee, J. (2023). The biotechnological application of bacteriophages: What to do and where to go in the middle of the post-antibiotic era. Microorganisms, 11(9), 2311.

[54] Yao, F., He, J., Nyaruaba, R., Wei, H., & Li, Y. (2025). Unveiling the role of phages in shaping the periodontal microbial ecosystem. Systems, 10(4), e00201–25.

[55] Liu, S., Lu, H., Zhang, S., Shi, Y., & Chen, Q. (2022). Phages against pathogenic bacterial biofilms and biofilm-based infections: A review. Pharmaceutics, 14(2), 427.

[56] Eghbalpoor, F., Gorji, M., Alavigeh, M. Z., & Moghadam, M. T. (2024). Genetically engineered phages and engineered phage-derived enzymes to destroy biofilms of antibiotics resistance bacteria. Heliyon, 10(15), e35666.

[57] Khambhati, K., Bhattacharjee, G., Gohil, N., Dhanoa, G. K., Sagona, A. P., Mani, I., Bui, N. L., Chu, T., Karapurkar, J. K., Jang, S. H., Chung, H. Y., Maurya, R., Alzahrani, K. J., Ramakrishna, S., & Singh, V. (2022). Phage engineering and phage-assisted CRISPR-Cas delivery to combat multidrug-resistant pathogens. Bioengineering & Translational Medicine, 8(2), e10381.

[58] Pacia, D. M., Brown, B. L., Minssen, T., & Darrow, J. J. (2024). CRISPR-phage antibacterials to address the antibiotic resistance crisis: Scientific, economic, and regulatory considerations. Journal of Law and the Biosciences, 11(1), lsad030.

[59] Brandt, L. J. et al. (2023). An overview of fecal microbiota transplantation: Techniques, indications, and outcomes. Gastrointestinal Endoscopy, 78, 240–249.

[60] Flores-Treviño, S., Bocanegra-Ibarias, P., Salas-Treviño, D., Ramírez-Elizondo, M. T., Pérez-Alba, E., & Camacho-Ortiz, A. (2025). Microbiota transplantation and administration of live biotherapeutic

products for the treatment of dysbiosis-associated diseases. Expert Opinion on Biological Therapy, 25(5), 507–520.

[61] Lindo, C. E., Sebastian, J., Kuntjoro, K. N., Halim, V. A., Tadjoedin, F. M., Kuswandani, S. O., & Sulijaya, B. (2024). Microbiota transplantation as an adjunct to standard periodontal treatment in periodontal disease: A systematic review. Medicina, 60(4), 672.

[62] Metwaly, A., Kriaa, A., Hassani, Z., Carraturo, F., Druart, C., Arnauts, K., Wilmes, P., Walter, J., Rosshart, S., Desai, M. S., Dore, J., Fasano, A., Blottiere, H. M., Maguir, E., & Haller, D. (2025). A consensus statement on establishing causality, therapeutic applications and the use of preclinical models in microbiome research. Nature Reviews Gastroenterology & Hepatology, 22(5), 343–356.

[63] Hajishengallis, G. (2023). Illuminating the oral microbiome and its host interactions: Animal models of disease. FEMS Microbiology Reviews, 47(3), fuad018.

[64] Han, Y., & Ding, H. (2025). Advancing periodontitis microbiome research: Integrating design, analysis, and technology. Frontiers in Cellular and Infection Microbiology, 15, 1616250.

[65] Lei, H., Liao, J., Lin, Y., Liu, T., Lei, W., & Gao, W. (2025). Application of metagenomic next-generation sequencing in treatment guidance for deep neck space abscess. BMC Microbiology, 25, 166.

[66] Sibley, C. D., Peirano, G., & Church, D. L. (2012). Molecular methods for pathogen and microbial community detection and characterization: Current and potential application in diagnostic microbiology. Infection, Genetics and Evolution, 12(3), 505.

[67] Ranjith, A., Nazimudeen, N. B., & Baiju, K. V. (2022). Probiotic mouthwash as an adjunct to mechanical therapy in the treatment of stage II periodontitis: A randomized controlled clinical trial. International Journal of Dental Hygiene, 20(2), 415–421.

[68] Nascimento, M. M., Alvarez, A. J., & Huang, X. et al. (2019). Metabolic profile of supragingival plaque exposed to arginine and fluoride. Journal of Dental Research, 98(11) 1245–1252.

Nada Tawfig Hashim, Sivan Padma Priya, Vivek Padmanabhan, and Md Sofiqul Islam

7 Artificial Intelligence in Diagnosis and Prognosis of Periodontal Disease

7.1 Introduction: The Convergence of Dentistry and Artificial Intelligence

The past decade has brought about a massive transformation in medical prognostic and diagnostic approaches that span across the diverse medical field [1]. The rapid advancement of medical science has been significantly accelerated through the growing adoption of artificial intelligence (AI) and machine learning (ML) technologies [2]. The specialist field of periodontology, which has historically relied on subjective clinical assessment and static radiographs for evaluation now, experiences an extraordinary transformation through AI technology [3]. The evolution introduces a new standard of accuracy and standardized practices and advanced predictive modeling capabilities that were previously unattainable [4] (Figure 7.1). The revolutionary technology demonstrates remarkable capabilities to analyze radiographic images while measuring bone loss extent and identifying anatomical landmarks precisely and risk stratification and treatment decision guidance, which will revolutionize periodontal diagnostics and therapeutic planning protocols beyond current expectations [5].

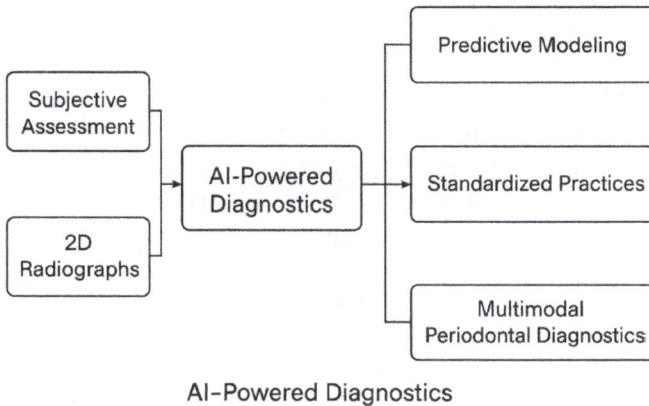

Figure 7.1: AI-powered diagnostics in periodontology. Traditional subjective assessments and 2D radiographs are integrated with AI systems to enable predictive modeling, standardized practices, and multimodal periodontal diagnostics. Figure created by the authors using Microsoft PowerPoint.

https://doi.org/10.1515/9783112219904-007

7.2 AI Technologies in Periodontology: Foundations and Classifications

An array of computational technologies forms the basis for the application of AI to the practice of periodontology, with each technology conferring unique strengths to diagnostic, prognostic, and decision-support application [6] (Figure 7.2). From among the core areas of AI, ML, and deep learning (DL) have high promise for clinical application [7]. ML comprised an ensemble of algorithms having the capability to extract patterns from structured data sets and thus permit predictions or classifications based on data [8]. Usual ML techniques, such as decision trees, support vector machines (SVMs), k-nearest neighbors, and random forests are adept to handle structured clinical predictors, such as pocket depth, bleeding on probing (BOP), plaque index, and gene polymorphisms [9]. These algorithms can be optimized to evaluate periodontal risk, predict disease progression, or even treatment responsiveness through the use of patient demographics, lifestyle factors, such as smoking and stress, and general system disease states [10].

Predictive modeling refers to analyzing data and identifying hidden patterns to predict event outcomes. ML models try to learn these patterns automatically by minimizing the dissimilarity of the input to the output and optimizing the result iteratively by adjusting weights [11]. Previous studies have used ML to predict periodontal tooth loss, but given tooth loss being a rare event, the resulting models have not reached clinical usefulness [12, 13].

DL, part of the ML category, applies multilayer neural networks to model high-dimensional, complicated data, such as convolutional neural networks (CNNs) for processing images [14, 15]. CNNs have become fundamental tools in periodontology for the analysis of periapical radiographs, panoramic radiographs, and cone beam-computed tomography (CBCT) images to enable automated detection and quantification of bone loss, anatomical features, furcation lesions, and defect structure [16]. These types of networks learn features from the hierarchy of pixels, edges, to high-level radiographic patterns, with the capability to match the accuracy of expert clinicians [17]. Another growth area is natural language processing (NLP) for reading and extracting meaningful information from unstructured documents, such as clinical notes, periodontal charting, or patient history stored in electronic health records (EHRs) [18]. NLP enables algorithms to interpret clinical vocabulary, identify disease patterns, analyze treatment history, and extract key contextual information to support decision-making and identify at-risk patients [19]. For instance, NLP can mine EHRs to correlate previous periodontal treatment outcomes with systemic risk factors, thereby facilitating more comprehensive and holistic risk assessment frameworks [20, 21]. Additionally, computer vision technologies – deeply integrated with DL enable real-time annotation, precise measurement, and recognition of 2D and 3D dental images [22]. As these AI subfields converge, hybrid systems are emerging that combine

CNN-based image analysis with ML-driven predictive models and NLP-derived text analytics [23]. This synergy is driving the development of robust multimodal AI platforms capable of advancing precision periodontics to unprecedented levels [24]. By understanding the underlying technologies and various AI approaches, clinicians and researchers are better positioned to evaluate their strengths, limitations, and future integration into modern periodontal care. Collectively, these tools transform clinical data into actionable insights, marking a shift from traditional reactive care to proactive, predictive strategies in periodontal disease management [25].

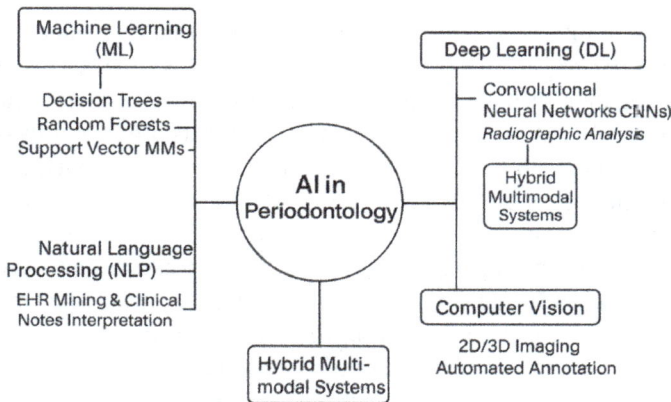

Figure 7.2: Artificial intelligence (AI) applications in periodontology. Machine learning, natural language processing, deep learning, and computer vision contribute to periodontal diagnostics, supported by hybrid multimodal systems. Figure created by the authors using Microsoft PowerPoint.

7.3 AI in Radiographic Diagnosis

Automation, accuracy, and consistency among the earliest and most prominent areas where AI has significantly influenced the field of periodontology is the interpretation of radiographs [26]. This area has been revolutionized through the unprecedented improvements in the accuracy and efficiency of diagnosis provided through CNNs. With large collections of labeled dental radiographs to draw upon, CNN-based algorithms have been found to match the performance of experienced clinicians to identify critical pathological features including horizontal and vertical alveolar bone loss, widening of the periodontal ligament space, furcation, and periapical radiolucencies [16, 27]. These systems have maintained impressive sensitivity and specificity rates rivaling – and even better at times – the skill of experienced periodontists, especially when it comes to detecting initial or subtle lesions often missed under manual examinations [28]. Among the strong features of the AI model is its impressive capability to precisely measure bone loss. Instead of simply doing the math to find the distance, in millimeters, from the alveolar crest to the cementoenamel junction, it provides the quantitative expression of bone loss in the form of root length ratio – a key element of the 2018 staging system for periodontitis [21, 26, 29]. This quantitative method not only supports automatic staging and grading of periodontitis but also allows for objective measures for continuous monitoring, promoting greater comparability among clinicians [21, 29]. More advanced DL models, such as U-Net, ResNet, and Mask R-CNN, have been used for anatomic and pathological feature segmentation [30]. U-Net, in particular, shows superior capability for segmentation at the pixel level of the cementoenamel junction, alveolar crest, furcation entrances, and root bifurcations, making it especially well-adapted for automatic contour mapping of the periodontal bone [31, 32]. These algorithms facilitate improved early diagnosis, aid treatment planning, and even provide surgical simulation through the provision of real-time overlays of bone loss or defect shape onto digital radiographs [17, 33]. In the context of three-dimensional imaging, especially with CBCT, AI programs now occupy the limelight to perform volumetric measurements of intrabony defects, dehiscence, fenestrations, and peri-implant bone loss [34]. The new technologies automate the segmentation of anatomical structures, such as the maxillary sinus, mandibular canal, and peri-implant interfaces significantly reducing the time and subjectivity involved with conventional manual reading of slices [35, 36]. Additionally, the integration of AI with CBCT analysis improves the accuracy of cortical bone integrity assessments, sinus lift needs, and the proximity of implants to vital structures, thus promoting safer and more predictable surgical results [37–39]. In addition, AI computer programs have become integrated into clinical radiographic platforms to the point where they automatically detect areas of interest, emphasize progressive changes between serial images, and offer diagnostic likelihoods – functioning virtually as an informed second opinion chairside [40]. These programs continually improve their diagnostic acumen through transfer learning and self-supervised update, resulting in enhanced diagnostic accuracy as they master the wide range of radiographic patterns from various patient populations [41].

In summary, the combination of AI with radiographic evaluation improves the sensitivity and specificity of the diagnosis of periodontal disease, and forms the critical imaging base for disease classification, treatment planning, and outcome evaluation – vital components of an evidence-based periodontal practice [42].

7.4 Periodontal Risk Assessment and Predictive Analytics

Historically, the periodontal risk assessment model and the model proposed by Lang and Tonetti [43] have relied on heuristic assessments. These models utilize a combination of clinical signs (e.g., probing pocket depth, BOP, and bone loss), behavioral risk factors (e.g., tobacco use), and systemic diseases (e.g., diabetes) [43]. Although such approaches are useful and clinically relevant, they have limitations owing to variabilty between evaluators, dependence on static measures, and failure to respond to changes in the patient's state over time [44].

AI through the use of ML algorithms enables substantial change through the provision of constant, data-directed, and personalized risk analysis. Instead of classifying risk into groups, AI techniques analyze intricate inputs of data to generate personalized, instant predictions of disease susceptibility, behaviors, and progression patterns [3].

The basis for assessing periodontal risk using AI lies in the application of supervised learning algorithms. These include a range of methods, including random forests, gradient boosting machines (GBM), SVMs, and more recently, deep neural networks (DNNs) [45]. These models are trained on large longitudinal databases comprising hundreds or thousands of clinical records [46]. The predictors often include:

- Clinical parameters include probing depth (PD), clinical attachment level (CAL), BOP, plaque index, and calculus score [47].
- Radiographic findings: Bone loss percentage, root proximity, furcation involvement [48].
- Behavioral risk factors: Smoking status (duration and intensity), stress level, oral hygiene compliance [49].
- Systemic conditions: HbA1c (Hemoglobin A1c) in diabetics, pregnancy status, immunocompromised states [50].
- Microbiological information: Quantitative evaluation of red complex bacteria (*Porphyromonas gingivalis*, *Treponema denticola*, and *Tannerella forsythia*) or the load of bacteria in saliva [51].
- Genetic and epigenetic susceptibility variants: Polymorphisms in IL-1β, TLR4, CD14, GLT6D1, and epigenetic markers like DNA methylation linked to genes involved in inflammatory mechanisms [52, 53].
- Salivary biomarkers: Interleukin-6 (IL-6), matrix metalloproteinase-8 (MMP-8), tumor necrosis factor-alpha (TNF-α), C-reactive protein (CRP), and miR-146a levels [54].

With the consolidation of this heterogeneous data set, algorithms created using AI identify personalized periodontal risk heat maps highlighting areas of increased risk for future deterioration, thus allowing clinicians to institute preventive treatment measures. These algorithms are especially useful in identifying "silent progressors" – patients with little clinical inflammation but progressive loss of attachment over time due to unrecognized genetic or microbial susceptibility [3, 55, 56].

Crucially, AI-powered predictive analytics are dynamic, not static. By leveraging reinforcement learning, these systems tune and revise their risk predictions based on new clinical information accrued at each visit – these can be new biomarker results, behavioral changes, or treatment responses [57]. This capability supports adaptive recall scheduling, allowing close follow-up for high-risk patients who need more intense monitoring, while enabling low-risk, stable patients to safely follow longer maintenance schedules [58]. Also, hybrid AI algorithms combining the information from periodontal history, saliva sensors, genomic data, and wearable healthcare technologies are gaining prominence. These algorithms have the ability not only to predict the progression of periodontal disease but also to evaluate the likelihood of increasing the risk factors systemically, such as the increased cardiovascular risks of untreated periodontitis and the risk for pregnancy complications among those with advanced gingivitis [3, 5, 59]. In addition, several cloud platforms today use ensemble methodologies of learning – combining the outputs of multiple models to enhance predictive accuracy. These methods are being researched for application to population-level screening programs and integration with national dental registries [60].

In future developments, AI-driven risk assessment tools embedded in dental software or mobile apps have the potential to give practitioners real-time decision support in patient treatment – enabling recommendations on the need for nonsurgical treatments, host modulation, microbiome rebalancing, or referrals to interdisciplinary specialists [61, 62].

The integration of predictive analytics in the field of AI is revolutionizing periodontology from a reactive specialty that treats problems after they have occurred to a preventive and proactive discipline, based on molecular insight and computational prowess. This shift lays the groundwork for greater accuracy in periodontics, where clinical decision-making is informed by predictive evidence that is carefully individualized to a patient's distinctive biological, behavioral, and environmental profile [63, 64].

7.5 Decision Support Systems and AI-Driven Treatment Planning

AI-driven clinical decision support systems (CDSS) are radically transforming how periodontal treatment planning is conceptualized by facilitating a level of care that is not only personalized but also informed by extensive data, ultimately going beyond the constraints of conventional heuristic models that have been in use for many decades [65, 66] (Figure 7.3). Such advanced systems are effectively amalgamating a broad range of multidimensional inputs, including key clinical parameters, such as PD, attachment loss, and bleeding index, along with crucial radiographic information, an analysis of microbial composition, detection of genetic polymorphisms, assessment of salivary biomarkers, as well as accounting for patient-specific risk factors – all of which synergize to yield extremely well-informed, evidence-based therapeutic suggestions that are specific to each patient's particular case [66, 67]. The fundamental strength of AI-based CDSS lies largely in its exceptional capacity to learn and adapt from large data sets, which enables it to steadily enhance its predictive precision with each additional clinical case that it is exposed to and processes. By utilizing a mix of both supervised and unsupervised ML algorithms, these high-end systems have the ability to classify different stages of disease, predict the likely progression of periodontal disease, and suggest the ideal interventions – all with a high degree of accuracy that serves to enrich the overall treatment experience for patients [68–70].

One of the genuinely groundbreaking and revolutionary features of AI in this specific area is its excellent capability to effectively prioritize treatment sites within the dentition [71, 72]. This is achieved by thorough and holistic analysis based on consideration of a plethora of absolutely necessary parameters, such as but not limited to severity of the disease, involvement of esthetic regions, the existence of systemic health comorbidities like diabetes and cardiovascular risk factors, and even cost-benefit analysis of complicated nature that weighs advantages and disadvantages [2, 55]. To take an example, imagine that you have a patient with generalized stage III periodontitis with another condition of uncontrolled diabetes; among such patients, the CDSS would recommend more conservative intervention of site-specific nature. Here, the importance of systemic stabilization is the key before any intervention involving greater regenerative therapy techniques is next undertaken. This is in complete contrast to patients who are younger and present with localized intrabony defects along with better regenerative potential; here, AI-driven algorithms can be of crucial use by assisting in the selection of optimal subjects for guided tissue regeneration (GTR), application of enamel matrix derivatives (EMDs), or array of combination therapy that can be more favorable in outcomes [42, 73, 74]. The selection is based on detailed assessments of radiographic morphology of the defects, with essential features, such as depth, width, and number of remaining walls [42, 73]. In addition to this, it factors in such significant molecular signatures, such as increased vascular endothelial growth factor (VEGF), or downregulation of MMP-8 in crevicular fluid, all of which are responsible in providing indispensable inputs to treatment planning [75].

Furthermore, it is important to note that AI algorithms, which have been carefully trained with large longitudinal data sets that provide details of treatment outcomes, have the potential to precisely predict the probability of major clinical events. The process of training involves exposing the AI system to a large amount of data, allowing it to learn and adapt its predictive capabilities. Such events may influence factors, such as regeneration of the tissue, maintenance of teeth, or the possibility of dental diseases recurring [68, 76, 77]. This great advantage is especially significant since it plays an important role in decreasing uncertainty while increasing confidence in the process of clinical decision-making [73, 74]. With regenerative periodontics as a specialty example, highly developed predictive analytics have been created to assess and determine the appropriateness of various grafting materials, unique compositions of scaffold, or biological adjuncts that might be used in various treatment protocols [74]. Furthermore, technology of AI is able to play a key role in matching patients with individualized treatment protocols or to appropriate clinical arms of trials. This is implemented by employing eligibility criteria that are based on detailed multi-omics profiling, including important factors, such as the gene expression profile of the host, salivary proteome composition, and appropriate epigenetic markers [73–75].

It is important to highlight the fact that CDSS, empowered by AI, can be seamlessly integrated with cloud-based EHRs and mobile applications [66, 78, 79]. This integration ensures the real-time delivery of recommendations during chairside consultations, enhancing the interaction between clinicians and their patients [80]. These advancements not only contribute to the standardization of treatments among different clinicians but also significantly improve patient education and involvement [66, 80]. By presenting data-driven therapy options in visually appealing and understandable formats, AI technology enhances patient understanding and engagement. Furthermore, with the continuous development and improvement of AI systems through the adoption of new techniques like reinforcement learning and federated learning paradigms, their adaptability and accuracy will be greatly enhanced. This ongoing process of improvement will provide periodontal treatment approaches with the best possible personalized, predictive, and preventive care strategies [81, 82].

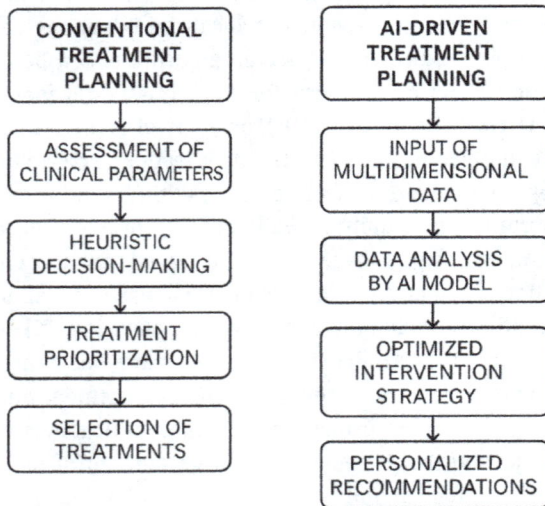

Figure 7.3: Comparison of conventional versus AI-driven treatment planning in periodontology. Conventional approaches rely on heuristic decision-making and treatment prioritization, while AI-based systems use multidimensional data analysis to optimize interventions and provide personalized recommendations. Figure created by the authors using Microsoft PowerPoint.

7.6 AI in Digital Periodontal Charting and Documentation

The field of AI is making tremendous strides that are progressively altering the way in which periodontal documentation is performed [59]. This is attained by the novel collaboration of state-of-the-art voice recognition systems with NLP [83]. Compared with this novel approach, traditional manual periodontal charting is not only time-consuming but also often yields variable and error-prone results due to operator dependency. However, the emergence of AI-driven digital charting systems has transformed this landscape [84]. These systems come with rich features of sophisticated voice recognition in real time. These systems have the awesome advantage of capturing voice observations by the clinician, such as pocket depth findings, signs of BOP, assessments of mobility, as well as estimates of gingival recession, and converting these voice inputs into structured electronic records in real time. This degree of technological sophistication not only streamlines the entire process of charting enormously, but it also allows clinicians to keep their eyes fixed on the patients uninterruptedly throughout examinations [63, 85]. As such, there is the distinct improvement in both the productivity of clinical tasks and the interaction between health care professionals and patients [63].

It is of paramount significance that advanced documentation systems powered by AI have the astounding capacity to automatically detect any disparities that may arise between the documented clinical parameters and the suggested treatment plans [2, 86]. For example, if a clinician records a diagnosis of generalized stage III periodontitis while, simultaneously, prescribing a treatment plan more suited to localized gingivitis, the advanced system can generate real-time alerts that either recommend a reevaluation of the scenario or offer a justification for the course of action that has been chosen [87, 88]. This astounding functionality tremendously bolster clinical accountability, while simultaneously enabling compliance with predefined best practice parameters that are integral in delivering quality care. In addition, the extensive structured data sets that are created through AI-enabled documentation workflows are incredibly valuable for a wide variety of applications that range from clinical studies and epidemiological research to quality assurance audits. These carefully crafted data sets provide strong data pipelines that can be successfully leveraged for retrospective studies or for training various AI models, eventually culminating in a remarkable refinement of healthcare practices as a whole [89, 90].

As these sophisticated technologies further mature and unfold over time, the synthesis of multimodal data input – an amalgamation of voice input, high-resolution radiographs, and extensive biometric sensor data – has the potential to facilitate the development of completely automated periodontal charting systems. Such novel systems could greatly minimize the administrative workload presently borne by dental clinicians, increase the fidelity of diagnostics, and offer priceless support for real-time, AI-supported clinical decision-making directly at the chairside during patient treatment [91, 92].

7.7 Integration of AI with Mobile Health and Teleperiodontics

The confluence of AI, and mobile health technologies, or mHealth, is both quickly and profoundly broadening the possibilities of both preventive care and remote monitoring of periodontal health [93]. This cutting-edge intersection yields a patient-centric model that encourages ongoing monitoring of periodontal health, enabling it to break free from the constraints of the classical clinical environment. Consequently, it efficiently resolves a number of pivotal issues that have long bedeviled the discipline, such as maintaining compliance with treatment protocols, enabling access to required care, and making possible the early detection and intervention of disease – issues that are particularly acute for underserved populations or those in far-flung areas with limited access to dental healthcare services [94, 95].

Smartphone applications based on sophisticated AI-powered image recognition capabilities now possess the capability to critically evaluate intraoral images, which typically are snapped by users in the guise of what can be described as dental selfies [96, 97]. These cutting-edge applications are calibrated to analyze visible signs of gingival inflammation, measure the deposition of plaque, and even identify early calculus formation in the mouth [97]. In order to be able to do this, such applications employ CNNs that have been carefully trained on large annotated data sets in order to categorize different features of gingival status, including redness, swelling, and bleeding [97]. Users are able to obtain immediate visual feedback that is both educational and enlightening in nature, along with targeted advice on how to better manage their dental hygiene habits [96, 97]. In addition, some platforms have gone the extra step to integrate features of gamification and behavioral nudges into their design, and this acts to profoundly amplify patient involvement and to induce the uptake of maintained oral health behaviors in the long term [98, 99].

Concurrently, wearable sensors of oral health have been creatively integrated into common items like toothbrushes, various dental devices, or even trendy smartwatches. These new devices are able to measure various biomechanical variables, including important measures like brushing time, frequency of brushing, force used in the process, and the particular motion patterns followed while brushing [100]. Complex AI models are programmed to analyze these disparate streams of data, offering important coaching feedback to individuals, detecting suboptimal brush techniques that are likely to be used during brushing, and issuing timely reminders in situations where brushing sessions might have been skipped entirely [101]. These highly sophisticated systems have shown great potential in increasing compliance with dental health regimens, particularly in populations including both children and the elderly, thus filling key health requirements within these targeted populations [100, 101].

In addition to this, there has been a significant trend towards the incorporation of AI-driven mHealth applications with teleperiodontics platforms, which are advanced systems specifically created for remote dental treatment [102]. Patients are able to upload several key documents and images, including radiographs, intraoral photos, and symptom questionnaires, through secure apps that are focused on their privacy and data safety [102]. On the clinician side of the process, state-of-the-art AI models are responsible for automatically extracting pathologic features from images that have been uploaded. This encompasses the identification of problems, such as horizontal or vertical bone loss, furcation involvement, and the presence of calculus deposits. These cutting-edge tools dramatically improve the capacities for remote screening, enabling initial diagnostics as well as offering valuable triage suggestions. This ultimately allows for a more effective system of scheduling appointments, enables prioritization of urgent cases, and permits timely medical interventions when they are needed [6, 103].

These platforms also serve a literally central role in the face of major public health crises, like pandemics, when customary in-person care can be drastically limited or even altogether inaccessible to patients [100–102]. AI-supported teleperiodontics supports and promotes continuity of care by making possible a variety of services, including asynchronous consultation, virtual follow-up, and extensive monitoring of both treatment results and the potential resurgence of disease [3, 104].

Looking forward into the future, it is envisioned that this genuinely extraordinary synergy of AI, next-generation mobile health technologies, and the newly developed discipline of teleperiodontics will slowly transform into sophisticated closed-loop precision monitoring systems. In this visionary and forward-looking paradigm, patient data – carefully collected in the comfort of patients' own homes – will not only be interpreted but also communicated effectively in real-time to healthcare clinicians, thus allowing them to provide proactive and personalized treatment that is highly responsive to the individualized characteristics and specific requirements of each and every patient [105]. Apart from this, the envisioned coupling of real-time biomarker sensing – made possible by the novel application of salivary biosensors or point-of-care diagnostic devices – into such revolutionary mobile platforms is expected to greatly improve their diagnostic return and clinical usefulness [106]. Such judicious integration will surely entrench and reinforce the priceless contributions of these next-generation technologies to the emerging ethos of digital periodontic treatment in the years to come.

7.8 Ethical, Legal, and Operational Considerations

The implementation of AI in periodontics faces multiple ethical and legal barriers despite its potential benefits [3]. The implementation of AI systems requires complete transparency about algorithm decisions and strict data privacy measures for biometric and genomic information and full compliance with regulatory standards [107]. The clinical practice should prevent total dependence on black-box models because AI systems should support human expertise instead of replacing it. Operationally, various challenges have to be resolved. The system requires standardized high-quality data sets that serve universal needs and seamless integration with dental EHRs and proper training for clinicians to interpret AI results effectively [108].

7.9 Future Directions and Research Horizons

AI in periodontology continues to experience a fast-paced transformation which will shape its future development [3]. The integration of clinical data with microbiological data and genetic data through revolutionary methods will produce advanced insights for periodontal disease phenotyping. Advanced biosensor-attached platforms will likely enable AI to perform real-time microbiome monitoring in the upcoming years. The system would simultaneously detect systemic complications linked to specific periodontal profiles while developing CRISPR-based therapy to control host responses [109].

The privacy-protecting feature of federated learning enables multiple dental centers to share AI benefits through model learning without revealing sensitive information [107, 108]. AI will evolve to transform both diagnosis and treatment methods while changing the fundamental philosophical approach of periodontal care from reactive to preventive and personalized.

7.10 Conclusion

The field of periodontology is experiencing its revolutionary rebirth through the advent of AI. By facilitating diagnostics that are not only objective and reproducible but also predictive in nature, AI provides an interface that is seamless between the traditional ways of clinical assessments and the emerging and new requirements imposed by precision medicine. The integration of AI in this field will be successful based on a culture of interdisciplinary collaboration among professionals, intense investment in ethical vision, and steadfast adherence to lifelong education and learning. As this revolution via digitization continues and reaches maturity, AI will evolve from being merely an ancillary tool to that of an invaluable partner in the ongoing pursuit of delivering biologically guided and patient-oriented treatment in periodontics.

References

[1]   Varnosfaderani, S. M., & Forouzanfar, M. (2024). The role of AI in hospitals and clinics: Transforming healthcare in the 21st century. Bioengineering, 11(4), 337.

[2]   Alowais, S. A., Alghamdi, S. S., & Alsuhebany, N. et al. (2023). Revolutionizing healthcare: The role of artificial intelligence in clinical practice. BMC Medical Education, 23, 689.

[3]   Sarakbi, R. M., Varma, S. R., Annamma, L. M., & Sivaswamy, V. (2025). Implications of artificial intelligence in periodontal treatment maintenance: A scoping review. Frontiers in Oral Health, 6, 1561128.

[4]   Shobanke, M., Bhatt, M., & Shittu, E. (2025). Advancements and future outlook of Artificial Intelligence in energy and climate change modeling. Advances in Applied Energy, 17, 100211.

[5]   Spartivento, G., Benfante, V., Ali, M., Yezzi, A., Di Raimondo, D., Tuttolomondo, A., Lo Casto, A., & Comelli, A. (2024). Revolutionizing periodontal care: The role of Artificial Intelligence in diagnosis, treatment, and prognosis. Applied Sciences, 15(6), 3295.

[6]   Roy, R., Chopra, A., Karmakar, S., & Bhat, S. G. (2025). Applications of Artificial Intelligence (AI) for diagnosis of periodontal/peri-implant diseases: A narrative review. Journal of Oral Rehabilitation, 6, 1193–1219.

[7]   Rahman, A., Debnath, T., Kundu, D., Islam Khan, M. S., Aishi, A. A., Sazzad, S., Sayduzzaman, M., & Band, S. S. (2024). Machine learning and deep learning-based approach in smart healthcare: recent advances, applications, challenges and opportunities. AIMS Public Health, 11(1), 58.

[8]   Sarker, I. H. (2021). Machine learning: Algorithms, real-world applications and research directions. SN Computer Science, 2(3), 160.

[9]   Zhu, Y., Du, M., Li, P., Lu, H., Li, A., & Xu, S. (2025). Prediction models for the complication incidence and survival rate of dental implants – a systematic review and critical appraisal. International Journal of Implant Dentistry, 11, 5.

[10] Walter, E., Brock, T., Lahoud, P., Werner, N., Czaja, F., Tichy, A., Bumm, C., Bender, A., Castro, A., Teughels, W., Schwendicke, F., & Folwaczny, M. (2025). Predictive modeling for step II therapy response in periodontitis – model development and validation. NPJ Digital Medicine, 8, 445.

[11] Shamout, F., Zhu, T., & Clifton, D. A. (2021). Machine learning for clinical outcome prediction. IEEE Reviews in Biomedical Engineering, 14, 116–126.

[12] Schwendicke, F. et al. (2018). Validation of multivariable models for predicting tooth loss in periodontitis patients. Journal of Clinical Periodontology, 45, 701–710.

[13] Schwendicke, F. et al. (2021). Association, prediction, generalizability: cross-center validity of predicting tooth loss in periodontitis patients. Journal of Dentistry, 109, 103662.

[14] Sarker, I. H. (2021). Deep learning: A comprehensive overview on techniques, taxonomy, applications and research directions. SN Computer Science, 2(6), 420.

[15] Taye, M. M. (2023). Theoretical understanding of convolutional neural network: Concepts, architectures, applications, future directions. Computation, 11(3), 52.

[16] Chen, I., Lin, C., Lee, M., Chen, T., Lan, T., Chang, C., Tseng, T., Wang, T., & Du, J. (2023). Convolutional-neural-network-based radiographs evaluation assisting in early diagnosis of the periodontal bone loss via periapical radiograph. Journal of Dental Sciences, 19(1), 550–559.

[17] Mall, P. K., Singh, P. K., Srivastav, S., Narayan, V., Paprzycki, M., Jaworska, T., & Ganzha, M. (2023). A comprehensive review of deep neural networks for medical image processing: Recent developments and future opportunities. Healthcare Analytics, 4, 100216.

[18] Wieland-Jorna, Y., Van Kooten, D., Verheij, R. A., de Man, Y., Francke, A. L., & Oosterveld-Vlug, M. G. (2024). Natural language processing systems for extracting information from electronic health records about activities of daily living: A systematic review. JAMIA Open, 7(2), ooae044.

[19] Demner-Fushman, D., Chapman, W. W., & McDonald, C. J. (2009). What can natural language processing do for clinical decision support?. Journal of Biomedical Informatics, 42(5), 760.

[20] Thyvalikakath, T. P., Padman, R., Vyawahare, K., Darade, P., & Paranjape, R. (2015). Utilizing dental electronic health records data to predict risk for periodontal disease. Studies in Health Technology and Informatics, 216, 1081.

[21] Ameli, N., Firoozi, T., Gibson, M., & Lai, H. (2024). Classification of periodontitis stage and grade using natural language processing techniques. PLOS Digital Health, 3(12), e0000692.

[22] Alharbi, S. S., & Alhasson, H. F. (2024). Exploring the applications of artificial intelligence in dental image detection: A systematic review. Diagnostics, 14(21), 2442.

[23] Khan, W., Daud, A., Khan, K., Muhammad, S., & Haq, R. (2023). Exploring the frontiers of deep learning and natural language processing: A comprehensive overview of key challenges and emerging trends. Natural Language Processing Journal, 4, 100026.

[24] Li, M., Jiang, Y., Zhang, Y., & Zhu, H. (2023). Medical image analysis using deep learning algorithms. Frontiers in Public Health, 11, 1273253.

[25] Vinayaka, A. M., & Laxmi, K. S. (2024). Artificial intelligence in periodontics: Transforming the future of periodontal care. IP International Journal of Maxillofacial Imaging, 10(3), 129–131.

[26] Tariq, A., Nakhi, F. B., Salah, F., Eltayeb, G., Abdulla, G. J., Najim, N., Khedr, S. A., Elkerdasy, S., Al-Rawi, N., Alkawas, S., Mohammed, M., & Shetty, S. R. (2023). Efficiency and accuracy of artificial intelligence in the radiographic detection of periodontal bone loss: A systematic review. Imaging Science in Dentistry, 53(3), 193.

[27] Samaranayake, L., Tuygunov, N., Schwendicke, F., Osathanon, T., Khurshid, Z., Boymuradov, S. A., & Cahyanto, A. (2025). The transformative role of artificial intelligence in dentistry: A comprehensive overview. part 1: Fundamentals of AI, and its contemporary applications in dentistry. International Dental Journal, 75(2), 383.

[28] Mathur, A., Pawar, S., Kamma, P. K., Obulareddy, V. T., Dash, K. S., Meto, A., & Mehta, V. (2025). Comparative evaluation of images of alveolar bone loss using panoramic images and artificial intelligence. Engineering Proceedings, 87(1), 80.

[29] Jundaeng, J., Chamchong, R., & Nithikathkul, C. (2025). Advanced AI-assisted panoramic radiograph analysis for periodontal prognostication and alveolar bone loss detection. Frontiers in Dental Medicine, 5, 1509361.

[30] Malhotra, P., Gupta, S., Koundal, D., Zaguia, A., & Enbeyle, W. (2022). Deep neural networks for medical image segmentation. Journal of Healthcare Engineering, 2022, 9580991.

[31] Punn, N. S., & Agarwal, S. (2022). Modality specific U-Net variants for biomedical image segmentation: A survey. Artificial Intelligence Review, 55(7), 5845.

[32] Yin, X., Sun, L., Fu, Y., Lu, R., & Zhang, Y. (2022). U-net-based medical image segmentation. Journal of Healthcare Engineering, 2022, 4189781.

[33] Widyaningrum, R., Candradewi, I., Ahmad Seno Aji, N. R., & Aulianisa, R. (2022). Comparison of multi-label U-net and mask R-CNN for panoramic radiograph segmentation to detect periodontitis. Imaging Science in Dentistry, 52(4), 383.

[34] Ahn, J., Nguyen, T. P., Kim, Y. J., Kim, T., & Yoon, J. (2022). Automated analysis of three-dimensional CBCT images taken in natural head position that combines facial profile processing and multiple deep-learning models. Computer Methods and Programs in Biomedicine, 226, 107123.

[35] Park, J. H., Hamimi, M., Choi, J. J. E., Figueredo, C. M. S., & Cameron, M. A. (2025). Comparisons of AI automated segmentation techniques to manual segmentation techniques of the maxilla and maxillary sinus for CT or CBCT scans – a systematic review. Dentomaxillofacial Radiology, twaf042, 54, 529–539.

[36] Macrì, M., Forte, M., Capodiferro, S., Favia, G., Alrashadah, A. O., García, V. D., & Festa, F. (2024). The role and applications of artificial intelligence in dental implant planning: A systematic review. Bioengineering, 11(8), 778.

[37] Meto, A., & Halilaj, G. (2024). The integration of cone beam computed tomography, artificial intelligence, augmented reality, and virtual reality in dental diagnostics, surgical planning, and education: A narrative review. Applied Sciences, 15(11), 6308.

[38] Shujaat, S., Alfadley, A., Morgan, N., Jamleh, A., Riaz, M., Aboalela, A. A., & Jacobs, R. (2024). Emergence of artificial intelligence for automating cone-beam computed tomography-derived maxillary sinus imaging tasks: A systematic review. *Clinical Implant Dentistry and Related Research, 26(5), 899–912.

[39] Morgan, N., Meeus, J., Shujaat, S., Cortellini, S., Bornstein, M. M., & Jacobs, R. (2023). CBCT for diagnostics, treatment planning and monitoring of sinus floor elevation procedures. Diagnostics, 13(10), 1684.

[40] Mao, K., Thu, K. M., Hung, K. F., Yu, O. Y., Tai-Chiu Hsung, R., & Yu-Hang Lam, W. (2025). Artificial intelligence in detecting periodontal disease from intraoral photographs: A systematic review. International Dental Journal, 75(5), 100883.

[41] Jundaeng, J., Chamchong, R., & Nithikathkul, C. (2025). Artificial intelligence-powered innovations in periodontal diagnosis: a new era in dental healthcare. Frontiers in Medical Technology, 6, 1469852.

[42] Patil, S., Joda, T., Soffe, B., Awan, K. H., Fageeh, H. N., Tovani-Palone, M. R., & Licari, F. W. (2023). Efficacy of artificial intelligence in the detection of periodontal bone loss and classification of periodontal diseases: A systematic review. Journal of the American Dental Association, 154(9), 795–804.e1.

[43] Lang, N. P., & Tonetti, M. S. (2003). Periodontal risk assessment (PRA) for patients in supportive periodontal therapy (SPT). Oral Health & Preventive Dentistry, 1(1), 7–16.

[44] Shah, E. B., Modi, B. B., Shah, M. A., & Dave, D. H. (2017). Patient centered outcomes in periodontal treatment – an evidenced based approach. Journal of Clinical and Diagnostic Research, 11(4), ZE05.

[45] Bashir, N. Z., Rahman, Z., & Chen, S. (2022). Systematic comparison of machine learning algorithms to develop and validate predictive models for periodontitis. Journal of Clinical Periodontology, 49(10), 958.

[46] Farhadian, M., Shokouhi, P., & Torkzaban, P. (2020). A decision support system based on support vector machine for diagnosis of periodontal disease. BMC Research Notes, 13, 337.

[47] Abreu, M. H., Bianchini, M. A., Magini, R. S., & Rösing, C. K. (2007). Clinical and radiographic evaluation of periodontal and peri-implant conditions in patients with implant-supported prosthesis. Acta Odontológica Latinoamericana, 20(2), 87–95.

[48] Renvert, S., & Persson, G. R. (2004). Patient-based assessments of clinical periodontal conditions in relation to alveolar bone loss. Journal of Clinical Periodontology, 31(3), 208–213.

[49] Genco, R. J., & Genco, F. D. (2014). Common risk factors in the management of periodontal and associated systemic diseases: The dental setting and interprofessional collaboration. Journal of Evidence Based Dental Practice, 14, 4–16.

[50] Gupta, S., Maharjan, A., Dhami, B., Amgain, P., Katwal, S., Adhikari, B., & Shukla, A. (2018). Status of tobacco smoking and diabetes with periodontal disease. JNMA: Journal of the Nepal Medical Association, 56(213), 818.

[51] Jiang, Y., Song, B., Brandt, B. W., Cheng, L., Zhou, X., Exterkate, R. A., Crielaard, W., & Deng, D. M. (2021). Comparison of red-complex bacteria between saliva and subgingival plaque of periodontitis patients: A systematic review and meta-analysis. Frontiers in Cellular and Infection Microbiology, 11, 727732.

[52] Cárdenas, A. M., Ardila, L. J., Vernal, R., & Hernández, H. G. (2021). Biomarkers of periodontitis and its differential DNA methylation and gene expression in immune cells: A systematic review. International Journal of Molecular Sciences, 23(19), 12042.

[53] Hashim, N. T., Linden, G. J., Ibrahim, M. E., Gismalla, B. G., Lundy, F. T., & Hughes, F. J. et al. (2015). Replication of the association of GLT6D1 with aggressive periodontitis in a Sudanese population. Journal of Clinical Periodontology, 42(4), 319–324.

[54] Ali, M., Taj, Y., Tanwir, F., Bakhat, S., & Ahmed, S. A. (2025). MMP-8, IL-6, and IL-1β: The most promising salivary biomarkers for early diagnosis of periodontitis. Journal of the College of Physicians and Surgeons Pakistan, 35(7), 825–829.

[55] Parihar, A. S., Narang, S., Tyagi, S., Narang, A., Dwivedi, S., Katoch, V., & Laddha, R. (2024). Artificial intelligence in periodontics: A comprehensive review. Journal of Pharmacy & Bioallied Sciences, 16 (Suppl 3), S1956.

[56] Reddy, K. S., Ghosh, S., & Kale, P. (2024). Exploring the synergy between artificial intelligence and periodontal treatment. IP International Journal of Periodontology and Implantology, 9(3), 128–131.

[57] Coronato, A., Naeem, M., De Pietro, G., & Paragliola, G. (2020). Reinforcement learning for intelligent healthcare applications: A survey. Artificial Intelligence in Medicine, 109, 101964.

[58] Górriz, J., Álvarez-Illán, I., Álvarez-Marquina, A., Arco, J., Atzmueller, M., Ballarini, F., & Ferrández-Vicente, J. (2023). Computational approaches to explainable artificial intelligence: Advances in theory, applications and trends. Information Fusion, 100, 101945.

[59] Scott, J., Biancardi, A. M., Jones, O., & Andrew, D. (2023). Artificial intelligence in periodontology: A scoping review. Dentistry Journal, 11(2), 43.

[60] Chakraborty, C., Bhattacharya, M., Pal, S., & Lee, S. (2023). From machine learning to deep learning: advances of the recent data-driven paradigm shift in medicine and healthcare. *current Research in Biotechnology*, 7, 100164.

[61] Zwiri, A., Jotish, R., Alam, M. K., Almuhanna, S., K., N., Alazmi, A. M., Bin Mohd Noor, N. F., & Islam, M. S. (2025). Exploration of AI-powered tools for risk assessment in general dentistry. Journal of Pharmacy & Bioallied Sciences, 17(Suppl 2), S1270.

[62] Bamashmous, M. (2025). The role of artificial intelligence in transforming dental public health: Current applications, ethical considerations, and future directions. Open Dentistry Journal, 19, e18742106363413.

[63] Chatzopoulos, G. S., Koidou, V. P., Tsalikis, L., & Kaklamanos, E. G. (2025). Clinical applications of artificial intelligence in periodontology: A scoping review. Medicina, 61(6), 1066.

[64] Pindi, V. (2019). AI-assisted clinical decision support systems: Enhancing diagnostic accuracy and treatment recommendations. International Journal of Innovations in Engineering Research and Technology, 6(10), 1–10.

[65] Akram, H. M. (2025). Artificial intelligence in dentistry: Advancements in periodontology and other specialties, diagnosis, treatment planning, and ethical considerations. Dentistry Review, 5(2), 100157.

[66] Elhaddad, M., & Hamam, S. (2024). AI-driven clinical decision support systems: An ongoing pursuit of potential. Cureus, 16(4), e57728.

[67] Butnaru, O., Tatarciuc, M., Luchian, I., Tudorici, T., Balcos, C., Budala, D. G., Sirghe, A., Virvescu, D. I., & Haba, D. (2025). AI efficiency in dentistry: Comparing artificial intelligence systems with human practitioners in assessing several periodontal parameters. Medicina, 61(4), 572.

[68] Krishnan, G., Singh, S., Pathania, M., Gosavi, S., Abhishek, S., Parchani, A., & Dhar, M. (2023). Artificial intelligence in clinical medicine: Catalyzing a sustainable global healthcare paradigm. Frontiers in Artificial Intelligence, 6, 1227091.

[69] Javed, H., El-Sappagh, S., & Abuhmed, T. (2025). Robustness in deep learning models for medical diagnostics: Security and adversarial challenges towards robust AI applications. Artificial Intelligence Review, 58, 12.

[70] Sloane, E. B., & Silva, R. J. (2019). Artificial intelligence in medical devices and clinical decision support systems, In: Clinical Engineering Handbook. 2nd ed, 556–568. https://doi.org/10.1016/B978-0-12-813467-2.00084-5.

[71] Karuppan Perumal, M. K., Rajan Renuka, R., Kumar Subbiah, S., & Manickam Natarajan, P. (2025). Artificial intelligence-driven clinical decision support systems for early detection and precision therapy in oral cancer: A mini review. Frontiers in Oral Health, 6, 1592428.

[72] Turkestani, N. A., Bianchi, J., Deleat-Besson, R., Le, C., Tengfei, L., Prieto, J. C., Cevidanes, S., & H, L. (2021). Clinical decision support systems in orthodontics: A narrative review of data science approaches. Orthodontics & Craniofacial Research, 24(Suppl 2), 26.

[73] Polizzi, A., Quinzi, V., Lo Giudice, A., Marzo, G., Leonardi, R., & Isola, G. (2024). Accuracy of artificial intelligence models in the prediction of periodontitis: A systematic review. JDR Clinical & Translational Research, 9(4), 312–324.

[74] Lakshmi, T., & Dheeba, J. (2022). Digital decision making in dentistry: Analysis and prediction of periodontitis using a machine learning approach. International Journal of Next Generation Computing, 13(3), https://doi.org/10.47164/ijngc.v13i3.614.

[75] Xiang, J., Huang, W., He, Y., Li, Y., Wang, Y., & Chen, R. (2022). Construction of artificial neural network diagnostic model and analysis of immune infiltration for periodontitis. Frontiers in Genetics, 13, 1041524.

[76] Arjmandmazidi, S., Heidari, H. R., Ghasemnejad, T., Mori, Z., Molavi, L., Meraji, A., & Montazersaheb, S. (2025). An in-depth overview of artificial intelligence tool utilization across diverse phases of organ transplantation. Journal of Translational Medicine, 23, 678.

[77] Saberian, E., Jenča, A., Zare-Zardini, H., Araghi, M., Petrášová, A., & Jenčová, J. (2024). Applications of artificial intelligence in regenerative dentistry: Promoting stem cell therapy and the scaffold development. Frontiers in Cell and Developmental Biology, 12, 1497457.

[78] Sutton, R. T., Pincock, D., Baumgart, D. C., Sadowski, D. C., Fedorak, R. N., & Kroeker, K. I. (2020). An overview of clinical decision support systems: Benefits, risks, and strategies for success. NPJ Digital Medicine, 3, 17.

[79] Marinescu, Ş. A., Oncioiu, I., & Ghibanu, A. (2024). The digital transformation of healthcare through intelligent technologies: A path dependence-augmented UTAUT model for clinical decision support systems. Healthcare, 13(11), 1222.

[80] Almadani, B., Kaisar, H., Thoker, I. R., & Aliyu, F. (2025). A systematic survey of distributed decision support systems in healthcare. Systems, 13(3), 157.

[81] Kovari, A. (2024). AI for decision support: Balancing accuracy, transparency, and trust across sectors. Information, 15(11), 725.

[82] Fröling, E., Rajaeean, N., & Hinrichsmeyer, K. S. et al. (2024). Artificial intelligence in medical affairs: A new paradigm with novel opportunities. Pharmaceutical Medicine, 38, 331–342.

[83] Khurana, D., Koli, A., & Khatter, K. et al. (2023). Natural language processing: State of the art, current trends and challenges. Multimedia Tools and Applications, 82, 3713–3744.

[84] Moufti, M., Talib, M. A., Mokdad, S. A., Alhouria, A., Alsaffarini, M., Almahmeed, N., & Nasir, Q. (2025). An artificial intelligence solution for automated dental inspection and charting. International Dental Journal, 75(4), 100849.

[85] Tan, M., Cui, Z., Li, Y., Fang, Y., Mei, L., Zhao, Y., Wu, X., Lai, H., Tonetti, M. S., & Shen, D. (2025). PerioAI: A digital system for periodontal disease diagnosis from an intra-oral scan and cone-beam CT image. *Cell Reports Medicine*, 6(6), 102186.

[86] Theriault-Lauzier, P., Cobin, D., Tastet, O., Langlais, E. L., Taji, B., Kang, G., & Avram, R. (2024). A responsible framework for applying artificial intelligence on medical images and signals at the point of care: The PACS-AI platform. Canadian Journal of Cardiology, 40(10), 1828–1840.

[87] Sanz, M., Herrera, D., Kebschull, M., Chapple, I., Jepsen, S., Berglundh, T., Sculean, A., & Tonetti, M. S. (2020). Treatment of stage I–III periodontitis – the EFP S3 level clinical practice guideline. Journal of Clinical Periodontology, 47(Suppl 22), 4.

[88] Sirinirund, B., Gianfilippo, R. D., Yu, H., Wang, L., & Kornman, K. S. (2021). Diagnosis of stage III periodontitis and ambiguities of the "gray zones" in between stage III and stage IV. Clinical Advances in Periodontics, 11(2), 111–115.

[89] Gupta, S., Kapoor, M., & Debnath, S. K. (2025). AI-based cybersecurity solutions for healthcare, In: Artificial Intelligence-Enabled Security for Healthcare Systems. Springer: Cham, 65–86.

[90]   Habli, I., Lawton, T., & Porter, Z. (2020). Artificial intelligence in health care: Accountability and safety. Bulletin of the World Health Organization, 98(4), 251.

[91]   Pfänder, L., Schneider, L., Büttner, M., Krois, J., Meyer-Lueckel, H., & Schwendicke, F. (2023). Multimodal deep learning for automated assembly of periapical radiographs. Journal of Dentistry, 135, 104588.

[92]   Camlet, A., Kusiak, A., Ossowska, A., & Świetlik, D. (2024). Advances in periodontal diagnostics: Application of multimodal language models in visual interpretation of panoramic radiographs. Diagnostics, 15(15), 1851.

[93]   Singh, B., & Kaunert, C. (2025). Uplifting digital technologies for preventive dentistry: catering needs of dental care in rural or remote areas, In: Next-Generation Dentistry Practices to Enhance Patient Outcomes. IGI Global, 239–266.

[94]   Wang Chau, R. C., Chung Cheng, A. C., Mao, K., Thu, K. M., Ling, Z., Tew, I. M., & Hang Lam, W. Y. (2025). External validation of an AI mHealth tool for gingivitis detection among older adults at daycare centers: A pilot study. International Dental Journal, 75(3), 1970.

[95]   Burrell, D. N. (2023). Dynamic evaluation approaches to telehealth technologies and artificial intelligence (AI) telemedicine applications in healthcare and biotechnology organizations. Merits, 3(4), 700–721.

[96]   Jayam, C., & Arun Babu, T. (2023). Dental selfie: An innovative teledentistry tool for safe dental examination of children during COVID-19 pandemic. Karnataka Paediatrics Journal, 38, 14–15.

[97]   Tobias, G., & Spanier, A. B. (2019). Modified gingival index (MGI) classification using dental selfies. Applied Sciences, 10(24), 8923.

[98]   Auf, H., Dagman, J., Renström, S., & Chaplin, J. (2021). Gamification and nudging techniques for improving user engagement in mental health and well-being apps. Proceedings of the Design Society, 1, 1647–1656.

[99]   Cencerrado, A. (2024). Gamification for mental health and health psychology: Insights at the first quarter mark of the 21st century. International Journal of Environmental Research and Public Health, 21(8), 990.

[100] Fahim, M., Sharma, V., & Duong, T. Q. (2022). A wearable-based preventive model to promote oral health through personalized notification. Proceedings of the IEEE EMBC, 2022, 4282–4285.

[101] Wang, K., Saragadam, A., Kaur, J., Dogra, A., Cao, S., Ghafurian, M., & Morita, P. P. (2025). A contactless method for recognition of daily living activities for older adults based on ambient assisted living technology. Internet of Things, 30, 101502.

[102] Li, Y., Wu, X., Liu, M., Deng, K., Tullini, A., Zhang, X., Shi, J., Lai, H., & Tonetti, M. S. (2024). Enhanced control of periodontitis by an AI-enabled multimodal-sensing toothbrush and targeted mHealth micromessages: A randomized trial. Journal of Clinical Periodontology, 51(12), 1632.

[103] Shetty, S., Talaat, W., AlKawas, S., Al-Rawi, N., Reddy, S., Hamdoon, Z., . . . David, L. R. (2024). Application of AI-based detection of furcation involvement in mandibular first molar using cone beam tomography images – a preliminary study. BMC Oral Health, 24(1), 1476.

[104] Batra, P., Tagra, H., & Katyal, S. (2022). Artificial intelligence in teledentistry. Discoveries, 10(3), 153.

[105] Prabhu, V. D., Saidath, K., Suvarna, N., Mohtesham, I., Shenoy, S., & Prabhu, R. V. (2025). Artificial intelligence and dentistry: The future. Journal of Pharmacy & Bioallied Sciences, 16(Suppl 5), S4257.

[106] Haji Mohammadi, M., Mulder, S., Khashayar, P., Kalbasi, A., Azimzadeh, M., & Aref, A. R. (2021). Saliva lab-on-a-chip biosensors: Recent novel ideas and applications in disease detection. Microchemical Journal, 168, 106506.

[107] Feng, Q. J., Harte, M., Carey, B., Alqarni, A., Monteiro, L., Fricain, C., & Albuquerque, R. (2024). The risks of artificial intelligence: A narrative review and ethical reflection from an oral medicine group. Oral Diseases, 31(2), 348.

[108] Williamson, S. M., & Prybutok, V. (2023). Balancing privacy and progress: A review of privacy challenges, systemic oversight, and patient perceptions in AI-driven healthcare. Applied Sciences, 14(2), 675.

[109] Sosnowski, K., Akarapipad, P., & Yoon, Y. (2020). The future of microbiome analysis: Biosensor methods for big data collection and clinical diagnostics. Medical Devices & Sensors, 3(5), e10085.

Nada Tawfig Hashim, Bakri Gobara, and Md Sofiqul Islam

8 Three-Dimensional Bioprinting and Regenerative Periodontics

8.1 Introduction

Periodontitis is a chronic inflammatory disease that results in gradual, progressive destruction of the periodontal ligament (PDL), cementum, and alveolar bone [1]. This debilitating disease continues to be one of the major causes of tooth loss globally, affecting millions of individuals [2]. Traditional regenerative approaches that have been attempted, including guided tissue regeneration, bone grafting procedures, and application of enamel matrix derivatives (EMDs), have met with only limited success in the reconstitution of complete periodontal health [3]. This is particularly true in treating complex or multi-tissue defects that pose formidable challenges to successful treatment and healing [4]. The introduction of 3D bioprinting has introduced a paradigm, offering heretofore unparalleled spatial precision in the creation of complex, patient-specific constructs that replicate native periodontal form and function [5].

3D bioprinting, defined as the layer-by-layer deposition of bioinks containing living cells, biomaterials, and signaling molecules, has traveled a considerable distance [6]. The technology has progressed from a proof-of-concept to a platform of tremendous significance for translational application in the specialized field of craniofacial tissue engineering [7]. Furthermore, its synergistic integration with the principles of stem cell biology, the engineering of bioactive scaffolds, and the personalized medicine paradigm firmly positions 3D bioprinting as a novel and disruptive tool in the field of periodontology [8].

8.2 Anatomical and Functional Challenges in Periodontal Regeneration

The **periodontium** is a complex system constituted by hierarchical structures with specialized functions in the maintenance of oral health. This complex structure comprises hard and soft tissues, each possessing unique cellular components as well as specific mechanical properties that are essential to their overall function [9]. In addition, these diverse tissues have different regenerative requirements that need to be fulfilled during regeneration. As such, the main challenge that is presented in the arena of periodontal regeneration is the simultaneous restoration and regeneration of cementum, PDL, and alveolar bone [10, 11]. These tissues have to function in complete harmony as an integrated structure in order to facilitate the optimal functioning

https://doi.org/10.1515/9783112219904-008

of the periodontium as a whole. The regeneration of these particular tissues demands an array of exacting biochemical and biomechanical signals, directional fiber alignment, and the inclusion of blood vessels, all of which are extremely significant factors that traditional scaffolds struggle to control and regulate in an optimal manner [12, 13]. Yet 3D bioprinting, renowned for its remarkable capacity to arrange complex cell types and biomaterials precisely in the positions required within a structure very closely similar to the arrangements of natural tissues, presents a highly optimistic answer to this extremely complex issue [14]. Not only does this novel technology enhance our understanding of tissue engineering but also introduce an element of hope and optimism for the future of periodontal tissue regeneration.

8.3 Bioprinting Technologies in Periodontics

Several bioprinting modalities have been explored for periodontal applications:
- Extrusion-based bioprinting: The most widely used technique due to its versatility. It enables the deposition of viscous bioinks loaded with cells, growth factors, and nanoparticles. Suitable for fabricating bone and ligament components with controlled porosity and alignment [15].
- Inkjet bioprinting: Utilizes thermal or piezoelectric forces to eject droplets of cell-laden bioinks. It allows high-resolution printing but is limited by bioink viscosity and cell density. It is often used for soft tissue regeneration or as a tool for growth factor patterning [16].
- Laser-assisted bioprinting (LAB): A non-contact, high-precision technique that uses laser energy to deposit bioinks onto a receiving substrate. LAB is especially useful for printing fragile cell types like stem cells or endothelial precursors [17, 18].
- Stereolithography (SLA): Employs photopolymerization of light-sensitive bioresins, offering ultrafine resolution. When used with photopolymerizable hydrogels, SLA is ideal for fabricating detailed scaffold architectures, including vascular channels [19, 20].

8.4 Scaffold Design and Bioink Composition

The design of scaffolds stands as a critical factor for achieving regenerative success [21]. Complex 3D-printed scaffolds function to replicate the native **extracellular matrix (ECM)** through controlled degradation and signaling processes for tissue regeneration [22]. Some recent developments include:
- **Multiphasic scaffolds:** The multiphasic scaffold design creates separate areas to simultaneously regenerate cementum and PDL and alveolar bone. The printing

process creates tissue-specific bioinks together with orientation markers which are placed in distinct compartments [23].

- **Hydrogel-based bioinks:** The natural hydrogels gelatin methacrylate (GelMA), alginate, collagen, and hyaluronic acid provide a cell-friendly microenvironment for survival because they act as hydrogel-based bioinks. The bioinks contain osteogenic or fibroblastic cells together with antimicrobial nanoparticles and angiogenic peptides [24].
- **Composite bioinks:** The combination of synthetic polymers, including polycaprolactone and polylactic-co-glycolic acid with composite bioinks enhances mechanical strength while allowing cells to attach and remodel tissue [25].
- **Gradient structures:** The scaffold's spatial axis benefits from gradient structures that mimic the natural signaling gradient that occurs during spontaneous tissue development [26].

8.5 Stem Cells in Bioprinted Constructs

The seeding of stem cells in 3D bioprinted scaffolds is a key determinant in enabling dynamic tissue remodeling and functional integration with host periodontal tissues [27]. One of the most widely utilized cell sources in periodontal bioprinting is periodontal ligament stem cells (PDLSCs), which are shown to be multipotent and possess inherent homing capacity to periodontal niches [28]. Their potential to differentiate into osteoblasts, cementoblasts, and fibroblasts makes them highly appropriate for compartmentalized scaffold printing [29]. Bone marrow, adipose tissue, or dental pulp-derived mesenchymal stem cells (MSCs) are also very common; they secrete trophic factors, have immunomodulatory function, and promote bone tissue engineering [30, 31]. Another promising candidate is induced pluripotent stem cells (iPSCs), which have unlimited proliferative capacity and multilineage differentiation. When directed to neural crest or mesodermal lineages, iPSCs are particularly valuable for craniofacial tissue regeneration [32, 33]. Their successful outcomes rely on the encapsulation of these stem cells in bioinks with cell viability, lineage specification, and matrix remodeling properties [34]. In addition, newer gene-editing tools, such as CRISPR/Cas9 are increasingly being employed to enhance the regenerative potential of these stem cells or deliver therapeutic genes pre-printing [35].

8.6 Role of Growth Factors and Bioactive Molecules

Controlled release of signaling molecules is a key factor in the successful modulation of the sequential phases in periodontal regeneration [36]. The bioprinted construct herein presents a highly flexible platform that facilitates controlled spatial and temporal delivery of key bioactive agents necessary for the regenerative process. These include bone morphogenetic proteins (BMP-2 and BMP-7) that induce osteogenesis and are typically designed in slow-release microparticles; platelet-derived growth factor (PDGF) that is accountable for inducing cellular proliferation and angiogenesis; and vascular endothelial growth factor (VEGF) that is necessary for neovascularization and is typically utilized in gradient setups to allow for precise angiogenic patterning [37, 38]. Also included are EMD for cementoblast differentiation and ECM formation [39]. The deliberate and layer-specific incorporation of these particular molecules within the architecture of multiphasic scaffolds achieves regenerative effects with specific targeting of different areas [40]. This strategy effectively recapitulates the native architecture and the dynamic mechanisms of healing associated with periodontal tissues [41].

8.7 Key Components and Translational Advances of 3D Bioprinting in Periodontal Regeneration

Three-dimensional bioprinting has emerged as a transformative approach in periodontal regeneration by enabling the precise fabrication of biomimetic constructs that integrate cells, bioactive molecules, and tailored scaffolding materials [42]. Bioinks, such as gelatin methacryloyl (GelMA), alginate-fibrin composites, and hyaluronic acid blends play a pivotal role as printable, hydrated matrices that not only encapsulate cells but also support angiogenesis and ECM mimicry, facilitating the creation of multilayered, tissue-mimetic scaffolds with exceptional spatial control [43]. Diverse cell sources, including PDLSCs, dental pulp stem cells, iPSC-derived mesenchymal cells, and bone marrow-derived MSCs, drive osteogenic, cementogenic, and ligamentous differentiation while modulating the local immune microenvironment, with both autologous and allogeneic stem cell integrations enhancing biocompatibility and regenerative outcomes [44, 45]. Growth factor incorporation, exemplified by BMP-2, PDGF-BB, and VEGF, enables controlled and sustained stimulation of bone regeneration, neovascularization, and fibroblast proliferation, ultimately accelerating defect healing and minimizing postoperative tissue loss [46-48]. Advanced bioprinting platforms, including extrusion-based techniques, SLA, and digital light processing, offer micron-scale resolution and allow the precise co-deposition of multiple cell types and biomaterials to create anatomically customized grafts for complex periodontal defects [49]. Functionalization strategies, such as nano-hydroxyapatite coating and ECM protein tethering (e.g., fibronectin and laminin), further enhance cell adhesion, mineralization, and host-tissue integration, significantly improving scaffold-host interfaces [50, 51]. Additionally, emerging immunomodulatory strategies, including CRISPR-engineered MSCs and miRNA-enriched scaffolds, aim to modulate macrophage polarization, attenuate local inflammation, and prevent fibrotic encapsulation, paving the way for next-generation immuno-regenerative constructs tailored to chronic inflammatory conditions like periodontitis [52, 53]. Clinically, 3D bioprinting holds substantial promise for addressing complex defects, such as class II furcation involvements, intrabony defects exceeding 3 mm, and vertical alveolar bone loss by generating spatially defined, compartmentalized constructs that simultaneously regenerate cementum, PDL, and alveolar bone [54, 55].

8.8 3D Bioprinting for Large and Irregular Craniofacial Defects

The reconstruction of maxillofacial deformities and large alveolar clefts has been achieved through bioprinting techniques [56]. The use of individualized CT-guided printing provides accurate anatomical matching and vascularized constructs improve both integration and survival rates. The main challenge of vascularization is being addressed through research on endothelial progenitor cells and microchannel printing techniques [57, 58].

8.9 Clinical Translation and Future Directions

Despite the fact that the majority of applications are still in the preclinical phase of development, some encouraging reports have emerged from recent pilot studies that have utilized printed scaffolds in primate models [59–61]. These have yielded encouraging results for alveolar bone filling, successful reattachment of functional ligaments, and remarkable reduction in inflammation. As a result of these findings, regulatory approval for initiation of human trials is expected to move forward at an accelerated pace [59–61]. This is expected to be fueled by consistent advancements being made in the area of biocompatible inks, scaffold sterilization methods, and automated systems used for bioprinting [62, 63]. Future directions in this vibrant and fast-evolving discipline entail a series of innovative approaches, including the current efforts on creating sophisticated smart scaffolds that are specifically tailored to release bioactive molecules in a targeted manner, particularly in response to local mechanical stress or inflammation within the body. Additionally, there is an intense emphasis on utilizing advanced 4D bioprinting technologies. These sophisticated technologies not only enable constructs to be printed with precision but also to adapt dynamically by changing their shape or function over time, in effect reacting to a variety of environmental stimuli present within the local environment [64, 65]. Another important advance is the integration of imaging-guided printing techniques, which utilize real-time intraoral scanning that is closely coupled to AI-empowered CAD/CAM platforms, enabling the swift and precise fabrication of scaffolds directly at the chair-side [66, 67]. Moreover, researchers are increasingly leveraging bioprinting-on-a-chip systems, which provide an excellent platform for conducting high-throughput testing of a variety of scaffold formulations under oral environment-mimicking conditions, and thus better understanding their performance and efficacy.

8.10 Conclusion

Three-dimensional bioprinting stands at the confluence of regenerative biology, bio-engineering, and precision dentistry. The innovative technology enables the precise placement of cells together with scaffolds and growth factors, which creates a revolu-tionary method to reconstruct complex periodontal and craniofacial defects. The mat-uration of this technology will revolutionize clinical regenerative periodontics by moving our practice from empirical to exact engineering and from general treatment approaches to highly individualized care that matches specific patient requirements.

References

[1]   Kinane, D. F., Stathopoulou, P. G., & Papapanou, P. N. (2017). Periodontal diseases. Nature Reviews Disease Primers, 3, 17038.
[2]   Al-Rafee, M. A. (2020). The epidemiology of edentulism and the associated factors: A literature review. Journal of Family Medicine and Primary Care, 9(4), 1841.
[3]   Alqahtani, A. M. (2023). Guided tissue and bone regeneration membranes: A review of biomaterials and techniques for periodontal treatments. Polymers, 15(16), 3355.
[4]   Wang, X., Guo, J., Yu, Q., Zhao, L., Gao, X., Wang, L., Wen, M., Yan, J., An, M., & Liu, Y. (2024). Decellularized matrices for the treatment of tissue defects: From matrix origin to immunological mechanisms. Biomolecules & Therapeutics, 32(5), 509.
[5]   Acharya, J. R., Kumar, S., Girdhar, G. A., Patel, S., Parekh, N. H., Patadiya, H. H., Zinjala, A. N., & Haque, M. (2025). 3D bioprinting: Shaping the future of periodontal tissue regeneration and disease management. Cureus, 17(4), e82432.
[6]   Tripathi, S., Mandal, S. S., Bauri, S., & Maiti, P. (2022). 3D bioprinting and its innovative approach for biomedical applications. MedComm, 4(1), e194.
[7]   Mao, J., Giannobile, W., Helms, J., Hollister, S., Krebsbach, P., Longaker, M., & Shi, S. (2006). Craniofacial tissue engineering by stem cells. Journal of Dental Research, 85(11), 966.
[8]   Latimer, J. M., Maekawa, S., Yao, Y., Wu, D. T., Chen, M., & Giannobile, W. V. (2021). Regenerative medicine technologies to treat dental, oral, and craniofacial defects. Frontiers in Bioengineering and Biotechnology, 9, 704048.
[9]   Nanci, A., & Bosshardt, D. D. (2006). Structure of periodontal tissues in health and disease. Periodontology, 2000, 40(1), 11–28.
[10] Liang, Y., Luan, X., & Liu, X. (2020). Recent advances in periodontal regeneration: A biomaterial perspective. Bioactive Materials, 5(2), 297–308.
[11] Galli, M., Yao, Y., Giannobile, W. V., & Wang, L. (2021). Current and future trends in periodontal tissue engineering and bone regeneration. Plastic and Aesthetic Research, 8, 3.

[12] Laurell, L., Bose, M., Graziani, F., Tonetti, M., & Berglundh, T. (2006). The structure of periodontal tissues formed following guided tissue regeneration therapy of intra-bony defects in the monkey. Journal of Clinical Periodontology, 33(8), 596–603.

[13] Chen, H., Song, G., Xu, T., Meng, C., Zhang, Y., Xin, T., Yu, T., Lin, Y., & Han, B. (2024). Biomaterial scaffolds for periodontal tissue engineering. Journal of Functional Biomaterials, 15(8), 233.

[14] Persaud, A., Maus, A., Strait, L., & Zhu, D. (2022). 3D bioprinting with live cells. Engineered Regeneration, 3(3), 292–309.

[15] Chen, X., Anvari-Yazdi, A. F., Duan, X., Zimmerling, A., Gharraei, R., Sharma, N., Sweilem, S., & Ning, L. (2023). Biomaterials / bioinks and extrusion bioprinting. Bioactive Materials, 28, 511–534. https://doi.org/10.1016/j.bioactmat.2023.06.006.

[16] Ghosh, E., Rego, G. P., & Ghosh, R. N. et al. (2025). Advances in in situ bioprinting: A focus on extrusion and inkjet-based bioprinting techniques. In: Regenerative Engineering and Translational Medicine. https://doi.org/10.1007//s40883-025-00420-1.

[17] Li, J., Chen, M., Fan, X., & Zhou, H. (2016). Recent advances in bioprinting techniques: Approaches, applications and future prospects. Journal of Translational Medicine, 14, 271.

[18] Guillemot, F., Souquet, A., Catros, S., & Guillotin, B. (2010). Laser-assisted cell printing: Principle, physical parameters versus cell fate and perspectives in tissue engineering. Nanomedicine (London), 5, 507–515.

[19] Li, W., Li, J., Pan, C., Lee, S., Kim, B. S., & Gao, G. (2024). Light-based 3D bioprinting techniques for illuminating the advances of vascular tissue engineering. Materials Today Bio, 29, 101286.

[20] Advincula, R. C., Dizon, J. R., Caldona, E. B., Viers, R. A., Siacor, F. D., & Maalihan, R. D. (2021). On the progress of 3D-printed hydrogels for tissue engineering. MRS Communications, 11(5), 539–553.

[21] Huang, D., Li, Z., Li, G., Zhou, F., Wang, G., Ren, X., & Su, J. (2025). Biomimetic structural design in 3D-printed scaffolds for bone tissue engineering. Materials Today Bio, 32, 101664.

[22] Do, V., Khorsand, B., Geary, S. M., & Salem, A. K. (2015). 3D printing of scaffolds for tissue regeneration applications. Advanced Healthcare Materials, 4(12), 1742–1762.

[23] Ivanovski, S., Vaquette, C., Gronthos, S., Hutmacher, D. W., & Bartold, P. M. (2014). Multiphasic scaffolds for periodontal tissue engineering. Journal of Dental Research, 93(12), 1212–1221.

[24] Fang, W., Yang, M., Wang, L., Li, W., Liu, M., Jin, Y., Wang, Y., Yang, R., Wang, Y., Zhang, K., & Fu, Q. (2023). Hydrogels for 3D bioprinting in tissue engineering and regenerative medicine: Current progress and challenges. International Journal of Bioprinting, 9(5), 759.

[25] Khoeini, R., Nosrati, H., Akbarzadeh, A., Eftekhari, A., Kavetskyy, T., Khalilov, R., Ahmadian, E., Nasibova, A., Datta, P., Roshangar, L., Deluca, D. C., Davaran, S., Cucchiarini, M., & Ozbolat, I. T. (2021). Natural and synthetic bioinks for 3D bioprinting. Advanced NanoBiomed Research, 1(8), 2000097.

[26] Xiong, Z., Hong, F., Wu, Z., Ren, Y., Sun, N., Heng, B., & Zhou, J. (2024). Gradient scaffolds for osteochondral tissue engineering and regeneration. Chemical Engineering Journal, 498, 154797.

[27] Santonocito, S., Ferlito, S., Polizzi, A., Ronsivalle, V., Reitano, G., & Lo Giudice, A. et al. (2023). Impact exerted by scaffolds and biomaterials in periodontal bone and tissue regeneration engineering: New challenges and perspectives for disease treatment. Exploration of Medicine, 4, 215–234.

[28] Meng, L., Wei, Y., Liang, Y., Hu, Q., & Xie, H. (2022). Stem cell homing in periodontal tissue regeneration. Frontiers in Bioengineering and Biotechnology, 10, 1017613.

[29] Zhao, Z., Liu, J., Weir, M. D., Schneider, A., Ma, T., Oates, T. W., Xu, H. H. K., Zhang, K., & Bai, Y. (2022). Periodontal ligament stem cell-based bioactive constructs for bone tissue engineering. Frontiers in Bioengineering and Biotechnology, 10, 1071472.

[30] Ayala-Cuellar, A. P., Kang, H., Jeung, B., & Choi, C. (2018). Roles of mesenchymal stem cells in tissue regeneration and immunomodulation. Biomolecules & Therapeutics, 27(1), 25–44.

[31] Ledesma-Martínez, E., Mendoza-Núñez, V. M., & Santiago-Osorio, E. (2016). Mesenchymal stem cells derived from dental pulp: A review. Stem Cells International, 2016, 4709572.

[32] Zhu, Q., Lu, Q., Gao, R., & Cao, T. (2016). Prospect of human pluripotent stem cell-derived neural crest stem cells in clinical application, Stem Cells International, 2016, 7695836.

[33] Soto, J., Ding, X., Wang, A., & Li, S. (2021). Neural crest-like stem cells for tissue regeneration. Stem Cells Translational Medicine, 10(5), 681–693.

[34] Panferov, E., Dodina, M., Reshetnikov, V., Ryapolova, A., Ivanov, R., Karabelsky, A., & Minskaia, E. (2024). Induced pluripotent (iPSC) and mesenchymal (MSC) stem cells for in vitro disease modeling and regenerative medicine. International Journal of Molecular Sciences, 26(12), 5617.

[35] Valenti, M. T., Serena, M., Dalle Carbonare, L., & Zipeto, D. (2019). CRISPR/Cas system: An emerging technology in stem cell research. World Journal of Stem Cells, 11(11), 937–956.

[36] Liu, G., Xue, J., Zhou, X., Gui, M., Xia, R., Zhang, Y., Cai, Y., Li, S., Shi, S., Mao, X., & Chen, Z. (2025). The paradigm shifts of periodontal regeneration strategy: From reparative manipulation to developmental engineering. Bioactive Materials, 49, 418–436.

[37] Wu, Y., Li, M., Su, H., Chen, H., & Zhu, Y. (2022). Up-to-date progress in bioprinting of bone tissue. International Journal of Bioprinting, 9(1), 628.

[38] Barati, D., Shariati, S. R. P., Moeinzadeh, S., Melero-Martin, J. M., Khademhosseini, A., & Jabbari, E. (2016). Spatiotemporal release of BMP-2 and VEGF enhances osteogenic and vasculogenic differentiation of human mesenchymal stem cells and endothelial colony-forming cells co-encapsulated in a patterned hydrogel. Journal of Controlled Release, 223, 126–136.

[39] Messenger, M. P., Raïf El, M., Seedhom, B. B., & Brookes, S. J. (2010). Enamel matrix derivative enhances tissue formation around scaffolds used for tissue engineering of ligaments. Journal of Tissue Engineering and Regenerative Medicine, 4(2), 96–104.

[40] Lin, X., Zhang, Y., Li, J., Oliver, B. G., Wang, B., Li, H., Yong, T., & Li, J. J. (2024). Biomimetic multizonal scaffolds for the reconstruction of zonal articular cartilage in chondral and osteochondral defects. Bioactive Materials, 43, 510–525.

[41] Xiang, C., Zhang, L., & Tao, E. (2025). Research progress of enamel matrix derivative on periodontal tissue regeneration: A narrative review. Frontiers in Dental Medicine, 6, 1611402.

[42] Acharya, J. R., Kumar, S., & Girdhar, G. A. et al. (2025). 3D bioprinting: Shaping the future of periodontal tissue regeneration and disease management. Cureus, 17(4), e82432.

[43] Asim, S., Tabish, T. A., Liaqat, U., Ozbolat, I. T., & Rizwan, M. (2023). Advances in gelatin bioinks to optimize bioprinted cell functions. Advanced Healthcare Materials, 12(17), e2203148.

[44] Huang, G. T., Gronthos, S., & Shi, S. (2009). Mesenchymal stem cells derived from dental tissues vs. those from other sources: Their biology and role in regenerative medicine. Journal of Dental Research, 88(9), 792–806.

[45] Ignacio, L., Elena, M., RG,, & Montesinos, J. J. (2023). Mesenchymal stromal cells derived from dental tissues: Immunomodulatory properties and clinical potential. International Journal of Molecular Sciences, 25(4), 1986.

[46] Kim, S. E., Yun, Y. P., Lee, J. Y., Shim, J. S., Park, K., & Huh, J. B. (2015). Co-delivery of platelet-derived growth factor (PDGF-BB) and bone morphogenic protein (BMP-2) coated onto heparinized titanium for improving osteoblast function and osteointegration. Journal of Tissue Engineering and Regenerative Medicine, 9(12), E219–E228.

[47] Galarraga-Vinueza, M. E., Barootchi, S., ML, N., Nevins, M., Miron, R. J., & Tavelli, L. (2024). Twenty-five years of recombinant human growth factors rhPDGF-BB and rhBMP-2 in oral hard and soft tissue regeneration. Periodontology, 2000, 94(1), 483–509.

[48] Chen, H., Wang, Y., Lai, Y., Meng, C., Ning, X., Xu, T., Song, G., Zhang, Y., Lin, Y., & Han, B. (2025). Advances of 3D bioprinting technology for periodontal tissue regeneration. iScience, 28(6), 112532.

[49] Shao, H., Wen, K., Liu, R., Ding, N., Gong, Y., Zhuang, Y., & He, Y. (2025). 3D printing of bioceramic multifunctional scaffolds for bone tissue engineering. Advanced Functional Materials, e09039. https://doi.org/10.1002/adfm.2025090939.

[50]   Zumbo, B., Guagnini, B., Medagli, B., Porrelli, D., & Turco, G. (2024). Fibronectin functionalization: A way to enhance dynamic cell culture on alginate/hydroxyapatite scaffolds. Journal of Functional Biomaterials, 15(8), 222.

[51]   Oliver-Cervelló, L., Martin-Gómez, H., & Mas-Moruno, C. (2021). New trends in the development of multifunctional peptides to functionalize biomaterials. Journal of Peptide Science, 28(1), e3335.

[52]   Wang, Y., Vizely, K., Li, C. Y., Shen, K., Shakeri, A., Khosravi, R., Smith, J R., Alteza, A. I., Zhao, Y., & Radisic, M. (2024). Biomaterials for immunomodulation in wound healing. Regenerative Biomaterials, 11, rbae032.

[53]   Chen, Y., Sun, W., Tang, H., Li, Y., Li, C., Wang, L., Chen, J., Lin, W., Li, S., Fan, Z., Cheng, Y., & Chen, C. (2022). Interactions between immunomodulatory biomaterials and immune microenvironment: Cues for immunomodulation strategies in tissue repair. Frontiers in Bioengineering and Biotechnology, 10, 820940.

[54]   Ostrovidov, S., Ramalingam, M., Bae, H., Orive, G., Fujie, T., Shi, X., & Kaji, H. (2023). Bioprinting and biomaterials for dental alveolar tissue regeneration. Frontiers in Bioengineering and Biotechnology, 11, 991821.

[55]   Sufaru, I., Macovei, G., Stoleriu, S., Martu, M., Luchian, I., & Solomon, S. M. (2022). 3D printed and bioprinted membranes and scaffolds for the periodontal tissue regeneration: A narrative review. Membranes, 12(9), 902.

[56]   Korn, P., Ahlfeld, T., Lahmeyer, F., Kilian, D., Sembdner, P., Stelzer, R., Pradel, W., Franke, A., Rauner, M., Range, U., Stadlinger, B., Lode, A., Lauer, G., & Gelinsky, M. (2020). 3D printing of bone grafts for cleft alveolar osteoplasty – in vivo evaluation in a preclinical model. Frontiers in Bioengineering and Biotechnology, 8, 217.

[57]   Li, S., Liu, S., & Wang, X. (2022). Advances of 3D printing in vascularized organ construction. International Journal of Bioprinting, 8(3), 588.

[58]   Kawai, T. (2025). Preclinical evaluation and advancements in vascularized bone tissue engineering. Biomimetics, 10(7), 412.

[59]   Thomas, C., Amsellem, P., Nascene, D., & Huang, Y. (2025). Orthopedic applications of 3D printing in canine veterinary medicine. Frontiers in Veterinary Science, 12, 1582720.

[60]   Hatt, L. P., Thompson, K., Helms, J. A., Stoddart, M. J., & Armiento, A. R. (2022). Clinically relevant preclinical animal models for testing novel cranio-maxillofacial bone 3D-printed biomaterials. Clinical and Translational Medicine, 12(2), e690.

[61]   Parsaee, F., Alizadeh, A., Rezaee, M., Alavi, O., & Alipour, H. (2023). Evaluation of the osteoconductive properties of scaffold containing platelet-enriched-fibrin (PRF) with three calcium phosphate (TCP) in the alveolar socket repair after tooth extraction: An animal study. Journal of Biomaterials Applications, 37, 1789–1800.

[62]   Rahimnejad, M., Makkar, H., Dal-Fabbro, R., Malda, J., Sriram, G., & Bottino, M. C. (2024). Biofabrication strategies for oral soft tissue regeneration. Advanced Healthcare Materials, 13(18), 2304537.

[63]   Budharaju, H., Sundaramurthi, D., & Sethuraman, S. (2024). Embedded 3D bioprinting – an emerging strategy to fabricate biomimetic & large vascularized tissue constructs. Bioactive Materials, 32, 356–384.

[64]   Arif, Z. U., Khalid, M. Y., Zolfagharian, A., & Bodaghi, M. (2022). 4D b printing of smart polymers for biomedical applications: Recent progress, challenges, and future perspectives. Reactive and Functional Polymers, 179, 105374.

[65]   Ramezani, M., & Ripin, Z. M. (2023). 4D printing in biomedical engineering: Advancements, challenges, and future directions. Journal of Functional Biomaterials, 14(7), 347.

[66] Richert, R., Goujat, A., Venet, L., Viguie, G., Viennot, S., Robinson, P., Farges, C., Fages, M., & Ducret, M. (2017). Intraoral scanner technologies: A review to make a successful impression. Journal of Healthcare Engineering, 2017, 8427595.

[67] Róth, I., Géczi, Z., Végh, D. C., Hegedüs, T., Pál, A., Hermann, P., & Schmalzl, J. (2025). The role of artificial intelligence in intraoral scanning for complete-arch digital impressions: An in vitro study. Journal of Dentistry, 156, 105717.

Mariam Elsheikh, Nada Tawfig Hashim, and Rasha Babiker

9 Periodontal Implications of Long COVID and Immune Dysregulation

9.1 Introduction

The SARS-CoV-2 pandemic has reshaped our understanding of chronic disease, extending its impact far beyond acute respiratory illness [1]. A substantial proportion of patients – regardless of the initial severity of infection – develop long COVID or post-acute sequelae of SARS-CoV-2 infection, a condition marked by persistent systemic inflammation, immune dysregulation, and multiorgan dysfunction [2]. This prolonged immunopathological state is characterized by an aberrant cytokine profile, endothelial damage, and impaired tissue repair mechanisms [3]. Within this systemic context, the oral cavity – and particularly the periodontium – emerges as a critical site of concern due to its delicate equilibrium between host defense and microbial challenge [4]. Long COVID, through its effects on immune surveillance, endothelial integrity, and wound healing, shares mechanistic pathways with periodontitis, a chronic inflammatory disease driven by unresolved immune responses and microbial dysbiosis [5]. Understanding these intersecting pathways provides valuable insights into how long COVID may exacerbate periodontal disease and highlights the importance of integrated diagnostic and therapeutic strategies targeting both oral and systemic health [6].

To appreciate the oral implications of long COVID, it is essential to first examine its underlying immunopathology – particularly the persistent systemic inflammation, immune dysregulation, and vascular dysfunction that directly influence periodontal tissues [7].

9.2 SARS-CoV-2 Tropism for Periodontal Tissues and Molecular Entry Mechanisms

SARS-CoV-2 is not limited to the respiratory tract; the oral cavity, and particularly the periodontium, has emerged as an important site of viral interaction [8]. The virus uses angiotensin-converting enzyme 2 (ACE2) receptors to enter cells, and these receptors are abundantly expressed in the gingival epithelium, periodontal ligament fibroblasts, and salivary gland acinar cells. To successfully invade, the viral spike protein must be "primed" by host proteases such as transmembrane protease serine 2 (TMPRSS2) and cathepsin B/L, which are also present in periodontal tissues [9, 10] (Figure 9.1).

https://doi.org/10.1515/9783112219904-009

Evidence from post-mortem studies has revealed traces of viral RNA and proteins within periodontal structures long after the virus is cleared from the nasopharynx [11, 12]. This suggests that the periodontium may act as a localized viral reservoir, capable of sustaining low-grade, chronic inflammation [12]. Persistent viral antigens at gingival sites could serve as a continuous immune stimulus, keeping cytokine levels elevated and fostering a pro-inflammatory environment that may worsen or reactivate underlying periodontal conditions [13].

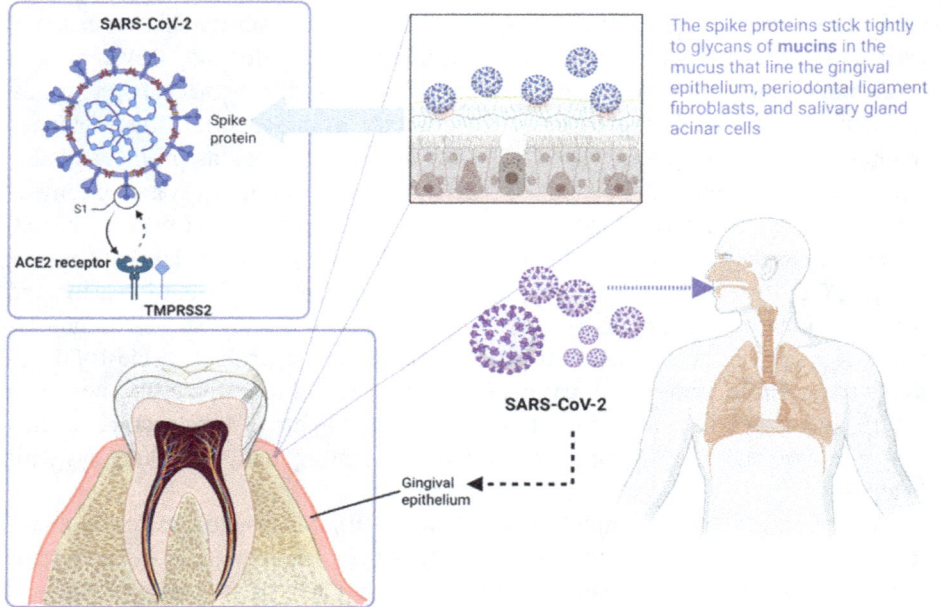

Figure 9.1: Interaction of SARS-CoV-2 with the oral cavity. The viral spike protein binds to ACE2 and TMPRSS2 receptors expressed in the gingival epithelium, periodontal ligament fibroblasts, and salivary gland acinar cells. Viral particles adhere to mucins in oral mucus, facilitating colonization and potential transmission to the respiratory tract. Created with Biorender.com.

9.3 Immune Dysregulation and Its Periodontal Ramifications

Long COVID represents a state of persistent immune imbalance, where both innate and adaptive immune responses fail to return to homeostasis [14]. Elevated levels of IL-6, TNF-α, and interferon-gamma (IFN-γ) dominate the systemic cytokine milieu, accompanied by sustained activation of the NLRP3 inflammasome. These features strongly parallel the inflammatory landscape observed in active periodontitis, suggesting shared pathogenic pathways that may amplify each other in susceptible individuals [15, 16].

One hallmark of this dysregulated immune response is the skewing of macrophages toward a pro-inflammatory M1 phenotype, with insufficient transition to the reparative M2 state [17]. In both long COVID and periodontitis, these M1 macrophages continuously release matrix metalloproteinases (MMPs), particularly MMP-8 and MMP-9, which degrade type I and III collagen. This not only accelerates soft tissue destruction but also hampers angiogenic remodeling, impairing the regenerative capacity of periodontal tissues [18, 19]. Equally significant is the phenomenon of T-cell exhaustion, a defining feature of long COVID. Exhausted T cells exhibit diminished IFN-γ production and overexpression of exhaustion markers such as PD-1 and TIM-3 [20]. Within the periodontium, this contributes to a disrupted Treg/Th17 balance, favoring IL-17-driven neutrophilic inflammation and osteoclast activation, which accelerate alveolar bone resorption [21]. Another critical immune dysfunction involves neutrophil extracellular traps (NETs). While NETosis plays a defensive role in pathogen containment, long COVID is characterized by exaggerated NET formation [22]. In the periodontal environment, this excess NETosis leads to epithelial injury, intensifies local oxidative stress, and generates autoantigens that perpetuate chronic inflammation [23]. Such persistent immune activation not only worsens periodontal tissue breakdown but may also create feedback loops that exacerbate systemic symptoms of long COVID [24] (Figure 9.2).

Collectively, the overlapping mechanisms of immune dysregulation – cytokine storms, impaired macrophage polarization, T-cell exhaustion, and excessive NETosis – position the periodontium as both a vulnerable target and a potential amplifier of post-viral sequelae [25]. Recognizing these shared immunopathological pathways underscores the need for integrated management approaches that address both systemic immune dysfunction and periodontal health.

9.4 Endothelial Dysfunction and Tissue Hypoxia

A hallmark of long COVID is widespread endothelial dysfunction, or endothelialitis, characterized by capillary rarefaction and the development of microthromboses across multiple organ systems [26]. In the context of the periodontium, these vascular changes have profound consequences. Compromised blood flow leads to reduced oxygen delivery, creating localized hypoxic environments that favor the proliferation of anaerobic periodontal pathogens such as *Porphyromonas gingivalis (P. gingivalis)* and *Tannerella forsythia (T. forsythia)*. This shift in microbial ecology can accelerate dysbiosis and drive inflammatory tissue destruction [27, 28] (Figure 9.3).

Under hypoxic conditions, the stabilization of hypoxia-inducible factor-1α (HIF-1α) becomes a critical regulatory event. While HIF-1α is designed to promote angiogenesis and restore oxygenation, it also induces the expression of MMPs, enzymes that degrade

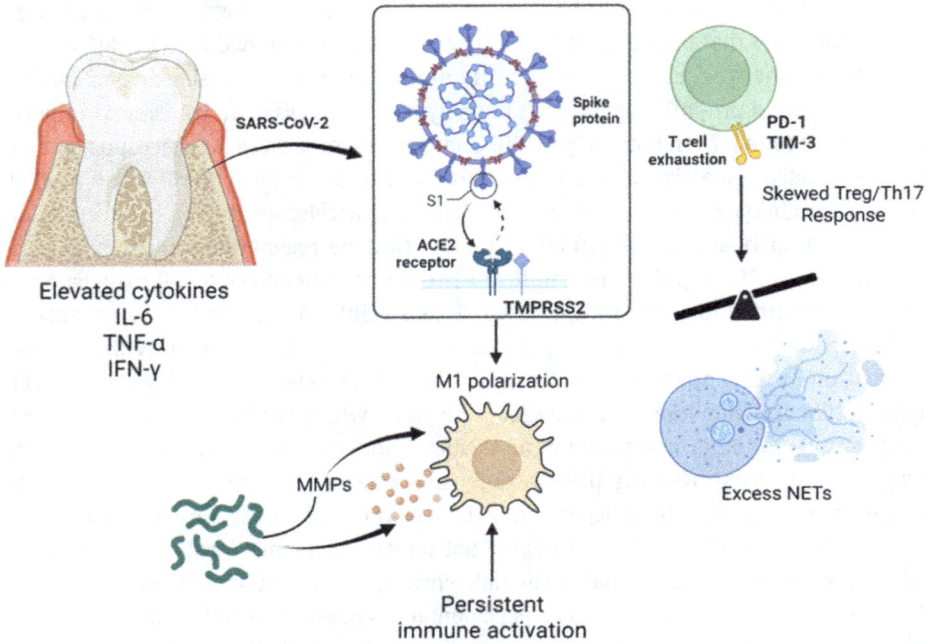

Figure 9.2: Immune dysregulation in the oral cavity during SARS-CoV-2 infection. Viral binding to ACE2/TMPRSS2 triggers elevated cytokine release (IL-6, TNF-α, IFN-γ), M1 macrophage polarization, excessive neutrophil extracellular traps (NETs), and persistent immune activation. T-cell exhaustion via PD-1/TIM-3 signaling and skewed Treg/Th17 responses further contribute to dysregulated immunity. Created with Biorender.com.

the extracellular matrix [29]. Paradoxically, this MMP-driven breakdown often occurs before effective vascular remodeling can take place, leading to further weakening of periodontal connective tissues [19]. As a result, long COVID-associated vascular injury not only undermines tissue repair but also creates a microenvironment that perpetuates inflammation and enhances periodontal disease progression [30].

9.5 Impaired Healing and Regeneration Post-COVID

Periodontal healing – particularly following surgical or regenerative interventions – relies on a finely tuned interplay of immune modulation, angiogenesis, extracellular matrix remodeling, and the recruitment of progenitor cells [31]. Long COVID exerts a profound influence on these processes, creating a biological environment that hinders predictable healing and regeneration [32] (Figure 9.4).

One major disruption occurs in vascular endothelial growth factor (VEGF) signaling. While VEGF is essential for microvessel formation and granulation tissue develop-

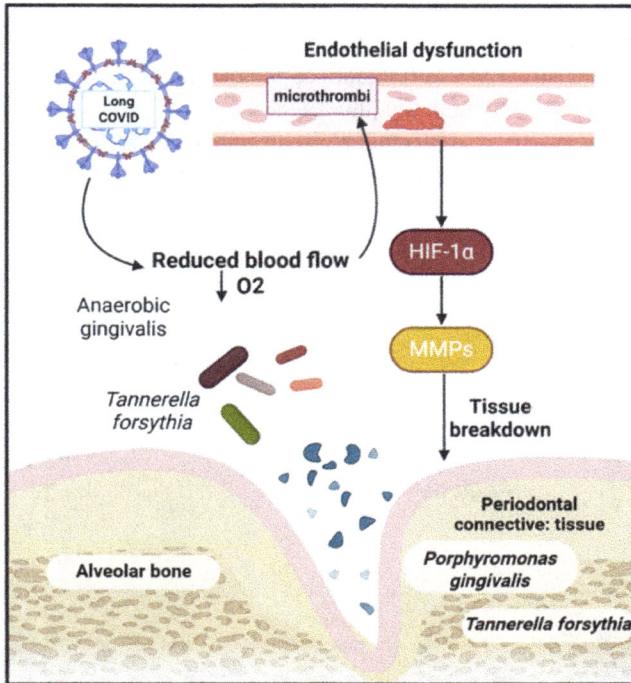

Figure 9.3: Mechanisms linking long COVID to periodontal breakdown. Endothelial dysfunction and microvascular damage reduce oxygen and blood flow, activating HIF-1α and matrix metalloproteinases (MMPs). These changes, combined with colonization by pathogens such as *Porphyromonas gingivalis* and *Tannerella forsythia*, promote connective tissue destruction and alveolar bone loss. Created with Biorender. com.

ment, its regulation becomes abnormal under the combined effects of chronic inflammation and hypoxia-induced feedback loops in long COVID [33]. Instead of promoting stable and functional neovessels, excessive or dysregulated VEGF drives the formation of immature and leaky vessels, contributing to defective angiogenesis and fibrotic scarring rather than true tissue repair [34].

Oxidative stress is another critical factor. Patients with long COVID experience persistently high oxidative stress due to mitochondrial dysfunction and a marked reduction in antioxidant defenses including diminished expression of key enzymes such as superoxide dismutase 2 and catalase [35, 36]. This pro-oxidative environment damages periodontal ligament stem cells, impairing both their proliferative capacity and osteogenic differentiation potential – two essential pillars of periodontal regeneration [37]. Furthermore, mesenchymal stem cells (MSCs) derived from post-COVID patients frequently exhibit signs of cellular senescence, with reduced colony-forming efficiency and increased expression of senescence markers like cyclin-dependent kinase inhibitor 2A (p16INK4A) and cyclin-dependent kinase inhibitor 1A (p21) [38]. Such alterations weaken the regenerative potential of MSC-based therapies and highlight the possible need for preconditioning strategies, antioxidant supplementation, or even genetic reprogramming to restore their functionality [39].

Collectively, these immune, vascular, and cellular impairments suggest that long COVID not only delays healing but also necessitates a re-evaluation of current regenerative protocols in periodontics [40].

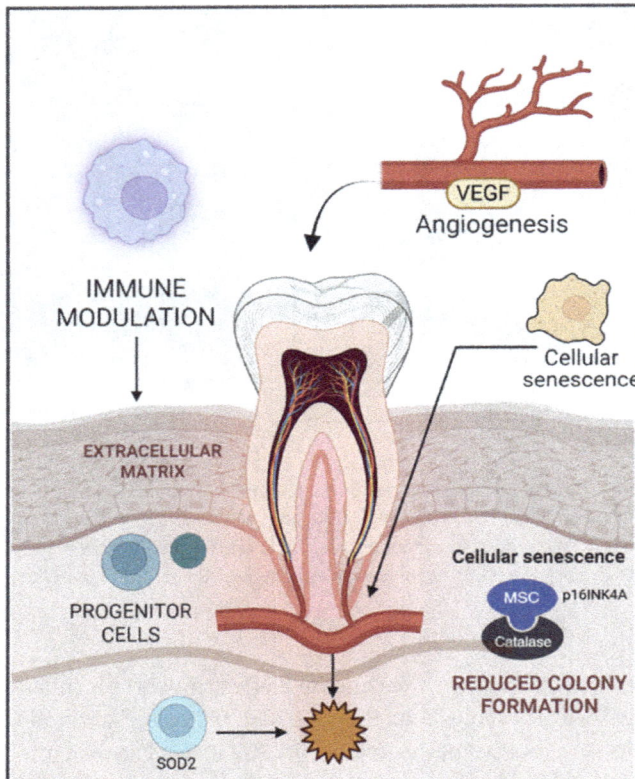

Figure 9.4: Long COVID-associated alterations in periodontal regeneration. Impaired immune modulation, increased cellular senescence, and reduced MSC colony formation compromise tissue repair. VEGF-driven angiogenesis and extracellular matrix disruption further hinder regenerative capacity in periodontal tissues. Created with Biorender.com.

9.6 Impact of Long COVID on Oral Microbiome and Dysbiosis

Long COVID significantly influences the **oral microbiome** through both systemic and local mechanisms [41]. Systemic immune imbalance, characterized by chronic inflammation and impaired mucosal immunity, disrupts the ecological balance of oral microbial communities. Additionally, frequent antibiotic use during COVID-19 treatment can deplete commensal bacterial populations, creating an environment conducive to dysbiosis [42, 43]. In this altered microbial landscape, there is a notable overgrowth of pathobionts such as *P. gingivalis* and *Fusobacterium nucleatum* (*F. nucleatum)*, which are key contributors to periodontal disease progression.

The persistent pro-inflammatory state further favors the proliferation of these pathogens, enhancing their ability to evade host defenses and form resilient biofilms [44] (Figure 9.5).

Moreover, emerging evidence suggests potential interactions between residual SARS-CoV-2 RNA in the oral mucosa and bacterial biofilms. Viral components may

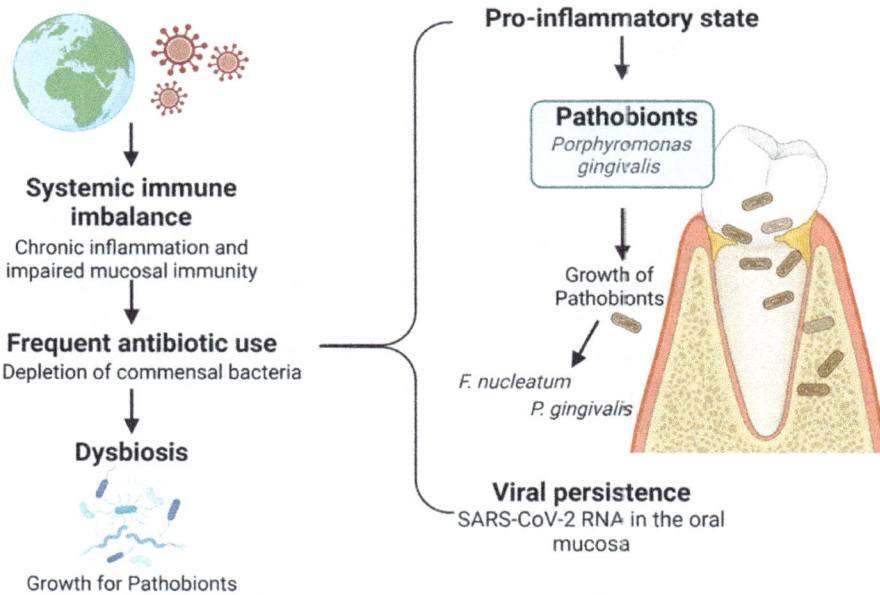

Figure 9.5: Links between systemic immune imbalance, dysbiosis, and viral persistence in the oral cavity. Chronic inflammation, impaired immunity, and frequent antibiotic use deplete commensal bacteria, favoring dysbiosis and the overgrowth of pathobionts such as *Porphyromonas gingivalis* and *Fusobacterium nucleatum*. This establishes a pro-inflammatory state and enables persistence of viral RNA in the oral mucosa. Created with Biorender.com.

alter epithelial barrier function or immune signaling, facilitating pathogen coloniza-tion and biofilm maturation. This interplay between viral persistence and bacterial dysbiosis may exacerbate periodontal inflammation and delay the restoration of a healthy oral microbiome post-COVID [13, 45].

9.7 Shared Mechanisms Between Periodontitis and Long COVID

9.7.1 Chronic Immune Activation

Both periodontitis and long COVID are marked by a failure in the resolution of inflam-mation, leading to prolonged tissue damage [46]. Key **pro-resolving** lipid mediators, such as resolvins and lipoxins, which normally promote the clearance of inflamma-tory cells and restoration of tissue homeostasis, are often deficient or functionally im-paired in both conditions [47, 48]. This deficiency perpetuates a cycle of neutrophil-driven tissue destruction and dysregulated immune responses, resulting in chronic in-flammation of the periodontium in periodontitis and persistent multisystem inflam-mation in long COVID [47, 48].

9.7.2 Oxidative Stress and Mitochondrial Dysfunction

SARS-CoV-2 infection induces mitochondrial damage, excessive production of reactive oxygen species, and impaired cellular bioenergeticsm [49]. These alterations closely resemble the oxidative stress-driven pathology of periodontitis, where mitochondrial dysfunction in gingival fibroblasts and immune cells leads to impaired collagen syn-thesis, extracellular matrix degradation, and heightened susceptibility to bacterial vir-ulence factors. The shared oxidative stress pathways further amplify local and sys-temic inflammatory cascades [50].

9.7.3 Systemic Spillover of Inflammatory Mediators

The "oral-systemic" axis underscores the bidirectional relationship between periodon-tal inflammation and systemic health. In periodontitis, pro-inflammatory cytokines (e.g., IL-6, TNF-α, and CRP) and bacterial endotoxins can enter systemic circulation, exacerbating chronic inflammatory states [4, 51, 52]. In the context of long COVID, this spillover may worsen systemic manifestations such as endothelial dysfunction, car-diovascular complications, and neuroinflammatory symptoms. Conversely, the systemic immune dysregulation of long COVID can intensify periodontal breakdown, creating a vicious cycle of mutual disease aggravation [53, 54].

9.8 Clinical Manifestations and Diagnostic Considerations

Long COVID presents a variety of oral manifestations that mirror systemic immune dysregulation and local tissue responses [7]. Patients commonly experience xerostomia, which may arise from salivary gland involvement or medication effects, and dysgeusia, often linked to viral-induced epithelial and neural damage [9, 55]. Additionally, recurrent or persistent mucosal lesions, gingival bleeding, and exacerbation of preexisting periodontitis are frequently observed due to impaired immune defense and persistent low-grade inflammation [56]. These findings underscore the importance of thorough periodontal and oral mucosal evaluations in individuals with post-COVID conditions.

9.9 Salivary and Crevicular Biomarkers of Post-COVID Inflammation

Saliva offers a unique, noninvasive medium for detecting both systemic and local inflammation in long COVID patients. Elevated levels of IL-6, IL-1β, MMP-8, C-reactive protein (CRP), and even viral RNA fragments have been associated with ongoing fatigue, musculoskeletal symptoms, and heightened periodontal disease activity ([57–60]). These biomarkers serve as valuable indicators for monitoring both systemic immune dysregulation and periodontal health, making saliva assays a dual-function diagnostic tool.

Advances in diagnostic technologies, such as CRISPR-based biosensors (e.g., SHER-LOCK) and electrochemical lab-on-chip platforms, now enable rapid detection of these molecular markers at the point of care. Integrating such systems into post-COVID dental practice could significantly enhance early intervention, personalized treatment planning, and continuous follow-up of patients at risk for both systemic and oral inflammatory complications [61, 62].

9.10 Therapeutic, Preventive, and Multidisciplinary Management Strategies

Managing periodontal health in post-COVID patients, especially those experiencing long COVID symptoms – requires a personalized and multidisciplinary approach due to their altered immune status and delayed healing capacity [63]. Conventional periodontal interventions, such as scaling and root planning, should be carefully tailored to minimize tissue trauma, with a preference for minimally invasive techniques. Adjunctive therapies, including laser treatment, offer added benefits by enhancing decontamination, reducing microbial load, and promoting biostimulatory effects that support tissue regeneration. Locally delivered antimicrobials and antiseptic rinses (e.g., chlorhexidine or essential oil-based formulations) may further control biofilm formation and prevent microbial dysbiosis in these susceptible patients [64–66].

A biomarker-driven risk stratification approach is essential for determining maintenance intervals, the need for adjunctive anti-inflammatory therapies, or the inclusion of host modulation strategies. Sub-antimicrobial dose doxycycline and omega-3 fatty acids, known for their dual benefits on periodontal inflammation and systemic immune regulation – can play a pivotal role in countering hyperinflammatory states [67, 68]. Additionally, advanced host modulation therapies, including nonsteroidal anti-inflammatory drugs, resolvins, and monoclonal antibodies targeting cytokines, such as IL-6 or TNF-α, may help limit tissue destruction while supporting systemic recovery [69].

Restoring immune homeostasis is equally critical. Probiotic and synbiotic supplementation can re-establish beneficial microbial communities, while nutritional strategies enriched with antioxidants, vitamins D and C, and polyphenols promote immune resilience and wound healing. These interventions, combined with personalized oral hygiene education, enhance both local periodontal stability and systemic health [70–72].

Given the complexity of long COVID, cross-referral networks involving periodontists, immunologists, primary care physicians, and infectious disease specialists are indispensable to ensure integrated care [73]. Tele-periodontics adds another layer of support by enabling remote monitoring, early detection of disease exacerbations, and real-time patient guidance through digital platforms. This hybrid care model, combining clinical, biochemical, and telehealth tools, ensures timely interventions, reduces chairside visits, and delivers a personalized continuum of care for high-risk patients [74, 75].

9.11 Conclusion and Future Directions

As our understanding of postviral syndromes evolves and becomes more sophisticated, there is an urgent need to clarify and determine if long COVID is a genuine modifier of periodontitis or an overlapping condition with the same immunopathological characteristics. To address this complex question in an effective way, future longitudinal investigations using multiomics platforms – transcriptomics, epigenomics, microbiomics, and metabolomics – are of absolute essence. These investigations will have a crucial role in delineating and recognizing disease-specific biomarkers and therapeutic targets that could result in improved therapies.

Moreover, preclinical studies that compare regenerative scaffolds loaded with anti-inflammatory cytokines or seeded with immuno-tolerized MSCs may unveil novel therapy for post-COVID periodontal regeneration. Finally, AI and machine learning systems that can integrate systemic inflammatory profiles, dental imaging, and patient-reported outcomes have the potential to revolutionize risk prediction and treatment personalization in this new cohort of post-COVID periodontal patients.

References

[1] Markov, P. V., Ghafari, M., & Beer, M. et al. (2023). The evolution of SARS-CoV-2. Nature Reviews Microbiology, 21, 361–379, https://doi.org/10.1038/s41579-023-00878-2.

[2] Tang, G., Bourgonje, A. R., & Hillebrands, L. (2025). Post-COVID-19 condition: Clinical phenotypes, pathophysiological mechanisms, pathology, and management strategies. The Journal of Pathology, 266(4–5), 369. https://doi.org/10.1002/path.6443.

[3] Gusev, E., & Sarapultsev, A. (2023). Exploring the pathophysiology of long COVID: The central role of low-grade inflammation and multisystem involvement. International Journal of Molecular Sciences, 25(12), 6389. https://doi.org/10.3390/ijms25126389.

[4] Martínez-García, M., & Hernández-Lemus, E. (2021). Periodontal inflammation and systemic diseases: An overview. Frontiers in Physiology, 12, 709438. https://doi.org/10.3389/fphys.2021.709438.

[5] Yekani, M., Dastgir, M., Fattahi, S., Shahi, S., Maleki, D. S., & Memar, M. Y. (2025). Microbiological and molecular aspects of periodontitis pathogenesis: An infection-induced inflammatory condition. Frontiers in Cellular and Infection Microbiology, 15, 1533658. https://doi.org/10.3389/fcimb.2025.1533658.

[6] Abdul-Azees, P., Marinkovic, M., Singh, B. B., Dean, D. D., Chen, D., Goldberg, M. P., Restrepo, M. I., Loomer, P. M., & Yeh, K. (n.d.). The impact of aging oral health on long COVID-19. Journal of Dental Research, https://doi.org/10.1177/00220345251349805.

[7] Schwartz, J., Capistrano, K., Hussein, H., Hafedi, A., Shukla, D., & Naqvi, A. (2025). Oral SARS-CoV-2 infection and risk for Long COVID. Reviews in Medical Virology, 35(2), e70029. https://doi.org/10.1002/rmv.70029.

[8] Tsuchiya, H. (2022). The oral cavity potentially serving as a reservoir for SARS-CoV-2 but not necessarily facilitating the spread of COVID-19 in dental practice. European Journal of Dentistry, 17(2), 310. https://doi.org/10.1055/s-0042-1757909.

[9] Okada, Y., Yoshimura, K., Toya, S., & Tsuchimochi, M. (2021). Pathogenesis of taste impairment and salivary dysfunction in COVID-19 patients. The Japanese Dental Science Review, 57, 111–122. https://doi.org/10.1016/j.jdsr.2021.07.001.

[10] Akagi, M., Ohta, K., Fukada, S., Sakuma, M., Naruse, T., Nakagawa, T., Ono, S., Nishi, H., Shigeishi, H., & Aikawa, T. (2024). ACE2 expression and spike S1 protein-mediated immune responses in oral mucosal cells. Oral Diseases, 30(4), 2293–2305. https://doi.org/10.1111/odi.14670.

[11] Servadei, F., Mauriello, S., Scimeca, M., Caggiano, B., Ciotti, M., Anemona, L., Montanaro, M., Giacobbi, E., Treglia, M., Bernardini, S., Marsella, L. T., Urbano, N., Schillaci, O., & Mauriello, A. (2021). Persistence of SARS-CoV-2 viral RNA in nasopharyngeal swabs after death: An observational study. Microorganisms, 9(4), 800. https://doi.org/10.3390/microorganisms9040800.

[12] Drozdzik, A. (2022). COVID-19 and SARS-CoV-2 infection in periodontology: A narrative review. Journal of Periodontal Research, https://doi.org/10.1111/jre.13034.

[13] Schwartz, J., Capistrano, K. J., Gluck, J., Hezarkhani, A., & Naqvi, A. R. (2024). SARS-CoV-2, periodontal pathogens, and host factors: The trinity of oral post-acute sequelae of COVID-19. Reviews in Medical Virology, 34(3), e2543. https://doi.org/10.1002/rmv.2543.

[14] Peluso, M. J., Abdel-Mohsen, M., Henrich, T. J., & Roan, N. R. (2024). Systems analysis of innate and adaptive immunity in long COVID. Seminars in Immunology, 72, 101873. https://doi.org/10.1016/j.smim.2024.101873.

[15] Hashim, N., Babiker, R., Mohammed, R., Rehman, M. M., Chaitanya, N. C., & Gobara, B. (2024). NLRP3 inflammasome in autoinflammatory diseases and periodontitis: Advance in the management. Journal of Pharmacy & Bioallied Sciences, 16(Suppl 2), S1110. https://doi.org/10.4103/jpbs.jpbs_1118_23.

[16] Kany, S., Vollrath, J. T., & Relja, B. (2018). Cytokines in inflammatory disease. International Journal of Molecular Sciences, 20(23), 6008. https://doi.org/10.3390/ijms20236008.

[17] Sica, A., Erreni, M., Allavena, P., & Porta, C. (2015). Macrophage polarization in pathology. Cellular and Molecular Life Sciences, 72(21), 4111–4126. https://doi.org/10.1007/s00018-015-1995-y.

[18] Zhao, T., Chu, Z., CH, C., Dong, S., Li, G., Wu, J., & Tang, C. (2023). Macrophages induce gingival destruction via Piezo1-mediated MMPs-degrading collagens in periodontitis. Frontiers in Immunology, 14, 1194662. https://doi.org/10.3389/fimmu.2023.1194662.

[19] Radzki, D., Negri, A., Kusiak, A., & Obuchowski, M. (2024). Matrix metalloproteinases in the periodontium – vital in tissue turnover and unfortunate in periodontitis. International Journal of Molecular Sciences, 25(5), 2763. https://doi.org/10.3390/ijms25052763.

[20] Kusnadi, A., Ramírez-Suástegui, C., Fajardo, V., Chee, S. J., Meckiff, B. J., Simon, H., Pelosi, E., Seumois, G., Ay, F., Vijayanand, P., & Ottensmeier, C. H. (2021). Severely ill COVID-19 patients display impaired exhaustion features in SARS-CoV-2-reactive CD8+ T cells. Science Immunology, 6(55), eabe4782. https://doi.org/10.1126/sciimmunol.abe4782.

[21] Tang, Z., Jin, L., & Yang, Y. (2025). The dual role of IL-17 in periodontitis regulating immunity and bone homeostasis. Frontiers in Immunology, 16, 1578635. https://doi.org/10.3389/fimmu.2025.1578635.

[22] Monsalve, D. M., Acosta-Ampudia, Y., Acosta, N. G., Celis-Andrade, M., Şahin, A., Yilmaz, A. M., Shoenfeld, Y., & Ramírez-Santana, C. (2025). NETosis: A key player in autoimmunity, COVID-19, and long COVID. Journal of Translational Autoimmunity, 10, 100280. https://doi.org/10.1016/j.jtauto.2025.100280.

[23] Wang, J., Zhou, Y., Ren, B., Zou, L., He, B., & Li, M. (2021). The role of neutrophil extracellular traps in periodontitis. Frontiers in Cellular and Infection Microbiology, 11, 639144. https://doi.org/10.3389/fcimb.2021.639144.

[24] Louisa, M., Anggraini, W., Putranto, R., Komala, O., & De Angelis, N. (2023). Periodontal disease markers among patients with long COVID: A case-control study. Open Dentistry Journal, 17, e187421062307030. http://dx.doi.org/10.2174/18742106-v17-230718-2023-53.

[25]   Vitkov, L., Knopf, J., Krunić, J., Schauer, C., Schoen, J., Minnich, B., Hannig, M., & Herrmann, M. (2022). Periodontitis-derived dark-NETs in severe COVID-19. Frontiers in Immunology, 13, 872695. https://doi.org/10.3389/fimmu.2022.872695.

[26]   Mondini, L., Confalonieri, P., Pozzan, R., Ruggero, L., Trotta, L., Lerda, S., Hughes, M., Bellan, M., Confalonieri, M., Ruaro, B., Salton, F., & Tavano, S. (2022). Microvascular alteration in COVID-19 documented by nailfold capillaroscopy. Diagnostics, 13(11), 1905. https://doi.org/10.3390/diagnostics13111905.

[27]   Luis, J., Israel, P., Stalin, M., Jafet, S., & Trinidad, P. (2025). Relationship between periodontitis, type 2 diabetes mellitus and COVID-19 disease: A narrative review. Frontiers in Cellular and Infection Microbiology, 15, 1527217. https://doi.org/10.3389/fcimb.2025.1527217.

[28]   Lloyd-Jones, G., Molayem, S., Pontes, C. C., & Chapple, I. (2021). The COVID-19 Pathway: A proposed oral-vascular-pulmonary route of SARS-CoV-2 infection and the importance of oral healthcare measures. Journal of Oral Medicine and Dental Research, 2(1), 1–25. https://doi.org/10.52793/JOMDR.2020.2(1)-13.

[29]   Gornostaeva, A., Buravkova, L., Lobanova, M., & Andreeva, E. (2024). HIFs in hypoxic regulation of the extracellular matrix: Focus on little-known player HIF-3. Biocell, 48, 677–692.

[30]   Carmona Loayza, D. A., & Lafebre, M. F. (2023). Periodontal disease and COVID-19: Prognosis and potential pathways of association in their pathogenesis. Canadian Journal of Dental Hygiene, 57(1), 44. https://pmc.ncbi.nlm.nih.gov/articles/PMC10032643/.

[31]   Cho, D., Kim, H., Lee, M., Ku, Y., & Seol, J. (2021). Periodontal wound healing and tissue regeneration: A narrative review. Pharmaceuticals, 14(5), 456. https://doi.org/10.3390/ph14050456.

[32]   Lin, C., Chiang, C., Lin, Y., Tseng, Y., Hsieh, T., Shieh, A., Huang, H., Tsai, T., Feng, W., Peng, Y., & Lee, T. (2023). Unraveling the link between periodontitis and COVID-19: Exploring pathogenic pathways and clinical implications. Biomedicines, 11(10), 2789. https://doi.org/10.3390/biomedicines11102789.

[33]   Lorenc, P., Sikorska, A., Molenda, S., Guzniczak, N., Dams-Kozlowska, H., & Florczak, A. (2024). Physiological and tumor-associated angiogenesis: Key factors and therapy targeting VEGF/VEGFR pathway. Biomedicine & Pharmacotherapy, 180, 117585. https://doi.org/10.1016/j.biopha.2024.117585.

[34]   Johnson, K. E., & Wilgus, T. A. (2014). Vascular endothelial growth factor and angiogenesis in the regulation of cutaneous wound repair. Advances in Wound Care, 3(10), 647–661. https://doi.org/10.1089/wound.2013.0517.

[35]   Valente Coronel, P. M., Dc, L. S. B., Espinoça, I. T., Campos, N. M., Nakano Ota, R. S., Ej, P., Filho, D. W., AR, C. M., Perdomo, R. T., & Parisotto, E. B. (2025). Involvement of oxidative stress in post-acute sequelae of COVID-19: Clinical implications. Redox Report, 30(1), 2471738. https://doi.org/10.1080/13510002.2025.2471738.

[36]   Tsermpini, E. E., Glamočlija, U., Ulucan-Karnak, F., Trampuž, S. R., & Dolžan, V. (2022). Molecular mechanisms related to responses to oxidative stress and antioxidative therapies in COVID-19: A systematic review. Antioxidants, 11(8), 1609. https://doi.org/10.3390/antiox11081609.

[37]   Jin, S., Jiang, H., Sun, Y., Li, F., Xia, J., Li, Y., Zheng, J., & Qin, Y. (2022). Osteogenic differentiation of periodontal membrane stem cells in inflammatory environments. Open Life Sciences, 17(1), 1240–1254. https://doi.org/10.1515/biol-2022-0474.

[38]   Elmi, F., Soltanmohammadi, F., Fayeghi, T., Farajnia, S., & Alizadeh, E. (2025). Preventing MSC aging and enhancing immunomodulation: Novel strategies for cell-based therapies. Regenerative Therapy, 29, 517–527. https://doi.org/10.1016/j.reth.2025.04.014.

[39]   Otani, M., & Fujimiya, M. (2019). p16INK4A-expressing mesenchymal stromal cells restore the senescence-clearance-regeneration sequence that is impaired in chronic muscle inflammation. EBioMedicine, 44, 86–97. https://doi.org/10.1016/j.ebiom.2019.05.012.

[40] Davis, H. E., McCorkell, L., Vogel, J. M., & Topol, E. J. (2023). Long COVID: Major findings, mechanisms and recommendations. Nature Reviews Microbiology, 21(3), 133–146. https://doi.org/10.1038/s41579-022-00846-2.

[41] Gang, J., Wang, H., Xue, X., & Zhang, S. (2022). Microbiota and COVID-19: Long-term and complex influencing factors. Frontiers in Microbiology, 13, 963488. https://doi.org/10.3389/fmicb.2022.963488.

[42] Smail, S. W., Albarzinji, N., Salih, R. H., Taha, K. O., Hirmiz, S. M., Ismael, H. M., Noori, M. F., Azeez, S. S., & Janson, C. (2025). Microbiome dysbiosis in SARS-CoV-2 infection: Implication for pathophysiology and management strategies of COVID-19. Frontiers in Cellular and Infection Microbiology, 15, 1537456. https://doi.org/10.3389/fcimb.2025.1537456.

[43] Rafiqul Islam, S. M., Foysal, M. J., Hoque, M. N., Mehedi, H. M., Rob, M. A., Salauddin, A., Tanzina, A. Y., Biswas, S., Noyon, S. H., Siddiki, A. M., Tay, A., & Mannan, A. (2022). Dysbiosis of oral and gut microbiomes in SARS-CoV-2 infected patients in Bangladesh: Elucidating the role of opportunistic gut microbes. Frontiers in Medicine, 9, 821777. https://doi.org/10.3389/fmed.2022.821777.

[44] EW, B., BM, B., Kusumaningrum, A., Sunarto, H., Soeroso, Y., Sulijaya, B., Theodorea, C. F., Pratomo, I. P., Efendi, D., Apriyanti, E., & Said, S. M. (2024). Association between dysbiotic perio-pathogens and inflammatory initiators and mediators in COVID-19 patients with diabetes. Heliyon, 10(2), e24089. https://doi.org/10.1016/j.heliyon.2024.e24089.

[45] Gomes, S. C., Fachin, S., Melchiors Angst, P. D., Lamers, M. L., & Nunes, L. N. (2021). Dental biofilm of symptomatic COVID-19 patients harbours SARS-CoV-2. Journal of Clinical Periodontology, 48(7), 880–885. https://doi.org/10.1111/jcpe.13471.

[46] Cai, W., Marouf, N., Said, K. N., & Tamimi, F. (2021). Nature of the interplay between periodontal diseases and COVID-19. Frontiers in Dental Medicine, 2, 735126. https://doi.org/10.3389/fdmed.2021.735126.

[47] Van Dyke, T. E. (2017). Pro-resolving mediators in the regulation of periodontal disease. Molecular Aspects of Medicine, 58, 21–36. https://doi.org/10.1016/j.mam.2017.04.006.

[48] Kumar, V., Yasmeen, N., Chaudhary, A. A., Alawam, A. S., Al-Zharani, M., Basher, N. S., Harikrishnan, S., Goud, M. D., Pandey, A., Lakhawat, S. S., & Sharma, P. K. (2023). Specialized pro-resolving lipid mediators regulate inflammatory macrophages: A paradigm shift from antibiotics to immunotherapy for mitigating COVID-19 pandemic. Frontiers in Molecular Biosciences, 10, 1104577. https://doi.org/10.3389/fmolb.2023.1104577.

[49] Shin, H. J., Lee, W., & Ku, K. B. et al. (2024). SARS-CoV-2 aberrantly elevates mitochondrial bioenergetics to induce robust virus propagation. Signal Transduction and Targeted Therapy, 9, 125, https://doi.org/10.1038/s41392-024-01836-x.

[50] Deng, Y., Xiao, J., Ma, L., Wang, C., Wang, X., Huang, X., & Cao, Z. (2023). Mitochondrial dysfunction in periodontitis and associated systemic diseases: Implications for pathomechanisms and therapeutic strategies. International Journal of Molecular Sciences, 25(2), 1024. https://doi.org/10.3390/ijms25021024.

[51] Amar, S., & Han, X. (2003). The impact of periodontal infection on systemic diseases. Medical Science Monitor, 9(12), RA291–RA299.

[52] Kim, M. Y., & Pang, E. K. (2025). Relationship between periodontitis and systemic health conditions: A narrative review. Ewha Medical Journal, 48(2), e27. https://doi.org/10.12771/emj.2025.00101.

[53] Gupta, G., Buonsenso, D., Wood, J., Mohandas, S., & Warburton, D. (2025). Mechanistic insights into long COVID: Viral persistence, immune dysregulation, and multi-organ dysfunction. Comprehensive Physiology, 15(3), e70019. https://doi.org/10.1002/cph4.70019.

[54] Sari, A., Dikmen, N. K., & Nibali, L. (2023). Association between periodontal diseases and COVID-19 infection: A case–control study with a longitudinal arm. Odontology, 111(4), 1009–1020. https://doi.org/10.1007/s10266-023-00797-x.

[55] Aliberti, A., Gasparro, R., Mignogna, M., Canfora, F., Spagnuolo, G., Sammartino, G., & Coppola, N. (2024). Unveiling the oral lesions, dysgeusia and osteonecrosis related to COVID-19: A comprehensive systematic review. Journal of Clinical Medicine, 14(4), 1267. https://doi.org/10.3390/jcm14041267.

[56] Roberto, J., Calixta, M., Monserrath, S., & M, L. (2021). Oral lesions associated with COVID-19 and the participation of the buccal cavity as a key player for establishment of immunity against SARS-CoV-2. International Journal of Environmental Research and Public Health, 19(18), 11383. https://doi.org/10.3390/ijerph191811383.

[57] Dongiovanni, P., Meroni, M., Casati, S., Goldoni, R., Thomaz, D. V., Kehr, N. S., Galimberti, D., Fabbro, M. D., & Tartaglia, G. M. (2023). Salivary biomarkers: Novel noninvasive tools to diagnose chronic inflammation. International Journal of Oral Science, 15, 27. https://do .org/10.1038/s41368-023-00231-6.

[58] Bachtiar, E., BM, B., Kusumaningrum, A., Sunarto, H., Soeroso, Y., Sulijaya, B., Apriyanti, E., Theodorea, C. F., Putra Pratomo, I., Yudhistira, Y., Efendi, D., & Lestari, W. (2024). The utility of salivary CRP and IL-6 as a non-invasive measurement evaluated in patients with COVID-19 with and without diabetes. F1000Research, 12, 419. https://doi.org/10.12688/f1000research.130995.3.

[59] Shakeeb, N., Varkey, P., & Hynse, A. et al. (2022). Saliva as a potential specimen to monitor IL-6, TNF-α and IL-10 in COVID-19 patients. Inflammation, 45, 2368–2374, https://doi.org/10.1007/s10753-022-01698-x.

[60] Kim, J., & Kim, H. (2020). Changes in inflammatory cytokines in saliva after non-surgical periodontal therapy: A systematic review and meta-analysis. International Journal of Environmental Research and Public Health, 18(1), 194. https://doi.org/10.3390/ijerph18010194.

[61] Hassan, Y. M., Mohamed, A. S., Hassan, Y. M., & El-Sayed, W. M. (2025). Recent developments and future directions in point-of-care next-generation CRISPR-based rapid diagnosis. Clinical and Experimental Medicine, 25(1), 33–50. https://doi.org/10.1007/s10238-024-01540-8.

[62] Kumaran, A., Serpes, N. J., Gupta, T., James, A., Sharma, A., Kumar, D., Nagraik, R., Kumar, V., & Pandey, S. (2023). Advancements in CRISPR-based biosensing for next-gen point-of-care diagnostic application. Biosensors, 13(2), 202. https://doi.org/10.3390/bios13020202.

[63] Abbas, A. H., Haji, M. R., Shimal, A. A., Kurmasha, Y. H., Aa, H. A., Azeez, Z. T., AR, S. A., HM, H. A., AR, A. A., Abdulhadi, N. A., AZ, H. A., MM, A., & Hussin, O. A. (2025). A multidisciplinary review of long COVID to address the challenges in diagnosis and updated management guidelines. Annals of Medicine and Surgery, 87(4), 2105. https://doi.org/10.1097/MS9.0000000000003066.

[64] Shirmohammadi, A. (2021). Post-COVID-19 tsunami of periodontal diseases. Journal of Advanced Periodontology & Implant Dentistry, 13(1), 1. https://doi.org/10.34172/japid.2021.009.

[65] Wang, M., Xu, Y., & Fang, W. et al. (2023). Impact of COVID-19 on patient follow-up during supportive periodontal therapy: A retrospective study based on phone call survey. BMC Oral Health, 23, 811, https://doi.org/10.1186/s12903-023-03539-1.

[66] Coulthard, P. (2020). Dentistry and coronavirus (COVID-19) – moral decision-making. British Dental Journal, 228(7), 503–505. https://doi.org/10.1038/s41415-020-1482-1.

[67] Qi, M., Sun, W., Wang, K., Li, W., Lin, J., Gong, J., & Wang, L. (2022). Periodontitis and COVID-19: Immunological characteristics, related pathways, and association. International Journal of Molecular Sciences, 24(3), 3012. https://doi.org/10.3390/ijms24033012.

[68] Mlachkova, A., & Maynalovska, H. (2024). Nanoparticles as strategies for modulating the host's response in periodontitis treatment. Nanomaterials, 15(7), 476. https://doi.org/10.3390/nano15070476.

[69] Golub, L. M., Lee, H., Bacigalupo, J., & Gu, Y. (2024). Host modulation therapy in periodontitis, diagnosis and treatment – status update. Frontiers in Dental Medicine, 5, 1423401. https://doi.org/10.3389/fdmed.2024.1423401.

[70] Kadyan, S., Park, G., Singh, T. P., Patoine, C., Singar, S., Heise, T., Domeier, C., Ray, C., Kumar, M., Behare, P. V., Chakrabarty, P., Efron, P., Sheffler, J., & Nagpal, R. (2025). Microbiome-based therapeutics towards healthier aging and longevity. Genome Medicine, 17, 75. https://doi.org/10.1186/s13073-025-01493-x.

[71] Bhatia, A., Sharma, D., Mehta, J., Kumarasamy, V., Begum, M. Y., Siddiqua, A., Sekar, M., Subramaniyan, V., Wong, L. S., & Izzati Mat Rani, N. N. (2025). Probiotics and synbiotics: Applications, benefits, and mechanisms for the improvement of human and ecological health. Journal of Multidisciplinary Healthcare, 18, 1493–1517. https://doi.org/10.2147/JMDH.S501056.

[72] Bazyar, H., Maghsoumi-Norouzabad, L., Yarahmadi, M., Gholinezhad, H., Moradi, L., Salehi, P., & Javid, A. Z. (2020). The impacts of synbiotic supplementation on periodontal indices and biomarkers of oxidative stress in type 2 diabetes mellitus patients with chronic periodontitis under non-surgical periodontal therapy: a double-blind, placebo-controlled trial. Diabetes, Metabolic Syndrome and Obesity: Targets and Therapy, 13, 19–27. https://doi.org/10.2147/DMSO.S230060.

[73] Barshikar, S., Laguerre, M., Gordon, P., & Lopez, M. (2023). Integrated care models for long coronavirus disease. Physical Medicine and Rehabilitation Clinics of North America, https://doi.org/10.1016/j.pmr.2023.03.007.

[74] Kemajou, P. M., Mbanya, A., & Coppieters, Y. (2024). Digital approaches in post-COVID healthcare: A systematic review of technological innovations in disease management. Biology Methods & Protocols, 9(1), bpae070. https://doi.org/10.1093/biomethods/bpae070.

[75] Avula, H. (2015). Tele-periodontics – oral healthcare at a grass-root level. Journal of Indian Society of Periodontology, 19(5), 589–593. https://doi.org/10.4103/0972-124X.157875.

Bakri Gobara, Nada Tawfig Hashim, Rasha Babiker, and Muhammed Mustahsen Rahman

10 Host Modulation Therapy in Periodontitis: Beyond NSAIDs

10.1 Introduction

Periodontitis is a multifactorial, chronic inflammatory disease in which a perpetual microbial challenge is joined by an abnormal host response that leads to connective tissue breakdown of the periodontium and alveolar bone [1]. A key aspect of the pathophysiology is the overproduction of inflammatory mediators – most importantly, prostaglandins, cytokines, and matrix metalloproteases (MMPs), which not only lead to local tissue destruction but are also engaged in systemic inflammation [2]. Of the various mediators, prostaglandin E2 (PGE$_2$), produced through the cyclooxygenase (COX) pathway, is a major player in inducing osteoclastic bone resorption and enhancing inflammation [3]. In this regard, nonsteroidal anti-inflammatory drugs (NSAIDs) have been traditionally employed as adjunct therapies for periodontitis because of their COX enzyme suppressive activity and thereby the inhibition of PGE$_2$ synthesis [4]. Early studies had demonstrated that NSAIDs like flurbiprofen, ibuprofen, and naproxen can reduce alveolar bone loss, reduce gingival inflammation, and lower prostanoid levels in gingival crevicular fluid (GCF) [5–9]. Nevertheless, the clinical usefulness in the practical environment of NSAIDs is marred by several significant limitations. In the first place, their action is mainly symptomatic, without any influence on underlying causes of inflammation or dysbiosis in the subgingival microbiome [10]. Second, long-term NSAID therapy is associated with gastrointestinal, renal, and cardiovascular adverse effects and thus is not suitable for long-term administration [11]. Third, discontinuation of NSAID treatment inevitably results in a rebound effect on inflammatory markers and bone resorption rates at or even above baseline – illustrating the need for more lasting solutions [12]. Lastly, NSAIDs exert nonselective immunosuppressive actions that may compromise healing and host defense, particularly in patients with comorbid systemic disease [13].

The challenges above have called for a paradigm shift in host modulation paradigms, from broad suppression to precision immunotherapeutics that effectively target the cytokine networks, signal transduction pathways, and epigenetic regulators orchestrating periodontal inflammation and tissue destruction. Host modulation therapy today comprises monoclonal antibodies (mAbs), pro-resolving lipid mediators, epigenetic agents, and phytochemicals, all aimed at restoring immune balance, enabling tissue repair, and inducing long-term disease remission with lower risks of systemic side effects [14].

https://doi.org/10.1515/9783112219904-010

10.2 Monoclonal Antibodies: Targeted Immunotherapeutics in Periodontitis

Monoclonal antibodies (mAbs) have proven to be effective agents for the selective modulation of hyperactive immune mechanisms central to periodontitis development [15]. Among the most attractive targets are pro-inflammatory cytokines such as tumor necrosis factor-alpha (TNF-α) and interleukin-6 (IL-6), both of which are implicated in osteoclastogenesis and matrix breakdown [16–18] (Figure 10.1).

Anti-TNF-α monoclonal antibodies (e.g., infliximab, adalimumab), originally developed for rheumatoid arthritis, inhibit the TNF receptor-mediated activation of NF-κB and AP-1 transcription factors in periodontal tissue [19]. Soluble and membrane-bound TNF-α are neutralized by these drugs, thereby inhibiting leukocyte recruitment, cytokine amplification, and osteoclast differentiation. In experimental periodontitis, local or systemic administration of anti-TNF mAbs have been shown in preclinical studies to lead to decreased alveolar bone loss and downregulated expression of MMP [20]. Therefore, tocilizumab, an anti-IL-6 receptor monoclonal antibody, disrupts IL-6/STAT3 signaling pathways implicated in periodontal inflammation and systemic metabolic dysregulation. Besides inhibiting neutrophil infiltration, this blockade also inhibits RANKL expression on osteoblasts and T-cells, thus restricting osteoclast activation [21]. Despite the infancy of the use of tocilizumab in dental practice, these agents have potential in immune-targeted adjunctive therapy for refractory periodontitis or periodontitis with associated systemic comorbidities.

10.3 Lipid Mediators: Pro-resolving Molecules in Inflammation Termination

Specialized pro-resolving lipid mediators (SPMs) represent a distinct class of bioactive molecules that include lipoxins, resolvins, protectins, and maresins [22]. These critical mediators are biosynthesized from omega-3 and omega-6 polyunsaturated fatty acids and play a pivotal role in orchestrating the active resolution phase of inflammation [23] (Figure 10.2). Unlike conventional anti-inflammatory agents, which primarily suppress immune responses, SPMs reprogram leukocytes and resident tissue cells to actively clear inflammation without inducing immunosuppression [24].

Resolvin E1 (RvE1), a metabolite of eicosapentaenoic acid (EPA), interacts with ChemR23 receptors on macrophages and neutrophils to enhance efferocytosis and inhibit neutrophil chemotaxis [25]. In experimental models of periodontitis, topical RvE1 application has demonstrated reductions in alveolar bone loss, inflammatory cytokines (IL-1β, TNF-α), and matrix MMPs, while simultaneously promoting periodontal tissue regeneration. Similarly, Lipoxin A4 (LXA4) exerts its pro-resolving action by in-

MONOCLONAL ANTIBODIES

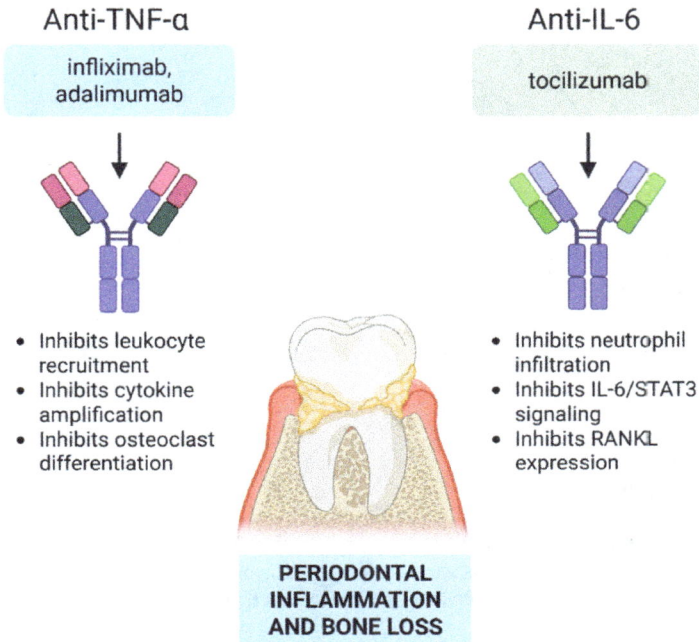

Anti-TNF-α

infliximab, adalimumab

- Inhibits leukocyte recruitment
- Inhibits cytokine amplification
- Inhibits osteoclast differentiation

Anti-IL-6

tocilizumab

- Inhibits neutrophil infiltration
- Inhibits IL-6/STAT3 signaling
- Inhibits RANKL expression

PERIODONTAL INFLAMMATION AND BONE LOSS

Figure 10.1: Monoclonal antibodies in periodontal therapy. Anti-TNF-α agents (infliximab, adalimumab) inhibit leukocyte recruitment, cytokine amplification, and osteoclast differentiation. Anti-IL-6 therapy (tocilizumab) reduces neutrophil infiltration, blocks IL-6/STAT3 signaling, and suppresses RANKL expression. Together, these biologics mitigate periodontal inflammation and bone loss. Created with Borender.com.

hibiting NF-κB signaling and attenuating the production of pro-inflammatory prosta-glandins and leukotrienes [26] (Figures 10.3 and 10.4).

Unlike conventional drugs that operate via direct cytokine inhibition, SPMs engage in a proactive termination of the inflammatory cascade and restore tissue homeostasis. This unique mechanism is critical in preventing chronic immune dysregulation, often associated with periodontal lesions, positioning SPMs as a key factor in maintaining oral health [27, 28].

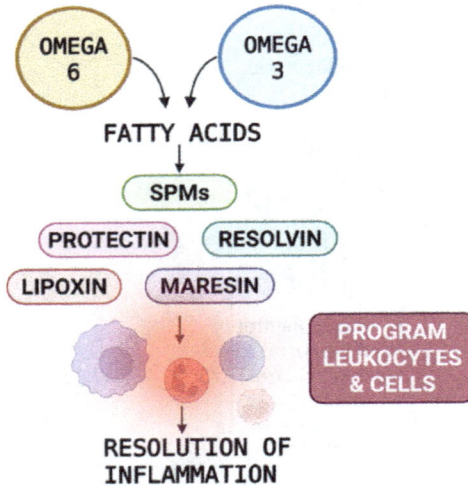

Figure 10.2: Specialized pro-resolving lipid mediators (SPMs) in periodontal inflammation. Derived from omega-3 and omega-6 fatty acids, mediators such as resolvins, protectins, lipoxins, and maresins reprogram leukocytes and cells to actively resolve inflammation and restore tissue homeostasis. Created with Biorender.com.

10.4 Plant-Derived Bioactive Compounds: Phytochemicals with Multi-target Modulatory Effects

Natural products with both anti-inflammatory and antioxidant properties have attracted increasing interest as adjunct therapy in the treatment of periodontal diseases. The interest has been motivated by their favorable safety profiles and their inherent polypharmacological nature, which allows them to exert several effects at a time [29, 30].

Curcumin, the bioactive polyphenol of turmeric (Curcuma longa), blocks several pathways involved in periodontitis, such as NF-κB, COX-2, and MAPK signaling. By inhibiting the expression of IL-1β, TNF-α, and MMPs, curcumin diminishes collagen degradation and bone resorption. In addition, it increases antioxidant defenses like HO-1 and SOD2, reversing oxidative stress, a principal driver of periodontal tissue breakdown [31, 32] (Figure 10.5).

Resveratrol, a stilbene found in grapes and berries, inhibits RANKL-induced osteoclastogenesis by modulating the SIRT1/NF-κB pathway [33]. It also restores Treg/

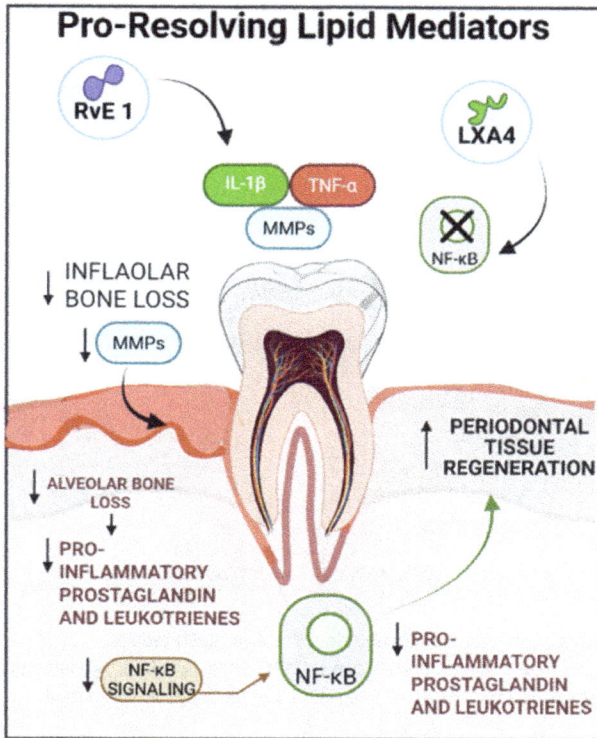

Figure 10.3: Actions of pro-resolving lipid mediators in periodontitis. Mediators such as resolvin (RvE1), lipoxin (LXA4), and maresin (MaR1) inhibit pro-inflammatory cytokines (IL-1β, TNF-α), reduce NF-κB signaling, and limit alveolar bone loss. These pathways promote periodontal tissue regeneration and restore homeostasis. Created with Biorender.com.

Th17 balance, a critical immunologic shift to remove chronic inflammation within periodontal pockets. Animal models demonstrate that resveratrol administration leads to reduced alveolar bone loss, decreased activity of MMP-8, and preservation of connective tissue attachment [34] (Figure 10.6).

Catechins in green tea, particularly epigallocatechin-3-gallate (EGCG), exhibit antimicrobial activity against *P. gingivalis* and inhibit inflammatory mediators through inhibition of Akt phosphorylation and STAT signaling. EGCG also boosts epithelial barrier function and fibroblast viability, promoting healing in periodontal tissues that are inflamed [35, 36] (Figure 10.6).

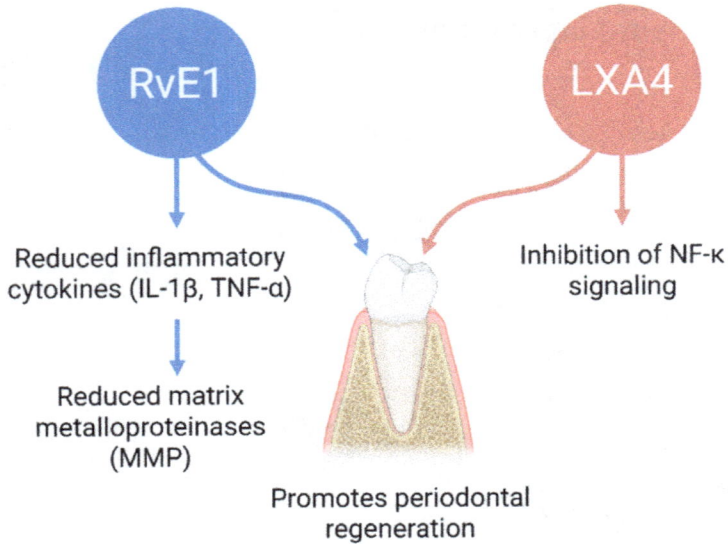

Plant-Derived Bioactive Compounds: Phytochemicals with Multi-Target Modulatory Effects

Figure 10.4: Pro-resolving lipid mediators in periodontal regeneration. Resolvin (RvE1) reduces inflammatory cytokines (IL-1β, TNF-α) and matrix metalloproteinases (MMPs), while lipoxin (LXA4) inhibits NF-κB signaling. Together, they promote periodontal tissue regeneration and modulate inflammation. Created with Biorender.com.

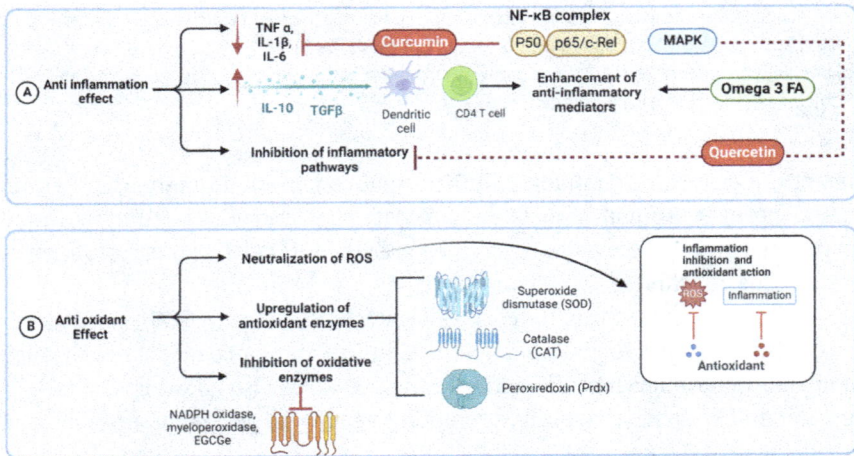

Figure 10.5: Anti-inflammatory and antioxidant effects of bioactive compounds in periodontal therapy. (A) Compounds such as curcumin, omega-3 fatty acids, and quercetin inhibit pro-inflammatory pathways, enhance anti-inflammatory mediators, and suppress NF-κB/MAPK signaling. (B) Antioxidant effects include neutralization of ROS, inhibition of oxidative enzymes, and upregulation of antioxidant enzymes such as SOD, catalase, and peroxiredoxin. Created with Biorender.com.

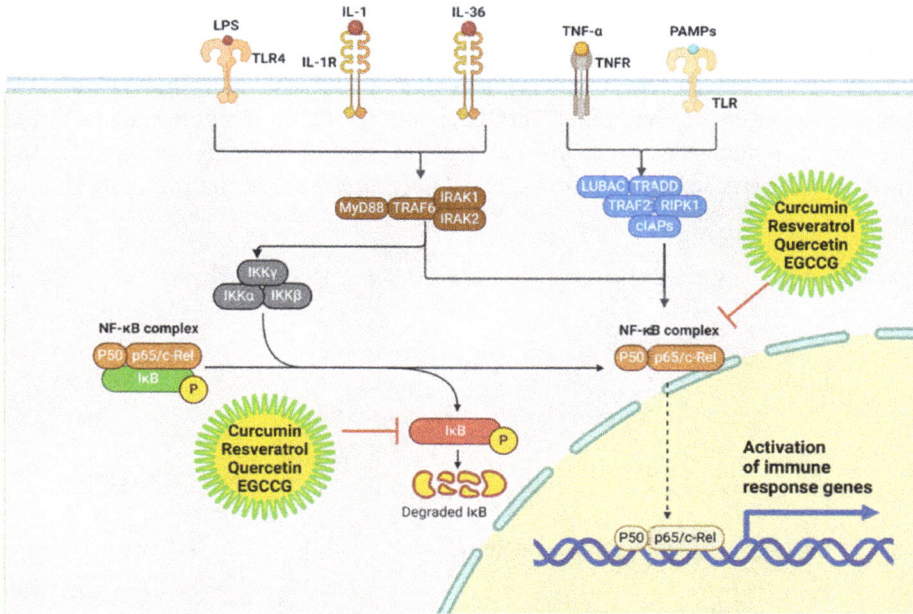

Figure 10.6: Modulation of NF-κB signaling by phytochemicals in periodontal inflammation. Bioactive compounds such as curcumin, resveratrol, quercetin, and EGCG inhibit NF-κB activation by blocking IκB degradation and interfering with upstream signaling pathways triggered by TLRs, IL-1R, and TNFR. These actions suppress pro-inflammatory cytokine expression and regulate immune response genes. Created with Biorender.com.

10.5 Epigenetic Modulators: Reprogramming Gene Expression for Inflammatory Control

Epigenetic changes, including significant processes such as DNA methylation, histone modification, and microRNA dysregulation, have been found to play central and critical roles in maintaining the chronicity of periodontitis. Furthermore, drugs that have the ability to reverse such epigenetic changes represent a novel and exciting group of modulators with potential therapeutic application [37] (Figure 10.7).

Histone deacetylase inhibitors (HDACi), such as suberoylanilide hydroxamic acid (SAHA) or valproic acid enhance the acetylation of histones, enhancing transcription of anti-inflammatory genes and inhibiting cytokines IL-6 and TNF-α. The agents also decrease the expression of MMP-13 and RANKL, limiting connective tissue and bone destruction [38, 39].

DNA methylation inhibitors, including the older drug 5-azacytidine, have been shown to have a profound impact on re-establishing the expression levels of important regulatory genes, including SOCS1 and IL-10, through the process of demethylating their respective promoters [40]. This therapeutic effect has the impact of reducing and attenuating the hyperinflammatory state that can occur in many diseases. While it should be stated that at this point clinical application of these drugs in the practice of periodontics remains largely theoretical, they do provide intriguing insights into the possibility of precision host modulation based upon broad epigenomic profiling [41].

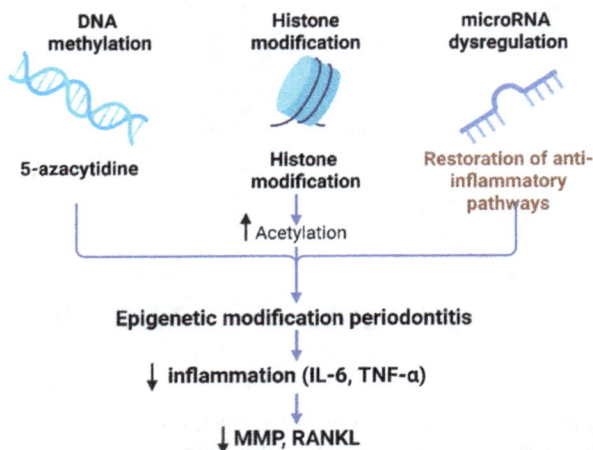

Figure 10.7: Epigenetic modulation in periodontitis. DNA methylation, histone modifications, and microRNA regulation influence inflammatory pathways. Agents such as 5-azacytidine restore anti-inflammatory signaling by reducing IL-6, TNF-α, MMPs, and RANKL expression, thereby attenuating periodontal tissue destruction. Created with Biorender.com.

10.6 Cytokine Receptor Antagonists: Disrupting Inflammatory Signal Reception

Cytokine receptor antagonists act by competitively inhibiting the process of cytokines attaching to their respective cell-surface receptors, a process which effectively inhibits the initiation of the downstream signaling cascades required for inflammation and tissue destruction [42] (Figure 10.8). Among the numerous agents that have been extensively investigated within this particular drug class, Anakinra is one of the most important, a recombinant interleukin-1 receptor antagonist, otherwise referred to as IL-1Ra [43].

In periodontitis, the cytokine IL-1β has a central and pivotal role in the regulation and orchestration of the neutrophil infiltration, fibroblast breakdown, as well as in the process of osteoclastogenesis. Anakinra acts by interfering with the interaction between IL-1β and its receptor (IL-1R1), and consequently effectively inhibits the activation of the MyD88–IRAK–TRAF6 signaling pathway that ultimately controls the transcription events regulated by NF-κB and AP-1 of pro-inflammatory mediators responsible for the disease [44, 45]. It has been demonstrated in preclinical studies that IL-1Ra can significantly reduce the inflammatory infiltrates, lead to a downregulation of MMP expression, as well as also provide protection to alveolar bone from the harmful effects of resorption [46–48].

In the same way, IL-6 receptor drugs such as tocilizumab successfully inhibit IL-6 binding with the gp130/JAK/STAT3 pathway of osteoblasts and gingival fibroblasts. By this action, the drugs induce a decrease in RANKL expression, which decreases downstream osteoclast activation via the signaling cascade [49, 50]. This mode of action is especially applicable to patients who suffer from systemic diseases such as diabetes or rheumatoid arthritis, where an overproduction of IL-6 accounts for increased loss of periodontal tissue [51].

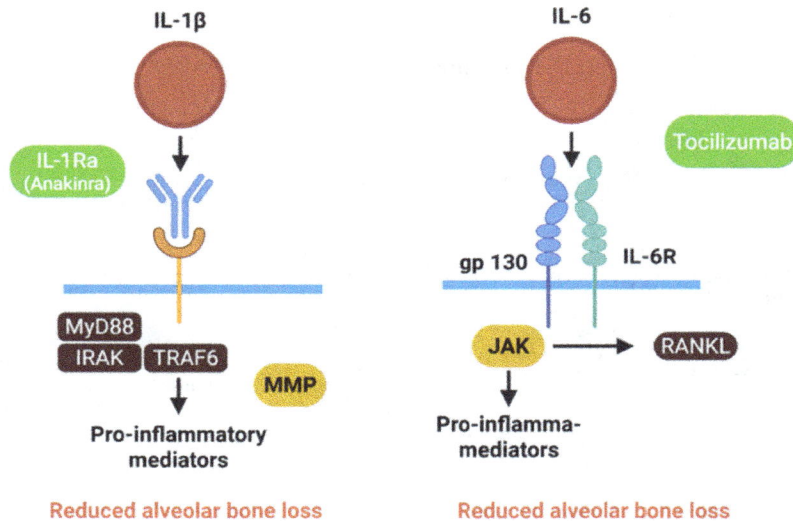

Cytokine inhibition in periodontitis

Figure 10.8: Cytokine inhibition in periodontitis. IL-1 receptor antagonist (IL-1Ra, anakinra) blocks IL-1β signaling via MyD88/TRAF6, reducing pro-inflammatory mediator and MMP activity. Tocilizumab inhibits IL-6/IL-6R–JAK/STAT3 signaling, lowering RANKL expression. Both pathways attenuate inflammation and reduce alveolar bone loss. Created with Biorender.com.

10.7 Microbiome-Targeted Immunomodulators: Balancing Immunity Without Sterilization

In contrast to antibiotics, which nonspecifically kill not only disease-causing organisms but also health-maintaining commensal microbes, microbiome-targeted immunomodulators are designed to selectively alter and reshape the host immune response [52]. Their primary goal is to promote microbial tolerance and maintain the delicate ecological balance of the gut and other microbiota. A new and exciting class of agents includes Toll-like receptor (TLR) antagonists, along with a variety of metabolites derived from the microbiota itself [53, 54].

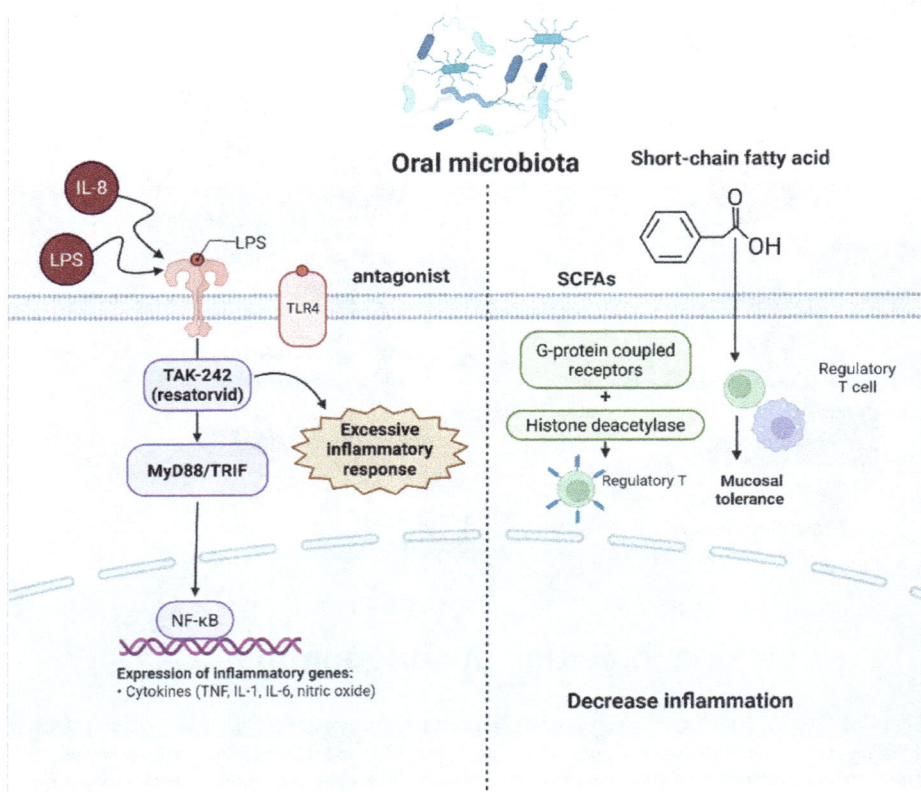

Figure 10.9: Oral microbiota-derived mechanisms in periodontal inflammation. On the left, IL-1β and LPS activate TLR4 signaling through MyD88/TRIF, inducing NF-κB and expression of pro-inflammatory cytokines. On the right, microbial short-chain fatty acids (SCFAs) act via G-protein-coupled receptors and histone deacetylase inhibition, enhancing regulatory T cell activity and promoting mucosal tolerance, thereby decreasing inflammation. Created with Biorender.com.

TLR4 antagonists such as TAK-242 (resatorvid) inhibit TLR4-MD2-LPS interactions and, consequently, inhibit the MyD88/TRIF pathways triggered by Gram-negative bacteria such as *P. gingivalis* [55]. This leads to decreased IL-1β, TNF-α, and nitric oxide production while preserving baseline immune surveillance. This "immune detuning" reduces excessive responses without inducing immunosuppression [56].

Additionally, short-chain fatty acids, or SCFAs, such as butyrate, are produced by gut commensal anaerobic bacteria. SCFAs exert their effects through the activation of G-protein-coupled receptors, specifically GPR41 and GPR43, as well as histone deacetylase inhibition [57]. Such induction fosters the generation of regulatory T cells and the promotion of anti-inflammatory macrophage phenotypes. The practice of supplementing with SCFAs or encouraging the growth of SCFA-producing bacteria, such as *Faecalibacterium prausnitzii* (*F. prausnitzii*), for instance, could significantly contribute to preserving mucosal tolerance in chronically inflamed areas [58] (Figure 10.9).

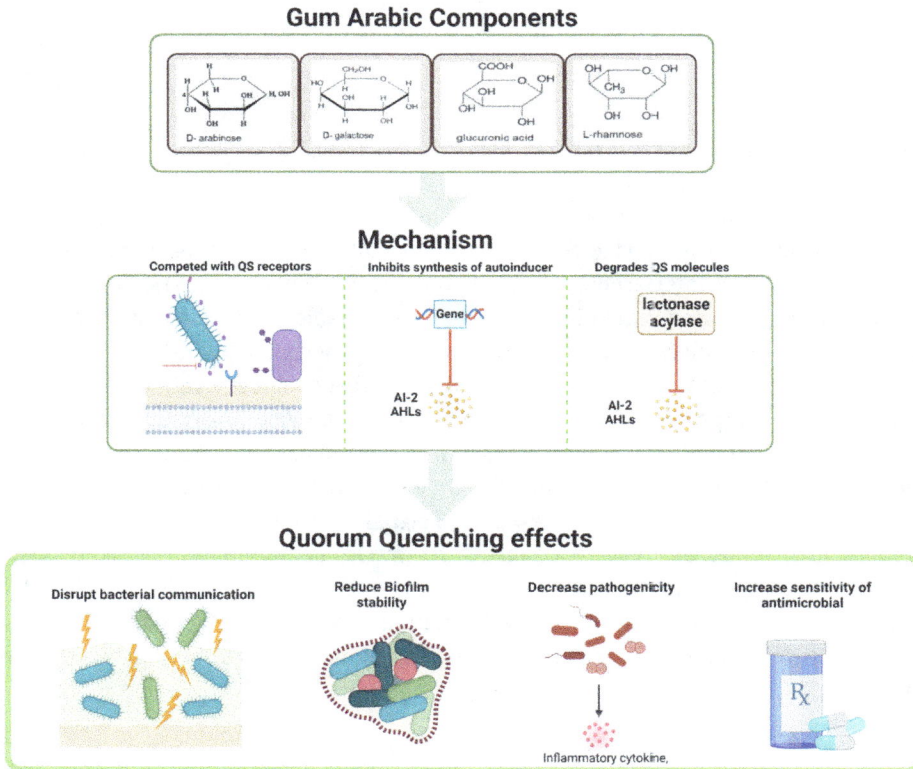

Figure 10.10: Quorum quenching effects of gum arabic in periodontal therapy. Gum arabic components act by disrupting bacterial communication, inhibiting quorum sensing pathways, and degrading signal molecules. These effects reduce biofilm stability, decrease pathogenic virulence, and increase antibiotic sensitivity. Created with Biorender.com.

Building on the role of SCFAs, gum arabic (GA) acts as a potent prebiotic that enhances the growth of butyrate-producing gut bacteria, which in turn exerts systemic and oral anti-inflammatory effects [59]. Butyrate generated from GA fermentation has been shown to upregulate host defense peptides such as LL-37 by inducing the CAMP gene, thereby strengthening the innate immune response in oral tissues [60]. In addition to its prebiotic effects, GA disrupts quorum sensing (QS) by inhibiting bacterial communication pathways like AI-2 signaling, leading to reduced biofilm formation and decreased bacterial virulence [61] (Figure 10.10). This dual action – through both butyrate-mediated immune modulation and QS interference – not only supports mucosal tolerance and healing but also reduces inflammatory cytokines within periodontal pockets, offering a comprehensive mechanism of immune regulation and tissue protection. Such pathways highlight the therapeutic promise of GA in maintaining periodontal homeostasis through gut–oral axis modulation and local biofilm control [61].

10.8 CRISPR-Cas-Based Immune Editing: Precision Modulation at the Genetic Level

The most promising future direction in host modulation through CRISPR-Cas systems involves using these systems to edit or silence pro-inflammatory genes in periodontal tissues [62]. CRISPR interference (CRISPRi) and CRISPR activation (CRISPRa) have recently emerged as gene regulation methods which enable reversible control of gene expression through mechanisms that do not alter DNA permanently [63] (Figure 10.11).

The use of CRISPRi to target TNF-α, MMP-9, or IL-6 promoters in gingival epithelial cells creates a physical barrier that prevents RNA polymerase from binding thus lowering cytokine and protease production in a controlled way. CRISPRa technology enables the activation of anti-inflammatory genes including IL-10 and A20 (TNFAIP3) which function as natural regulators of NF-κB signaling [64, 65].

The RNA-guided Cas13 system enables the precise degradation of cytokine transcripts in inflamed tissues through its mRNA-targeting mechanism which provides detailed immune system control. The development of lipid nanoparticles and viral vectors and hydrogel-based local delivery systems makes this technology ready for localized periodontal application in the upcoming years [66–68].

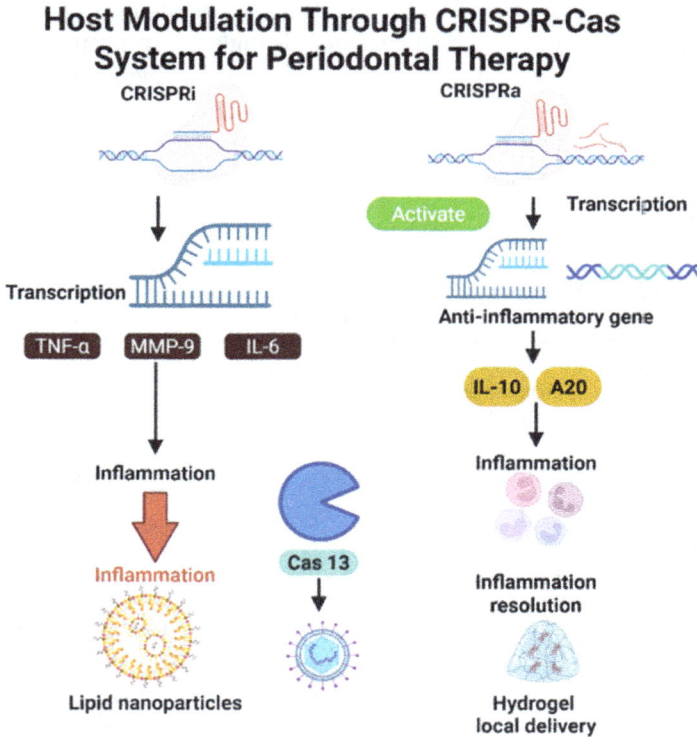

Figure 10.11: Host modulation through CRISPR-Cas systems for periodontal therapy. CRISPRi suppresses pro-inflammatory genes (TNF-α, MMP-9, IL-6), while CRISPRa activates ant -inflammatory genes (IL-10, A20). These approaches regulate inflammation using delivery methods such as lipid nanoparticles and hydrogel-based local therapy, offering precision host modulation. Created with Biorender.com.

10.9 Conclusion

Together, these novel approaches to host response modulation represent a stark paradigm shift away from the traditional approach of broad-spectrum suppression typically associated with NSAIDs. Instead, this new paradigm focuses on selective, mechanism-based modulation of the inflammation processes. Whether through targeted blockade of individual cytokines, utilization of pro-resolving mediators, epigenetic reprogramming, or even advanced gene editing techniques, the ultimate goal is clear. It is not so much a matter of blunting or inhibiting the activities of the immune system but resetting it in such a way as to promote resolution, facilitate repair, and aid regeneration of tissues and body systems. The future success we can expect in this field will be predicated, to a large extent, on the successful integration of biomarker-driven diagnostics with pharmacogenomics and advanced delivery technologies, all acting in concert for the tailored, individualized, and highly controlled modulation over an extended duration. The landscape of periodontal treatment is undergoing a rapid and dramatic transformation – the territory that was previously the sole domain of conventional methods such as mechanical debridement and antibiotics is now transforming into an era of advanced molecular periodontics.

This table illustrates emerging modulation therapies in periodontitis – mechanisms, targets, and therapeutic potential.

Therapy class	Representative agents	Mechanism of action	Targeted pathways	Delivery mode	Clinical relevance
NSAIDs (traditional)	Ibuprofen and diclofenac	Inhibit cyclooxygenase enzymes (COX-1/2), reducing prostaglandin synthesis	COX-PGE2 axis	Systemic/ topical	Reduces inflammation and bone resorption in early stages
Lipid mediators	Resolvin E1 and lipoxin A4	Promote resolution of inflammation and restore neutrophil clearance and macrophage balance	SPM pathways (ALX/FPR2 receptor)	Local injection/gel	Enhances healing; shifts macrophage phenotype to M2
Monoclonal antibodies	Anti-TNF-α and anti-IL-1β (canakinumab)	Neutralize pro-inflammatory cytokines	TNF-α/IL-1β	Systemic (injection)	May benefit refractory periodontitis and systemic comorbidities
Matrix metalloproteinase inhibitors	Sub-antimicrobial doxycycline and synthetic MMP inhibitors	Inhibit MMP activity to prevent collagen breakdown	MMP-8, MMP-9, and MMP-13	Systemic/local release	Approved adjunct (SDD); helps maintain attachment levels
Epigenetic modifiers	Histone deacetylase inhibitors (e.g., vorinostat), miRNA mimics	Modulate chromatin remodeling and gene expression in inflammation	NF-κB, IL-6, and miR-146a	Nanoparticles/ oral	Under investigation; precision modulation of host response
Plant-derived compounds	Curcumin, resveratrol, and baicalin	Antioxidant, NF-κB inhibition, and inflammasome modulation	Nrf2, NF-κB, and NLRP3	Local/oral rinse/gel	Safe adjunctive use; promising in chronic periodontitis

(continued)

Therapy class	Representative agents	Mechanism of action	Targeted pathways	Delivery mode	Clinical relevance
Probiotic modulators	*L. reuteri* and *Streptococcus salivarius*	Rebalance oral microbiome and reduce inflammatory cytokines	IL-10 and TGF-β	Oral tablet/ lozenges	Used in maintenance; supports ecological biofilm shift
RNA-based therapies	miRNA-155/146a inhibitors, siRNA	Silence pathogenic gene expression post-transcriptionally	NF-κB, TLR4, and STAT3	GCF-targeted microcarriers	Preclinical; offers highly specific host modulation
JAK/STAT pathway inhibitors	Tofacitinib and ruxolitinib	Inhibit JAK-mediated phosphorylation, blocking inflammatory gene transcription	JAK1/2-STAT3 pathway	Systemic/ topical	Under evaluation for autoimmune-mediated periodontitis

References

[1]   Kwon, T., Lamster, I. B., & Levin, L. (2021). Current concepts in the management of periodontitis. International Dental Journal, 71(6), 462–476. doi: 10.1111/idj.12630.

[2]   Neurath, N., & Kesting, M. (2024). Cytokines in gingivitis and periodontitis: From pathogenesis to therapeutic targets. Frontiers in Immunology, 15, 1435054. doi: 10.3339/fimmu.2024.1435054.

[3]   Båge, T., Kats, A., Lopez, B. S., Morgan, G., Nilsson, G., Burt, I., Korotkova, M., Corbett, L., Knox, A. J., Pino, L., Jakobsson, J., Modéer, T., & Yucel-Lindberg, T. (2011). Expression of prostaglandin e synthases in periodontitis: Immunolocalization and cellular regulation. The American Journal of Pathology, 178(4), 1676. doi: 10.1016/j.ajpath.2010.12.048.

[4]   Ren, J., Fok, M. R., Zhang, Y., Han, B., & Lin, Y. (2023 Feb 25).The role of non-steroidal anti-inflammatory drugs as adjuncts to periodontal treatment and in periodontal regeneration. Journal of Translational Medicine, 21(1). 149. 1186/s12967-023-03990-2. doi: 1C.

[5]   Farahmand, A., Sayar, F., Omidali, Z., Soleimani, M., & Esfahani, B. J. (2019). Efficacy of 2% ibuprofen subgingival irrigation as an adjunct to non-surgical therapy in the treatment of chronic periodontitis: A randomized controlled, split-mouth, clinical trial. Journal of Advanced Periodontology & Implant Dentistry, 11(2), 69. doi: 10.15171/japid.2019.012.

[6]   Elkhouli, A. M. (2011). The efficacy of host response modulation therapy (omega-3 plus low-dose aspirin) as an adjunctive treatment of chronic periodontitis (clinical and biochemical study. Journal of Periodontal Research, 46, 261–268. 1111/j.1600-0765.2010.01336.x. doi: 10.

[7]   Abd Rahman, F., Mohd Ali, J., Abdullah, M., Abu Kasim, N. H., & Musa, S. (2016). Aspirin enhances osteogenic Potential of Periodontal Ligament Stem Cells (PDLSCs) and modulates the expression profile of growth factor-associated genes in PDLSCs. Journal of Periodontal Research, 87, 837–847. 1902/jop.2016.150610. doi: 10.

[8]   Oduncuoglu, B. F., Kayar, N. A., Haliloglu, S., Serpek, B., Ataoglu, T., & Alptekin, N. O. (2018 May). Effects of a cyclic NSAID regimen on levels of gingival crevicular fluid prostaglandin E2and Interleukin-1β: a 6-month randomized controlled clinical trial. Nigerian Journal of Clinical Practice, 21(5), 658–666.

[9]   Kumar, A. K., Reddy, N. R., Babu, M., Kumar, P. M., Reddy, V. S., & Chavan, C. V. (2013). Estimation of prostaglandin E2 levels in gingival crevicular fluid in periodontal health, disease and after treatment. Contemporary Clinical Dentistry, 4(3), 303. doi: 10.4103/0976-237X.118354.

[10]   Bindu, S., Mazumder, S., & Bandyopadhyay, U. (2020). Non-steroidal anti-inflammatory drugs (NSAIDs) and organ damage: A current perspective. Biochemical Pharmacology, 180, 114147. doi: 10.1016/j.bcp.2020.114147.

[11]   Showande, S. J., & Akinbode, T. E. (2024). Nonsteroidal anti-inflammatory drug use by patients: Impact of modular educational training on pharmacists' questioning, counselling and risk assessments. Exploratory Research in Clinical and Social Pharmacy, 15, 100494. doi: 10.1016/j.rcsop.2024.100494.

[12]   Doux, J. D., Bazar, K. A., Lee, P. Y., & Yun, A. J. (2005).Can chronic use of anti-inflammatory agents paradoxically promote chronic inflammation through compensatory host response?. Medical Hypotheses, 65(2). 389–91. 1016/j.mehy.2004.12.021. doi: 10.

[13]   Zhao-Fleming, H., Hand, A., Zhang, K., Polak, R., Northcut, A., Jacob, D., Dissanaike, S., & Rumbaugh, K. P. (2018). Effect of non-steroidal anti-inflammatory drugs on post-surgical complications against the backdrop of the opioid crisis. Burns & Trauma, 6, 25. doi: 10.1186/s41038-018-0128-x.

[14]   Zumla, A., Rao, M., Wallis, R. S., Kaufmann, E., H., S., Rustomjee, R., Mwaba, P., Vilaplana, C., Yeboah-Manu, D., Chakaya, J., Ippolito, G., Azhar, E., Hoelscher, M., & Maeurer, M. (2016). Host-directed therapies for infectious diseases: Current status, recent progress, and future prospects. The Lancet, Infectious Diseases, 16(4), e47. doi: 10.1016/S1473-3099(16.

[15]   Posner, J., Barrington, P., Brier, T., & Datta-Mannan, A. (2019). Monoclonal antibodies: Past, present and future. Handbook of Experimental Pharmacology, 260, 81–141. 1007/164_2019_323. doi: 10.

[16]   Aboul-Ella, H., Gohar, A., Ali, A. A., Ismail, L. M., El-Regal Mahmoud, A. E., Elkhatib, W. F., & Aboul-Ella, H. (2024). Monoclonal antibodies: From magic bullet to precision weapon. Molecular Biomedicine, 5, 47. doi: 10.1186/s43556-024-00210-1.

[17]   Travan, S., Li, F., Slate, E. H., & Kirkwood, K. L. (2013). Differential expression of mitogen activating protein kinases in periodontitis. Journal of Clinical Periodontology, 40(8), 757. doi: 10.1111/jcpe.12123.

[18]   Kirkwood, K. L., Cirelli, J. A., Rogers, J. E., & Giannobile, W. V. (2007). Novel host response therapeutic approaches to treat periodontal diseases. Periodontology 2000, 43, 294. doi: 10.1111/j.1600-0757.2006.00166.x.

[19]   Abunemer, R. M., Shaheen, R. S., & Alghamdi, R. A. (2023). Correlation of anti-TNF-a biological therapy with periodontal conditions and osteonecrosis in autoimmune patients: A systematic review. The Saudi Dental Journal, 35(7), 785. doi: 10.1016/j.sdentj.2023.07.006.

[20]   TJ, D. V., Yousovich, J., Schoenmaker, T., Scheres, N., & Everts, V. (2016 Apr). Tumor necrosis factor-α antagonist infliximab inhibits osteoclast formation of peripheral blood mononuclear cells but does not affect periodontal ligament fibroblast-mediated osteoclast formation. Journal of Periodontal Research, 51(2), 186–95. 1111/jre.12297. doi: 10.

[21]   Kobayashi, T., Ito, S., Kobayashi, D., Kojima, A., Shimada, A., Narita, I., Murasawa, A., Nakazono, K., & Yoshie, H. (2015). Interleukin-6 receptor inhibitor tocilizumab ameliorates periodontal inflammation in patients with rheumatoid arthritis and periodontitis as well as tumor necrosis factor inhibitors. Clinical and Experimental Dental Research, 1(2), 63. doi: 10.1002/cre2.11.

[22]   Bannenberg, G., & Serhan, C. N. (2010). Specialized pro-resolving lipid mediators in the inflammatory response: An update. Biochimica et Biophysica Acta, 1801(12), 1260. doi: 10.1016/j.bbalip.2010.08.002.

[23] Calder, P. C. (2010). Omega-3 fatty acids and inflammatory processes. Nutrients, 2(3), 355. doi: 10.3390/nu2030355.

[24] Freire, M. O., & Van Dyke, T. E. (2013). Natural resolution of inflammation. Periodontology 2000, 63(1), 149. doi: 10.1111/prd.12034.

[25] Gyurko, R., & Van Dyke, T. E. (2014). The role of polyunsaturated ω-3 fatty acid Eicosapentaenoic acid–derived Resolvin E1 (RvE1) in bone preservation. Critical Reviews in Immunology, 34(4), 347. doi: 10.1615/critrevimmunol.2014009982.

[26] Ali, M., Yang, F., Plachokova, A. S., Jansen, J. A., & Walboomers, X. F. (2021). Application of specialized pro-resolving mediators in periodontitis and peri-implantitis: A review. European Journal of Oral Sciences, 129(1), e12759. doi: 10.1111/eos.12759.

[27] Basil, M. C., & Levy, B. D. (2015). Specialized pro-resolving mediators: Endogenous regulators of infection and inflammation. Nature Reviews, Immunology, 16(1), 51. doi: 10.1038/nri.2015.4.

[28] Julliard, W. A., Aung Myo, Y. P., Perelas, A., Jackson, P. D., Thatcher, T. H., & Sime, P. J. (2022). Specialized pro-resolving mediators as modulators of immune responses. Seminars in Immunology, 59, 101605. doi: 10.1016/j.smim.2022.101605.

[29] Malcangi, G., Inchingolo, A. M., Casamassima, L., Trilli, I., Ferrante, L., Inchingolo, F., Palermo, A., Inchingolo, A. D., & Dipalma, G. (2024). Effectiveness of herbal medicines with Anti-Inflammatory, Antimicrobial, and Antioxidant properties in improving oral health and treating Gingivitis and Periodontitis: A systematic review. Nutrients, 17(5), 762. doi: 10.3390/nu17050762.

[30] Pasupuleti, M. K., Nagate, R. R., Alqahtani, S. M., Penmetsa, G. S., Gottumukkala, S., V., N., Ramesh, V., & S, K. (2023). Role of medicinal herbs in periodontal therapy: A systematic review. Journal of International Society of Preventive & Community Dentistry, 13(1), 9. doi: 10.4103/jispcd.JISPCD_210_22.

[31] Ridho, F. M., Syachputra, A. J., Ulfah, K., Faqih, M., & Nurhuda, A. (2024). Pre-clinical and clinical efficacy of curcumin as an anti-inflammatory agent for periodontitis. A systematic review. Revista Científica Odontológica, 12(4), e222. doi: 10.21142/2523-2754-1204-2024-222.

[32] Hashim, N. T., Babiker, R., Chaitanya, N. C., Mohammed, R., Priya, S. P., Padmanabhan, V., Ahmed, A., Dasnadi, S. P., Islam, M. S., Gismalla, B. G., & Rahman, M. M. (2024). new insights in natural bioactive compounds for periodontal disease: Advanced molecular mechanisms and therapeutic potential. Molecules, 30(4), 807. doi: 10.3390/molecules30040807.

[33] He, X., Andersson, G., Lindgren, U., & Li, Y. (2010 Oct 22).Resveratrol prevents RANKL-induced osteoclast differentiation of murine osteoclast progenitor RAW 264.7 cells through inhibition of ROS production. Biochemical and Biophysical Research Communicatons, 401(3). 356–62. 1016/j.bbrc.2010.09.053. Epub 2010 Sep 17. PMID: 20851107. doi: 10.

[34] Casati, M. Z., Algayer, C., Cardoso da Cruz, G., Ribeiro, F. V., Casarin, R. C., Pimentel, S. P., & Cirano, F. R. (2013 Oct).Resveratrol decreases periodontal breakdown and modulates local levels of cytokines during periodontitis in rats. Journal of Periodontology, 84(10). e58–64. 1902/jop.2013.120746. Epub 2013 Mar 14. PMID: 23489233. doi: 10.

[35] Cai, Y., Chen, Z., Liu, H., Xuan, Y., Wang, X., & Luan, Q. (2015 Dec). Green tea epigallocatechin-3-gallate alleviates Porphyromonas gingivalis-induced periodontitis in mice. International Immunopharmacology, 29(2), 839–845. 1016/j.intimp.2015.08.033. Epub 2015 Sep 7. PMID: 26359545. doi: 10.

[36] Li, Y., Cheng, L., & Li, M. (2024). Effects of green tea extract Epigallocatechin-3-Gallate on oral diseases: A narrative review. Pathogens, 13(8), 634. doi: 10.3390/pathogens13080634.

[37] Huang, J., & Zhou, Y. (2022). Emerging role of epigenetic regulations in periodontitis: a literature review. American Journal of Translational Research, 14(4), 2162.

[38] Zhang, S., Zhang, L., Wen, R., Yang, N., & Zhang, T. (2024). Histone deacetylases and their inhibitors in inflammatory diseases. Biomedicine and Pharmacotherapy, 179, 117295. doi: 10.1016/j.biopha.2024.117295.

[39] Cantley, M. D., Bartold, P. M., Marino, V., Fairlie, D. P., Le, G. T., Lucke, A. J., & Haynes, D. R. (2011). Histone deacetylase inhibitors and periodontal bone loss. Journal of Periodontal Research, 46(6), 697–703. doi: 10.1111/j.1600-0765.2011.01392.x.

[40] Liu, R., Zhao, E., & Yu, H. et al. (2023). Methylation across the central dogma in health and diseases: new therapeutic strategies. Signal Transduction and Targeted Therapy, 8, 310. doi: 10.1038/s41392-023-01528-y.

[41] Liu, L., Xiao, Z., Ding, W., Wen, C., Ge, C., Xu, K., & Cao, S. (2022). Relationship between microRNA expression and inflammatory factors in patients with both type 2 diabetes mellitus and periodontal disease. American Journal of Translational Research, 14(9), 6627.

[42] Megha, K., Joseph, X., Akhil, V., & Mohanan, P. (2021). Cascade of immune mechanism and consequences of inflammatory disorders. Phytomedicine, 91, 153712. doi: 10.1016/j.phymed.2021.153712.

[43] Fleishmann, R. M. (2002 Sep-Oct). Safety of anakinra, a recombinant interleukin-1 receptor antagonist (r-metHuIL-1ra), in patients with rheumatoid arthritis and comparison to anti-TNF-alpha agents. Clinical and Experimental Rheumatology, 20(5 Suppl 27), S35–41.

[44] Papathanasiou, E., Conti, P., Carinci, F., Lauritano, D., & Theoharides, T. C. (2020). IL-1 superfamily members and periodontal diseases. Journal of Dental Research, doi: 10.1177/0022034520945209.

[45] Steemers, E., Talbi, W. M. I., Hogervorst, J. M. A., Schoenmaker, T., & de Vries, T. J. (2025 Feb 28).IL-1 Receptor Antagonist Anakinra inhibits the effect of IL-1β- Mediated Osteoclast Formation by Periodontal Ligament Fibroblasts. Biology (Basel), 14(3). 250. 3390/biology14030250. doi: 10.

[46] Dinarello, C. A. (2011). Interleukin-1 in the pathogenesis and treatment of inflammatory diseases. Blood, 117(14), 3720. doi: 10.1182/blood-2010-07-273417.

[47] Fatemi, K., Rezaee, S. A., & SA, B. et al. (2020). Importance of MMP-8 in salivary and gingival crevicular fluids of periodontitis patients. Iranian Journal of Immunology, 17(3), 236–243. 22034/iji.2020.81170.1512. doi: 10.

[48] Gonçalves, P. F., Huang, H., & McAninley, S. et al. (2013). Periodontal treatment reduces matrix metalloproteinase levels in localized aggressive periodontitis. Journal of Periodontology, 84(12), 1801–1808. 1902/jop.2013.130002. doi: 10.

[49] Jones, S. A., Scheller, J., & Rose-John, S. (2011). Therapeutic strategies for the clinical blockade of IL-6/gp130 signaling. The Journal of Clinical Investigation, 121(9), 3375. doi: 10.1172/JCI57158.

[50] Axmann, R., Böhm, C., Krönke, G., Zwerina, J., Smolen, J., & Schett, G. (2009 Sep).Inhibition of interleukin-6 receptor directly blocks osteoclast formation in vitro and in vivo. Arthritis & Rheumatology, 60(9). 2747–56. 1002/art.24781. doi: 10.

[51] Klinder, A., Sellin, M., Wolfien, M., Prehn, F., & Bader, R. (2022). Effects of the Interleukin-6 receptor blocker Sarilumab on metabolic activity and differentiation capacity of primary human Osteoblasts. Pharmaceutics, 14(7), 1390. doi: 10.3390/pharmaceutics14071390.

[52] Mazziotta, C., Tognon, M., Martini, F., Torreggiani, E., & Rotondo, J. C. (2023). Probiotics mechanism of action on immune cells and beneficial effects on human health. Cells, 12(1), 184. doi: 10.3390/cells12010184.

[53] Chen, L., Zhang, L., Hua, H., Liu, L., Mao, Y., & Wang, R. (2024). Interactions between toll-like receptors signaling pathway and gut microbiota in host homeostasis. Immunity, Inflammation and Disease, 12(7), e1356. doi: 10.1002/iid3.1356.

[54] Panwar, R. B., Sequeira, R. P., & Clarke, T. B. (2021). Microbiota-mediated protection against antibiotic-resistant pathogens. Genes and Immunity, 22(5), 255–267. doi: 10.1038/s41435-021-00129-5.

[55] Díaz-Dinamarca, D. A., Salazar, M. L., Escobar, D. F., Castillo, B. N., Valdebenito, B., Díaz, P., Manubens, A., Salazar, F., Troncoso, M. F., Lavandero, S., Díaz, J., Becker, M. I., & Vásquez, A. E. (2023). Surface immunogenic protein from Streptococcus agalactiae and Fissurella

latimarginata hemocyanin are TLR4 ligands and activate MyD88- anc TRIF dependent signaling pathways. Frontiers in Immunology, 14, 1186188. doi: 10.3389/fimmu.2023.1186188.

[56] Kuzmich, N. N., Sivak, K. V., Chubarev, V. N., Porozov, Y. B., N., T., & Peri, F. (2017). TLR4 signaling pathway modulators as potential Therapeutics in Inflammation and Sepsis. Vaccines, 5(4), 34. doi: 10.3390/vaccines5040034.

[57] Ney, M., Wipplinger, M., Grossmann, M., Engert, N., Wegner, V. D., & Mosig, A. S. (2023). Short chain fatty acids: key regulators of the local and systemic immune response in inflammatory diseases and infections. Open Biology, 13(3), 230014. doi: 10.1098/rsob.230014.

[58] Facchin, S., Bertin, L., Bonazzi, E., Lorenzon, G., De Barba, C., Barberio, B., Zingone, F., Maniero, D., Scarpa, M., Ruffolo, C., Angriman, I., & Savarino, E. V. (2024). Short-chain fatty acids and human health: From metabolic pathways to current therapeutic implications. Life, 14(5), 559. doi: 10.3390/life14050559.

[59] Babiker, R., Kaddam, L., & Mariod, A. (2022). The role of Gum Arabic as an anti-inflammatory, antioxidant, and immune modulator in COVID-19: a review. Functional Food Sci, 2, 242–57. 31989/ffs.v2i10.1019. doi: 10.

[60] Siednamohammeddeen, N., Badi, R., Mohammeddeen, T., Enan, K., & Amal, S. (2022). The effect of Gum Arabic supplementation on cathelicidin expression in monocyte-derived macrophages in mice. BMC Complementary Medicine and Therapies, 22, 149. 1186/s12906-022-03627-9. doi: 10.

[61] Hashim, N. T., Babiker, R., Rahman, M. M., Chaitanya, N. C., Mohammed, R., Dasnadi, S. P., & Gismalla, B. G. (2024). Gum Arabic as a potential candidate in quorum quenching and treatment of periodontal diseases. Frontiers in Oral Health, 5, 1459254. doi: 10.3389/froh.2024.1459254.

[62] Chopra, A., Bhuvanagiri, G., Natu, K., & Chopra, A. (2024). Role of CRISPR-Cas systems in periodontal disease pathogenesis and potential for periodontal therapy: A review. Molecular Oral Microbiology, 40(1), 1. doi: 10.1111/omi.12483.

[63] Soong Karlson, C. K., Mohd-Noor, S. N., Nolte, N., & Tan, B. C. (2021). CRISPR/dCas9-based systems: Mechanisms and applications in plant sciences. Plants, 10(10), 2055. doi: 10.3390/plants10102055.

[64] Woo, H. N., Cho, Y. J., Tarafder, S., & Lee, C. H. (2021). The recent advances in scaffolds for integrated periodontal regeneration. Bioactive Materials, 6(10), 3328–3342. doi: 10.1016/j.bioactmat.2021.03.012.

[65] Farhang, N., Brunger, J. M., Stover, J. D., Thakore, P. I., Lawrence, B., Guilak, F., Gersbach, C. A., Setton, L. A., & Bowles, R. D. (2017). CRISPR-based Epigenome editing of Cytokine receptors for the promotion of cell survival and tissue deposition in inflammatory environments. Tissue Engineering, Part A:23(15–16), 738. doi: 10.1089/ten.tea.2016.0441.

[66] Jia, S., Liang, R., Chen, J., Liao, S., Lin, J., & Li, W. (2024). Emerging technology has a brilliant future: The CRISPR-Cas system for senescence, inflammation, and cartilage repair in osteoarthritis. Cellular & Molecular Biology Letters, 29, 64. doi: 10.1186/s11658-024-00581-x.

[67] Kim, E. H., Teerdhala, S. V., Padilla, M. S., Joseph, R. A., Li, J. J., Haley, R. M., & Mitchell, M. J. (2024). Lipid nanoparticle-mediated RNA delivery for immune cell modulation. European Journal of Immunology, 54(12), 2451008. doi: 10.1002/eji.202451008.

[68] Tu, Z., Zhong, Y., Hu, H., Shao, D., Haag, R., Schirner, M., Lee, J., Sullenger, B., & Leong, K. W. (2022). Design of therapeutic biomaterials to control inflammation. Nature Reviews, Materials, 7(7), 557. doi: 10.1038/s41578-022-00426-z.

Nallan C. S. K. Chaitanya, Nada Tawfig Hashim,
and Muhammed Mustahsen Rahman

11 Pharmacogenomics in Periodontal Therapy

11.1 Introduction to Pharmacogenomics in Periodontics

Pharmacogenomics, a highly technical science dedicated to probing the complex ways in which individual genetics may influence the response to various drugs, is revolutionizing the entire landscape of personalized medicine [1]. Pharmacogenetics, which has a vital role in dental care, uses information about an individual genome to choose drugs and drug doses that likely to work best for particular individual unique genetic profile – a departure from the one-drug/one-dosage-fits-all approach.

Pharmacoepigenomics target treatment that may reduce or reverse epigenetic effects in diseases. Clinical applications of pharmacoepigenomic interventions have increased and shown promise for treating oral and craniofacial diseases that result from a combination of genomic, metabolic, epigenomic, and environmental factors [2, 3]. An example of progress in which genetic strategies may be particularly valuable is a targeted approach aimed at the tumor suppressor p53 protein that shows promise in sensitizing head and neck cancer stem cells to chemotherapy [4].

In the branch of periodontology, a science in which responses to drug treatments are far too commonly beset with variability; in large measure because of the complex interactions among the genetic inputs and the vast diversity of microbials, pharmacogenomics provides the unprecedented chance to intervene [5, 6]. With this approach, clinicians are able to create pharmacological interventions exactly tailored to the unique individual patient genotype profile [7, 8]. Through the use of this focused strategy, we are in a position to drastically enhance the effectiveness of medicine, reduce adverse effects, and achieve more certain clinical outcomes that are ultimately of greater benefit to the patients [8]. As precision periodontics becomes increasingly evolved, the incorporation of knowledge extracted through the use of pharmacogenomics into the process of clinical decision-making represents a step-change. It is a profound departure from empiricism and a move toward molecular-based, evidence-based approaches [9].

https://doi.org/10.1515/9783112219904-011

11.2 Antibiotic Metabolism and Host-Microbial Interactions

Genetic factors influence the pharmacodynamics and pharmacokinetics of antibiotics used for the treatment of periodontitis [10]. Genetic variation in the SLCO1B1 gene, coding for hepatic drug transport, governs the systemic clearance of macrolide drugs such as azithromycin [11, 12]. Variation in the CYP3A5 gene causes variation in the metabolism of antibiotics and their effectiveness [13]. Genetic polymorphisms within host defense-regulatory genes, such as *IL1B* and *TLR4*, exert a profound influence on the colonization patterns of periodontal microorganisms and the immune-inflammatory response that governs disease progression and therapeutic outcomes [14]. Variants in these genes can modulate cytokine expression, toll-like receptor sensitivity, and downstream signaling cascades, ultimately altering the host's ability to recognize and eliminate pathogens effectively [15]. This genetic predisposition not only affects the baseline microbial composition but also shapes the efficacy of adjunctive antimicrobial therapies [16, 17]. Emerging evidence suggests that such host genetic factors may interact with microbial genomic adaptations to promote antibiotic resistance by creating an ecological niche favoring resistant strains [18]. For instance, chronic inflammation driven by hyperactive *IL1B* alleles can enhance biofilm resilience and reduce antibiotic penetration, facilitating the persistence of keystone pathogens such as *Porphyromonas gingivalis* (*P. gingivalis*) [19, 20].

Pharmacogenomics is now emerging as a powerful tool to personalize periodontal therapy by integrating the individual genetic background with drug metabolism and microbial resistance profiles [6]. Variations in genes encoding drug-metabolizing enzymes (e.g., CYP450 family) and drug transporters (e.g., ABC transporters) can influence the pharmacokinetics and bioavailability of commonly prescribed antibiotics such as amoxicillin or metronidazole, leading to suboptimal therapeutic outcomes or unintended microbial shifts [21, 22]. Furthermore, genetic factors affecting host immunity may indirectly drive selective pressure on microbial communities, accelerating the emergence of resistant phenotypes [23]. By combining pharmacogenomic screening with microbial susceptibility testing, clinicians can identify the most effective drug regimens and dosages for individual patients while minimizing resistance development [24]. Future approaches may involve the integration of multi-omics platforms, where host genetics, microbial genomics, and metabolomic profiles are jointly analyzed to predict antibiotic efficacy, reduce collateral damage to commensal flora, and enhance the precision of adjunct antimicrobial strategies in periodontal care.

11.3 Host Modulation Therapy and Genetic Determinants

Host modulation therapy represents a significant approach that is aimed directly at controlling and managing the underlying inflammatory pathways within the disease process, as opposed to simply treating the microbial insult alone [25]. One such example of this novel approach includes the application of sub-antimicrobial dose doxycycline, which plays a fundamental role in the inhibition of matrix metalloproteinases (MMPs); these enzymes are key players in both tissue remodeling and inflammation [26]. It is important to note that the metabolism of doxycycline can be affected by genetic polymorphisms within the CYP3A4 and CYP2D6 genes, which can have potentially profound effects on both its bioavailability and overall efficacy in terms of therapeutic effect [27]. Aside from these metabolic issues, genetic variations that arise within cytokine-related genes, such as TNFA and IL-6, can have a significant impact on the severity of the inflammatory response, which in turn influences the extent of benefits that may be derived from the use of immunomodulatory agents [28]. Moreover, in the case of biologics that are engineered to act against proinflammatory molecules like TNF-α or IL-6, the patient's specific genetic polymorphisms in the relevant genes could have a central role in determining not only the degree to which the pa-

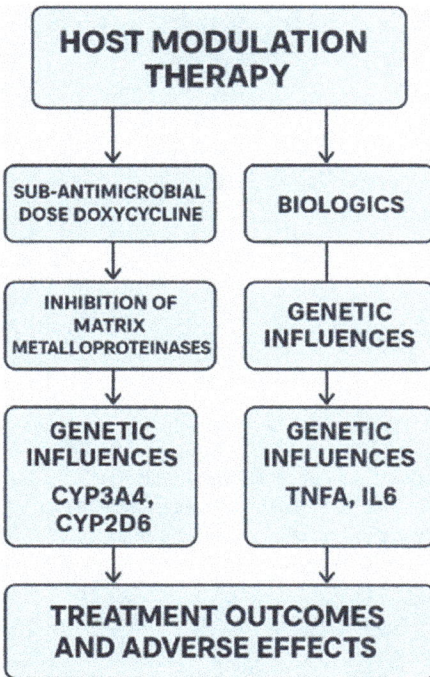

Figure 11.1: Host modulation therapy in periodontitis. Approaches include sub-antimicrobial dose doxycycline, biologics, and genetic influences. Doxycycline inhibits matrix metalloproteinases, while biologics target cytokines such as TNF-α and IL-6. Genetic polymorphisms (CYP3A4, CYP2D6) influence drug metabolism and treatment outcomes, highlighting variability in efficacy and adverse effects.

tient responds to therapy but also the respective risk profiles for the development of adverse effects [29–31] (Figure 11.1).

11.4 Genetic Variability in NSAID Response

Nonsteroidal anti-inflammatory drugs (NSAIDs) are important pharmacological agents in the treatment of periodontal diseases, alleviating pain and inflammation [32]. However, variability in individual response to NSAIDs is significantly influenced by polymorphisms in the metabolic enzymes, especially those belonging to the cytochrome P450 family [33]. Polymorphisms in the CYP2C9 and CYP2C8 genes can alter the metabolic breakdown of NSAIDs like ibuprofen and celecoxib. Poor metabolizers could exhibit increased plasma levels, thus posing a risk for gastrointestinal or renal toxicity, while rapid metabolizers could fail to achieve the desired therapeutic concentrations [34] (Figure 11.2). Additionally, polymorphisms in PTGS2, which codes for the COX-2 enzyme, affect the anti-inflammatory efficacy of selective COX-2 inhibitors, highlighting the need for genotype-guided NSAID prescriptions [35, 36].

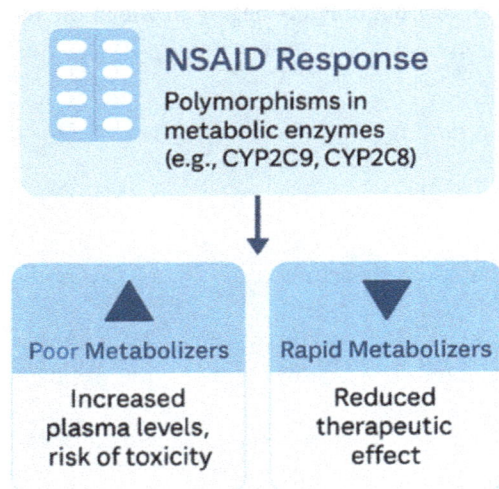

NSAID Response
Polymorphisms in
metabolic enzymes
(e.g., CYP2C9, CYP2C8)

▲
Poor Metabolizers
Increased
plasma levels,
risk of toxicity

▼
Rapid Metabolizers
Reduced
therapeutic
effect

Figure 11.2: Pharmacogenomic influence on NSAID response in periodontitis. Polymorphisms in metabolic enzymes (CYP2C9 and CYP2C8) alter drug metabolism. Poor metabolizers experience higher plasma levels and risk of toxicity, whereas rapid metabolizers show reduced therapeutic effect, underscoring the need for personalized NSAID therapy.

11.5 Adverse Drug Reactions and the Genetic Risk Factors That Contribute to Them

Pharmacogenomics, which is fundamentally the examination and research into the way in which genes affect and contribute to the reaction of the individual to medicines, has a vital and extremely important role not just in the prediction but even in the active prevention of dangerous and debilitating adverse drug reactions [6] (Figure 11.3). As an example, patients with the HLA-B*58:01 allele, for example, have been shown to display a considerably increased risk for developing hypersensitivity to the drug allopurinol, a drug that has been the subject of extensive study for its antioxidant activity, especially in the course of periodontal treatment [37, 38]. Similarly, a deficiency in the presence of the enzyme thiopurine methyltransferase (TPMT), as a direct outcome of certain varieties of the respective gene, puts the individuals bearing this deficiency at considerable risk for myelosuppression following the administration of azathioprine, a drug that is, at times, used for immune-mediated periodontal disorders [39]. Identifying and recognizing these genetic hazards ahead of time allow healthcare professionals to take preventive steps to steer clear of prescribing potentially toxic medicines, and this enhances the safety of patients and overall medical outcomes considerably.

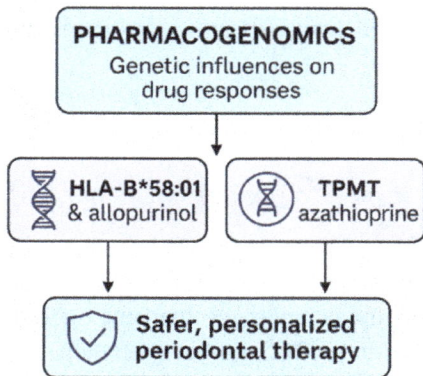

Figure 11.3: Pharmacogenomics in periodontal therapy. Genetic variations such as HLA-B*58:01 (linked to allopurinol hypersensitivity) and TPMT polymorphisms (affecting azathioprine metabolism) influence drug responses. Incorporating pharmacogenomic testing enables safer, personalized periodontal therapy.

11.6 Biomarker-Guided Therapeutic Stratification

The interaction between crevicular and salivary biomarkers and pharmacogenomics generates new paradigms for monitoring and stratification of treatment [40]. Patients with the IL1 composite genotype incorporating polymorphisms in IL1A and IL1B have elevated inflammatory indices at baseline and reduced response to conventional care [41]. High levels of MMPs, IL-6, or miR-146a in patients with this genotype may be a sign for adjunctive early treatment or prolonged maintenance [42–44]. The incorporation of genotypic data with real-time biomarker measurement has the capacity for a dynamic, personalized approach to modifying the therapy for optimal outcomes.

11.7 Future Perspectives and the Translation into Clinical Practice

Although the use of pharmacogenomics in the field of periodontology is currently in its early developmental stages, there is a sizeable and continually expanding repository of active research activity [6]. Furthermore, there are new clinical tools being developed and tested actively to seamlessly close the translational divide that has emerged in this domain. The advent of new point-of-care genotyping platforms, the incorporation of comprehensive genetic data into electronic health records, and the use of artificial intelligence for augmenting clinical decision-making processes are all critical phenomena currently driving and shaping the future of personalized medicine in the field of periodontology [45–47]. Furthermore, the routine incorporation of pharmacogenomic screening methods is expected to become a standard integral part of a comprehensive and extensive periodontal assessment in the not too distant future. Such a development would enable clinicians to take more informed, risk-adjusted, and patient-specified therapeutic decisions tailored to individual patient circumstances and requirements.

11.8 Conclusion

Pharmacogenomics offers an incredibly promising and exciting avenue whereby the precision and predictability of periodontal treatment can be dramatically increased and refined to new heights. By fully explaining the complex mechanisms through which multiple genetic polymorphisms manifest their effects on the metabolism of drugs, therapeutic response, and the profiles of possible side effects, clinicians will be in a position to move toward genuinely individualized treatment strategies that are precisely suited to address each patient's distinctive genetic profile. As scientific knowledge in this key field continues to grow and technology proceeds at a breathtaking rate, pharmacogenomics will certainly take its place as a keystone foundation in the advancement of periodontics. This change will signal a move away from the empiric care regimens of the past and toward a framework of evidence-based customization in the management of individual patients.

References

[1]   Sadee, W., Wang, D., Hartmann, K., & Toland, A. E. (2023). Pharmacogenomics: Driving personalized medicine. Pharmacological Reviews, 75(4). 789. https://doi.org/10.1124/pharmrev.122.000810.

[2]   Teijido, O., & Cacabelos, R. (2018). Pharmacoepigenomic interventions as novel potential treatments for Alzheimer's and Parkinson's diseases. International Journal of Molecular Sciences, 19(10). 3199.

[3]   Jones, P. A., Ohtani, H., Chakravarthy, A., & De Carvalho, D. D. (2019). Epigenetic therapy in immune-oncology. Nature Reviews Cancer, 19(3). 151–161.

[4]   Rodriguez-Ramirez, C., & Nör, J. E. (2018). p53 and cell fate: sensitizing head and neck cancer stem cells to chemotherapy. Critical Reviews in Oncogenesis, 23(3–4). 173–187.

[5]   Loos, B. G., & Van Dyke, T. E. (2020). The role of inflammation and genetics in periodontal disease. Periodontology 2000, 83(1). 26. https://doi.org/10.1111/prd.12297.

[6]   Oates, J., & Lopez, D. (2018). Pharmacogenetics: An important part of drug development with a focus on its application. International Journal of Biomedical Investigation, 1(2). 111. https://doi.org/10.31531/2581-4745.1000111.

[7]   Hashim, N. T., Babiker, R., Priya, S. P., Mohammed, R., Chaitanya, N. C., Padmanabhan, V., El Bahra, S., Rahman, M. M., & Gismalla, B. G. (2024). Microbial dynamics in periodontal regeneration: Understanding microbiome shifts and the role of antifouling and bactericidal materials: A narrative review. Current Issues in Molecular Biology, 46(11). 12196–12213. https://doi.org/10.3390/cimb46110724.

[8]   Hippman, C., & Nislow, C. (2019). Pharmacogenomic testing: Clinical evidence and implementation challenges. Journal of Personalized Medicine, 9(3). 40. https://doi.org/10.3390/jpm9030040.

[9]   Rakic, M., Pejcic, N., Perunovic, N., & Vojvodic, D. (2021). A roadmap towards precision periodontics. Medicina, 57(3). 233. https://doi.org/10.3390/medicina57030233.

[10] Kapoor, A., Malhotra, R., Grover, V., & Grover, D. (2012). Systemic antibiotic therapy in periodontics. Dental Research Journal, 9(5). 505. https://doi.org/10.4103/1735-3327.104866.

[11] Principi, N., Petropulacos, K., & Esposito, S. (2024). Genetic variations and antibiotic-related adverse events. Pharmaceuticals, 17(3). 331. https://doi.org/10.3390/ph17030331.

[12] Ramsey, L. B., Gong, L., Wagner, J. B., Zhou, X., Sangkuhl, K., Adams, S. M., Straka, R. J., Empey, P. E., Boone, E. C., Klein, T. E., Niemi, M., & Gaedigk, A. (2022). PharmVar GeneFocus: SLCO1B1. Clinical Pharmacology and Therapeutics, 113(4). 782. https://doi.org/10.1002/cpt.2705.

[13] Zhang, Y., Wang, Z., Wang, Y., Jin, W., Zhang, Z., Jin, L., Qian, J., & Zheng, L. (2024). CYP3A4 and CYP3A5: The crucial roles in clinical drug metabolism and the significant implications of genetic polymorphisms. PeerJ, 12, e18636. https://doi.org/10.7717/peerj.18636.

[14] Ferrara, E., D'Albenzio, A., Rapone, B., Mastrocola, F., & Murmura, G. (2025). Genetic polymorphisms associated with periodontitis in Japanese populations: A comprehensive review of pathways, interactions, and clinical implications. Infection, Genetics and Evolution, 133, 105781. https://doi.org/10.1016/j.meegid.2025.105781.

[15] Li, W., Cao, X., He, L., Meng, H., Yang, B., & Liao, Y. (2019). TLR4 polymorphisms may increase susceptibility to periodontitis in Pg-positive individuals. PeerJ, 7, e7823. https://doi.org/10.7717/peerj.7828.

[16] Haubek, D., Ennibi, O., Poulsen, K., Væth, M., Poulsen, S., & Kilian, M. (2008). Risk of aggressive periodontitis in adolescent carriers of the JP2 clone of Aggregatibacter (Actinobacillus) actinomycetemcomitans in Morocco: A prospective longitudinal cohort study. The Lancet, 371(9608). 237–242. https://doi.org/10.1016/S0140-6736(08)60135-X.

[17] Laforgia, A., Inchingolo, A. D., Piras, F., Colonna, V., Giorgio, R. V., Carone, C., Rapone, B., Malcangi, G., Inchingolo, A. M., Inchingolo, F., Palermo, A., & Dipalma, G. (2024). Therapeutic strategies and genetic implications for periodontal disease management: A systematic review. International Journal of Molecular Sciences, 25(13). 7217. https://doi.org/10.3390/ijms25137217.

[18] Łasica, A., Golec, P., Laskus, A., Zalewska, M., Gędaj, M., & Popowska, M. (2024). Periodontitis: Etiology, conventional treatments, and emerging bacteriophage and predatory bacteria therapies. Frontiers in Microbiology, 15, 1469414. https://doi.org/10.3389/fmicb.2024.1469414.

[19] Uruén, C., Chopo-Escuin, G., Tommassen, J., Mainar-Jaime, R. C., & Arenas, J. (2020). Biofilms as promoters of bacterial antibiotic resistance and tolerance. Antibiotics, 10(1). 3. https://doi.org/10.3390/antibiotics10010003.

[20] Hajishengallis, G., Darveau, R. P., & Curtis, M. A. (2012). The keystone pathogen hypothesis. Nature Reviews. Microbiology, 10(10). 717. https://doi.org/10.1038/nrmicro2873.

[21] Ahmed, S., Zhou, Z., Zhou, J., & Chen, Q. (2016). Pharmacogenomics of drug metabolizing enzymes and transporters: Relevance to precision medicine. Genomics, Proteomics & Bioinformatics, 14(5). 298. https://doi.org/10.1016/j.gpb.2016.03.008.

[22] Pinto, N., & Dolan, M. E. (2011). Clinically relevant genetic variations in drug metabolizing enzymes. Current Drug Metabolism, 12(5). 487. https://doi.org/10.2174/138920011795495321.

[23] Gomez, A., Espinoza, J. L., Harkins, D. M., Leong, P., Saffery, R., Bockmann, M., Torralba, M., Kuelbs, C., Kodukula, R., Inman, J., Hughes, T., Craig, J. M., Highlander, S. K., Jones, M. B., Dupont, C. L., & Nelson, K. E. (2017). Host Genetic control of the oral microbiome in health and disease. Cell Host & Microbe, 22(3). 269. https://doi.org/10.1016/j.chom.2017.08.013.

[24] Qahwaji, R., Ashankyty, I., Sannan, N. S., Hazzazi, M. S., Basabrain, A. A., & Mobashir, M. (2024). Pharmacogenomics: A genetic approach to drug development and therapy. Pharmaceuticals, 17(7). 940. https://doi.org/10.3390/ph17070940.

[25] Golub, L. M., Lee, M., Bacigalupo, J., & Gu, Y. (2024). Host modulation therapy in periodontitis, diagnosis and treatment – status update. Frontiers in Dental Medicine, 5, 1423401. https://doi.org/10.3389/fdmed.2024.1423401.

[26] Lee, H. M., Ciancio, S. G., Tüter, G., Ryan, M. E., Komaroff, E., & Golub, L. M. (2004 Mar). Subantimicrobial dose doxycycline efficacy as a matrix metalloproteinase inhibitor in chronic periodontitis patients is enhanced when combined with a non-steroidal anti-inflammatory drug. Journal of Periodontology, 75(3), 453–463. doi: 10.1902/jop.2004.75.3.453.

[27] Saiz-Rodríguez, M., Almenara, S., Navares-Gómez, M., Ochoa, D., Román, M., Zubiaur, P., Koller, D., Santos, M., Mejía, G., Borobia, A. M., Rodríguez-Antona, C., & Abad-Santos, F. (2020). Effect of the most relevant CYP3A4 and CYP3A5 polymorphisms on the pharmacokinetic parameters of 10 CYP3A substrates. Biomedicines, 8(4). 94. https://doi.org/10.3390/biomedicines8040094.

[28] Neurath, N., & Kesting, M. (2024). Cytokines in gingivitis and periodontitis: from pathogenesis to therapeutic targets. Frontiers in Immunology, 15, 1435054. https://doi.org/10.3389/fimmu.2024.1435054.

[29] Scheller, J., Chalaris, A., Schmidt-Arras, D., & Rose-John, S. (2011). The pro- and anti-inflammatory properties of the cytokine interleukin-6. Biochimica et Biophysica Acta (BBA) – Molecular Cell Research, 1813(5). 878–888. https://doi.org/10.1016/j.bbamcr.2011.01.034.

[30] Zlendić, M., Vrbanović Đuričić, E., Gall Trošelj, K., Tomljanović, M., Vuković Đerfi, K., & Alajbeg, I. Z. (2023). Genetic influences of proinflammatory cytokines on pain severity in patients with temporomandibular disorders. International Journal of Molecular Sciences, 25(16). 8730. https://doi.org/10.3390/ijms25168730.

[31] Mlachkova, A., Kotsilkov, K., & Maynalovska, H. (2025). The multifaceted role of IL-35 in periodontal disease and beyond: From genetic polymorphisms to biomarker potential. Genes, 16(8). 891. https://doi.org/10.3390/genes16080891.

[32] Ren, J., Fok, M. R., Zhang, Y., Han, B., & Lin, Y. (2023). The role of non-steroidal anti-inflammatory drugs as adjuncts to periodontal treatment and in periodontal regeneration. Journal of Translational Medicine, 21, 149. https://doi.org/10.1186/s12967-023-03990-2.

[33] Krasniqi, V., Dimovski, A., Domjanović, I. K., Bilić, I., & Božina, N. (2016 Mar). How polymorphisms of the cytochrome P450 genes affect ibuprofen and diclofenac metabolism and toxicity. Arh Hig Rada Toksikol, 67(1), 1–8. doi: 10.1515/aiht-2016-67-2754.

[34] Bagher, A. M. (2023). Association of CYP2C9*3 and CYP2C8*3 non-functional alleles with Ibuprofen-induced upper gastrointestinal toxicity in a Saudi patient. Case Reports in Medicine, 2023, 6623269. https://doi.org/10.1155/2023/6623269.

[35] Makar, K. W., Poole, E. M., Resler, A. J., Seufert, B., Curtin, K., Kleinstein, S. E., Duggan, D., Kulmacz, R. J., Hsu, L., Whitton, J., Carlson, C. S., Rimorin, C. F., Caan, B. J., Baron, J. A., Potter, J. D., Slattery, M. L., & Ulrich, C. M. (2013). COX-1 (PTGS1) and COX-2 (PTGS2) polymorphisms, NSAID interactions, and risk of colon and rectal cancer in two independent populations. Cancer Causes & Control: CCC, 24(12). 2059. https://doi.org/10.1007/s10552-013-0282-1.

[36] Domiati, S., & Ghoneim, A. (2015). Celecoxib for the right person at the right dose and right time: An updated overview. Springer Science Reviews, 3, 137–140. https://doi.org/10.1007/s40362-015-0034-6.

[37] Chong, H. Y., Lim, Y. H., Prawjaeng, J., & Tassaneeyakul, W. et al. (2018). Cost-effectiveness analysis of HLA-B*58: 01 genetic testing before initiation of allopurinol therapy to prevent allopurinol-induced Stevens-Johnson syndrome/toxic epidermal necrolysis in a Malaysian population. Pharmacogenet Genomics, 28(2). 56–67.

[38] Low, D. E., Nurul-Aain, A. F., Tan, W. C., & Tang, J. J. et al. (2020). HLA-B*58: 01 association in allopurinol-induced severe cutaneous adverse reactions: the implication of ethnicity and clinical phenotypes in multiethnic Malaysia. Pharmacogenet Genomics, 30(7). 153–160.

[39] Colombel, J. F., Ferrari, N., Debuysere, H., Marteau, P., Gendre, J. P., Bonaz, B., Soulé, J. C., Modigliani, R., Touze, Y., Catala, P., Libersa, C., & Broly, F. (2000 Jun) Genotypic analysis of thiopurine S-methyltransferase in patients with Crohn's disease and severe myelosuppression during azathioprine therapy. Gastroenterology, 118(6), 1025–1030, doi: 10.1016/s0016-5085(00)70354-4.

[40] Lauschke, V. M., Milani, L., & Ingelman-Sundberg, M. (2018). Pharmacogenomic biomarkers for improved drug therapy – recent progress and future developments AAPS Journal, 20(4), https://doi.org/10.1208/s12248-017-0161-x.

[41] Huynh-Ba, G., Lang, N. P., Tonetti, M. S., & Salvi, G. E. (2007 Apr). The association of the composite IL-1 genotype with periodontitis progression and/or treatment outcomes: A systematic review. Journal of Clinical Periodontology, 34(4), 305–317, doi: 10.1111/j.1600-051X.2007.01055.x.

[42] Sattari, M., Taheri, R. A., ArefNezhad, R., & Motedayyen, H. (2021). The expression levels of MicroRNA-146a, RANKL and OPG after non-surgical periodontal treatment. BMC Oral Health, 21, 523. https://doi.org/10.1186/s12903-021-01883-8.

[43] Fumimoto, C., Yamauchi, N., Imai, K., Nakamura, Y., Azuma, H., Kato, H., Taguchi, Y., & Umeda, M. (2024). The role of miR-146a in the anti-inflammatory and antioxidant effects of Shikonin on Gingival Fibroblasts. Applied Sciences, 15(4). 2019. https://doi.org/10.3390/app15042019.

[44] Zhao, L., Zhou, Y., Xu, Y., Sun, Y., Li, L., & Chen, W. (2011). Effect of non-surgical periodontal therapy on the levels of Th17/Th1/Th2 cytokines and their transcription factors in Chinese chronic periodontitis patients. Journal of Clinical Periodontology, 38(6). 509–516. https://doi.org/10.1111/j.1600-051X.2011.01712.x.

[45] Mendez, K. M., Reinke, S. N., Kelly, R. S., Chen, Q., Su, M., McGeachie, M., Weiss, S., Broadhurst, D. I., & Lasky-Su, J. A. (2025). A roadmap to precision medicine through post-genomic electronic medical records. Nature Communications, 16, 1700. https://doi.org/10.1038/s41467-025-56442-4.

[46] Marques, L., Costa, B., Pereira, M., Silva, A., Santos, J., Saldanha, L., Silva, I., Magalhães, P., Schmidt, S., & Vale, N. (2024). Advancing precision medicine: A review of innovative in Silico approaches for

drug development. Clinical Pharmacology and Personalized Healthcare. Pharmaceutics, 16(3). 332. https://doi.org/10.3390/pharmaceutics16030332.

[47] Rehm, H. L., Page, A. J., Smith, L., Adams, J. B., Alterovitz, G., Babb, L. J., Barkley, M. P., Baudis, M., Beauvais, M. J., Beck, T., Beckmann, J. S., Beltran, S., Bernick, D., Bernier, A., Bonfield, J. K., Boughtwood, T. F., Bourque, G., Bowers, S. R., Brookes, A. J., & Birney, E. (2021). GA4GH: International policies and standards for data sharing across genomic research and healthcare. Cell Genomics, 1(2). 100029. https://doi.org/10.1016/j.xgen.2021.100029.

Vivek Padmanabhan and Nada Tawfig Hashim

12 Enhancing Patient Safety in Periodontal Treatment

12.1 Introduction

Patient safety during periodontal therapy extends beyond preventing procedural accidents and complications to encompass a broader scope [1]. The safety approach encompasses multiple dimensions which thoroughly address drug stewardship and surgical care attention and infection control measures and advanced technology integration and patient-centered care practices [2] (Figure 12.1). In the field of periodontology, treatment is often an array of advanced and complicated procedures that may range from flap surgery, regenerative grafting procedures, placement of dental implants, to the administration of drugs either systemically or locally [3–7]. This chapter is dedicated to addressing contemporary approaches that are employed, comprehensive safety guidelines that are available, and the innovative advances that synergistically function to significantly minimize risks and thus optimize overall treatment efficacy in the practice of periodontal therapy.

12.2 Risk Assessment and Stratification

The foundation of safety begins with conducting thorough patient assessments [8, 9]. A complete medical and dental history requires information about diabetes mellitus, cardiovascular disease, bleeding disorders, anticoagulant and bisphosphonate medications, smoking and alcohol consumption, and stress levels [10]. The American Society of Anesthesiologists (ASA) classification and individualized periodontal risk calculators, including the Lang and Tonetti model, help healthcare providers determine patient risk levels for surgical and systemic complications [11, 12] (Table 12.1). The assessment process becomes more accurate and specific when multiple salivary and genetic biomarkers, including IL-1β, CRP, and matrix metalloproteinase-8 (MMP-8), are integrated at the beginning [13].

12.3 Infection Control and Antimicrobial Stewardship

Given the polymicrobial and biofilm-mediated nature of periodontal infection, indiscriminate use of broad-spectrum antibiotics obviously constitutes a significant patient

https://doi.org/10.1515/9783112219904-012

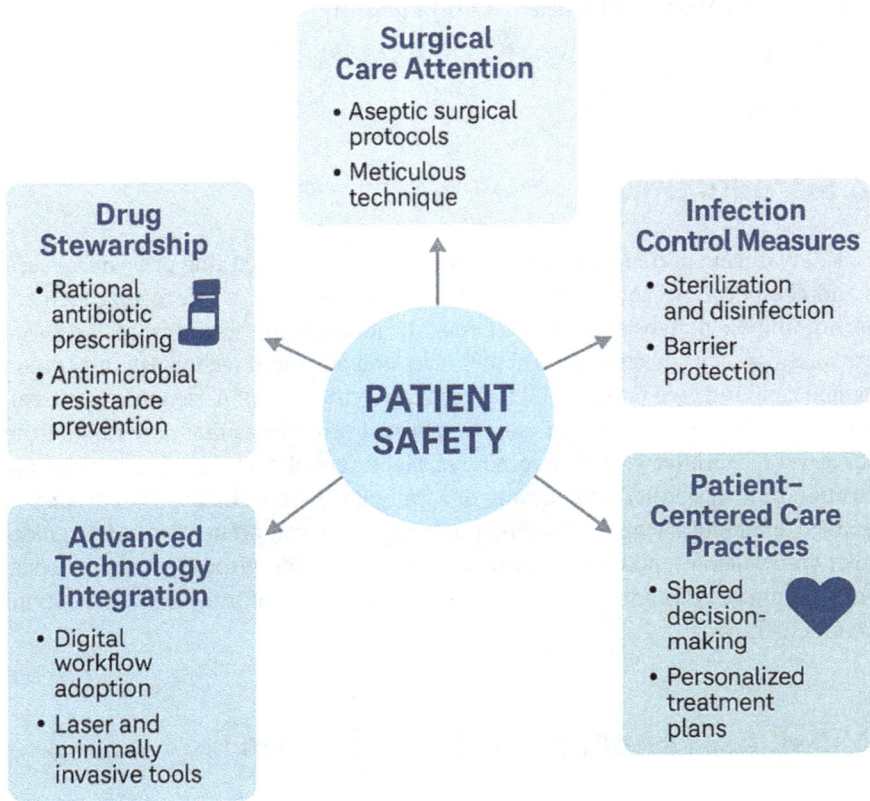

Figure 12.1: Key pillars of patient safety in periodontology. Core elements include drug stewardship (rational prescribing and resistance prevention), advanced technology integration (digital workflow and laser innovations), surgical care attention (aseptic protocols and meticulous technique), infection control measures (sterilization and barrier protection), and patient-centered care practices (shared decision-making and personalized treatment).

Table 12.1: A summary of two widely used clinical tools for evaluating patient risk: The ASA classification, which assesses systemic health and perioperative risk, and the Lang and Tonetti model, which stratifies periodontal disease risk based on clinical, systemic, and behavioral factors.

Tool	Purpose	Scope	Key features
ASA classification (American Society of Anesthesiologists)	Systemic risk stratification	General medical condition assessment	Ranges from ASA I (healthy) to ASA VI (brain-dead organ donor); helps assess surgical and anesthesia-related risk
Lang and Tonetti Periodontal Risk Assessment Model	Periodontal risk stratification	Dental and periodontal history	Factors include pocket depth, bleeding on probing, tooth loss, systemic conditions (e.g., diabetes), and environmental factors (e.g., smoking)

Both models guide tailored treatment planning and risk mitigation in periodontal care.

safety issue [14]. Excessive use of systemic antibiotics is a major driver of the global issue of antimicrobial resistance, in addition to causing the delicate balance of the oral and gut microbiome to be disrupted [15]. This, in turn, has the potential to result in the emergence of opportunistic infections, induce dysbiosis, and create long-term systemic health consequences [15]. Therefore, as a step toward enhancing patient safety in periodontal therapy, it becomes essential that we shift our focus to precision-based antimicrobial treatments [16]. One such innovative and efficient method in dentistry is the utilization of sophisticated microbial DNA analysis tests, for example, qPCR-based testing. The sophisticated approach facilitates targeted antimicrobial treatment by accurately identifying individual periodontal pathogens responsible for periodontal disease, which include *Porphyromonas gingivalis* (*P. gingivalis*), *Aggregatibacter actinomycetemcomitans* (*A. actinomycetemcomitans*), and *Tannerella forsythia* (*T. forsythia*) [17, 18]. Through the provision of this critical diagnostic insight, clinicians are in a position to prescribe narrow-spectrum antibiotics only when they are truly required, and this, in turn, translates to immense decrease in unnecessary utilization of broad-spectrum antibiotics that would otherwise result in resistance [19]. Furthermore, local delivery systems of antimicrobials such as doxycycline hyclate gels and minocycline microspheres yield high-dose, site-specific therapy with low-systemic absorption.

These drugs are most effective when administered adjunctively in periodontal pockets after debridement or surgical treatment. They not only increase microbial control but also augment clinical results such as pocket reduction and attachment gain with systemic safety [20, 21].

In addition, the rigid compliance with stringent infection control guidelines is strictly non-negotiable in the surgical treatment of periodontal disease [22]. It is of paramount value that there is complete adherence to the set standards promulgated by the CDC and OSHA including proper instrument sterilization, careful utilization of PPE, and careful maintenance of a sterile field [23–25]. This adherence is particularly imperative during regeneration procedures and implant placements, as any contamination of these delicate procedures risks markedly detracting from osseointegration and the general wound healing.

One of the newer techniques that is gaining significant traction and is proving to be more and more beneficial in this specific setting is laser-assisted periodontal therapy. Lasers utilized for dental treatment, i.e., Er:YAG, or erbium-doped yttrium aluminum garnet, and Nd:YAG, or neodymium-doped yttrium aluminum garnet, present a wide array of benefits [26, 27]. These advanced laser systems are capable of performing soft tissue ablation and pocket decontamination, and they also exhibit quite remarkable antimicrobial properties. They achieve this by effectively disrupting the complex structure of the bacterial biofilm that has a tendency to form in periodontal pockets, ultimately leading to a remarkable reduction in the total bacterial burden in these locations [28]. Furthermore, research has established that laser therapy effectively minimizes collateral tissue damage, reduces postoperative pain, and enhances wound healing. It is, therefore, a safer and useful adjunctive treatment in the nonsurgical and surgical treatment of periodontal diseases [29, 30].

Together, these carefully coordinated strategies encourage the development of a safer, evidence-based protocol for periodontal therapy (Figure 12.2). The approach not only honors the sophistication of microbial communities but also assists in ensuring patient health protection and achievement of acceptable therapeutic results.

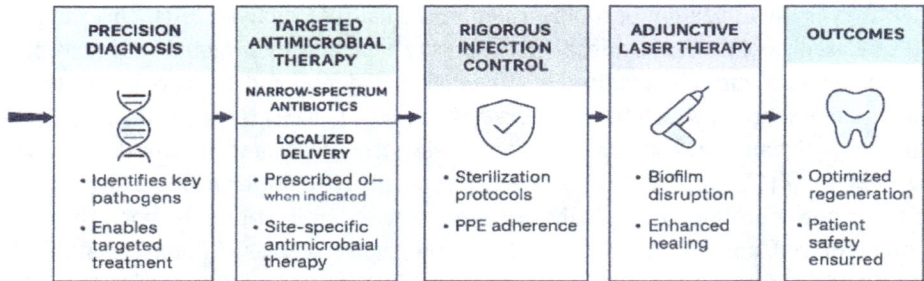

Figure 12.2: Integrated periodontal treatment pathway. Precision diagnosis identifies pathogens and enables targeted therapy. Antimicrobial therapy is tailored through narrow-spectrum antibiotics and site-specific delivery. Rigorous infection control ensures sterilization and PPE adherence. Adjunctive laser therapy aids in biofilm disruption and enhanced healing. The outcome is optimized regeneration with patient safety ensured.

12.4 Pharmacological Considerations and Drug Safety

The use of **NSAIDs** for postoperative pain management in periodontics has been extensive but their ability to block prostaglandin synthesis through COX-1 and COX-2 pathways interferes with healing processes and interacts with cardiovascular medications [31]. The safer options for pain management include acetaminophen with controlled dosing to minimize systemic side effects and celecoxib as a selective COX-2 inhibitor for patients with low cardiac risk [32, 33]. Preoperative povidone-iodine or chlorhexidine rinses are generally recommended to reduce microbial load without promoting resistance [34]. For regenerative treatments, clinicians are now favoring the use of platelet-rich fibrin with biologic agents such as enamel matrix derivatives and recombinant growth factors like rhPDGF-BB. The reason for such a trend is mainly to promote healing in a nonsystemic immunosuppressive way, as is common with corticosteroid use [35].

In the patient who has received head and neck radiation, especially doses in excess of 50–60 Gy, there is a great risk for the development of osteoradionecrosis (ORN) due to compromised vascularity and imperfect remodeling of the bone [36].

Periodontal procedures like extractions, flap surgeries, and implant placement can potentially start bone necrosis in such patients. Hence, meticulous preradiation dental assessment is necessary so that teeth that are nonrestorable or of poor prognosis can be removed before the start of therapy [37]. After radiation, invasive procedures must be avoided whenever feasible, and when unavoidable, must be performed prophylactically with antibiotics, atraumatically, and in consultation with the patient's oncologist or radiation specialist [38].

Similarly, patients receiving bisphosphonate (oral or IV) or denosumab are in danger of developing medication-related osteonecrosis of the jaw (MRONJ), particularly after invasive periodontal surgery. It is heightened with intravenous preparations, prolonged drug treatment, or concomitant corticosteroid therapy [39, 40]. Prior to initiating such drugs, patients should undergo rigorous periodontal evaluation and required dental treatment to stabilize the oral cavity. In patients already receiving therapy, nonsurgical periodontal treatment is optimal, and surgeries must be postponed carefully [41]. Drug holidays are contentious and must be decided in consultation with the treating doctor, especially as bisphosphonates exhibit prolonged half-lives in bone. To mitigate these risks, periodontists must implement [42, 43]:

- extensive medical history evaluations to identify high-risk patients;
- radiologic and clinical tests to evaluate bone density and vascular health;
- minimally invasive techniques and antimicrobial protocols use;
- interdisciplinary collaboration with oncologists, hematologists, and pharmacists for the planning of procedures safely.

Patient education regarding the risks and early signs of ORN and MRONJ, including exposed bone, persistent pain, and delayed wound healing, is essential to facilitate prompt reporting and timely intervention (Table 12.2). Integrating these considerations into clinical guidelines ensures that the unique vulnerabilities of oncology patients and those receiving antiresorptive therapy are appropriately addressed, thereby significantly enhancing patient safety during periodontal treatment [44].

Table 12.2: Considerations and management strategies for patients at risk of medication-related osteonecrosis of the jaw (MRONJ).

Aspect	Details
High-risk medications	– Bisphosphonates (oral and intravenous) – Denosumab – Antiangiogenic agents
Risk factors	– Intravenous administration – Prolonged duration of therapy – Concomitant corticosteroid use – Pre-existing periodontal or periapical infection

Table 12.2 (continued)

Aspect	Details
Pretreatment measures	– Comprehensive periodontal and dental evaluation – Radiographic assessment to detect pathology – Completion of extractions or necessary invasive treatments before initiation of antiresorptive therapy
Management during therapy	– Emphasis on nonsurgical periodontal treatment (scaling and root planning) – Avoid elective invasive procedures whenever possible – Employ minimally invasive surgical techniques if surgery is unavoidable
Drug holiday considerations	– Controversial: decisions individualized in consultation with the prescribing physician – Not uniformly recommended due to bisphosphonates' prolonged bone half-life
Preventive measures	– Antimicrobial mouth rinses (e.g., chlorhexidine) – Prophylactic antibiotics in selected cases – Careful wound closure if surgery is needed
Interdisciplinary collaboration	– Close coordination with oncologists, hematologists, pharmacists, and primary care physicians to balance oncologic/osteoporosis treatment needs with oral health
Patient education	– Inform patients about the risk and early signs of MRONJ: exposed bone, delayed healing, infection, and pain – Encourage prompt reporting of any suspicious symptoms
Follow-up and monitoring	– Regular periodontal maintenance visits – Periodic radiographic review of bone status – Documentation of all treatments and patient instructions

12.5 Surgical Safety and Minimally Invasive Techniques

Risks in periodontal surgery are hemorrhage, nerve damage, and postsurgical infection. Newer surgical procedures with the introduction of smaller incisions and minimally invasive approaches have minimized the procedure to safer limits by creating less damage to soft tissues and blood vessels, leading to decreased postsurgical complications and improved visibility with the aid of devices like magnifying glasses [45] (Table 12.3). The three-dimensional imaging method, which is attained using cone-beam computed tomography, significantly enhances the visibility of the anatomical structures in an extremely detailed manner. Additionally, the utilization of digital planning software is crucial to enable practitioners to stay at the proper and safe distance from vital anatomical regions such as the inferior alveolar nerve or the maxillary sinus in order to ensure safety for patients during procedures [46, 47].

Table 12.3: Risk factors, mechanisms, and safety measures in periodontal treatment.

Clinical risk	Underlying mechanism	Potential consequences	Recommended safety strategy
Excessive tissue trauma during instrumentation	Use of dull instruments, poor angulation, and excessive force	Delayed healing, post-op pain, and gingival recession	Use sharpened instruments, follow ergonomic protocols, and ensure adequate visibility
Local anesthetic overdose or allergy	High dosage or hypersensitivity to amide/ester compounds	Systemic toxicity and anaphylaxis	Dose calculation by weight, aspirate before injection, and consider allergy testing
Inadvertent root surface damage	Aggressive scaling, p	Hypersensitivity and compromised regenerative response	Apply gentle tactile pressure and use of ultrasonic scalers with adaptive power settings
Postsurgical infection	Poor aseptic technique and systemic immunosuppression	Delayed wound healing and abscess formation	Preoperative antisepsis, systemic evaluation, and proper suture technique
Bleeding complications	Anticoagulant/ antiplatelet use and coagulopathy	Intraoperative or delayed bleeding	Medical history review, INR/PT checks, and local hemostatic agents
Allergic reactions to materials	Hypersensitivity to latex, chlorhexidine, or resorbable membranes	Urticaria, mucosal sloughing, and anaphylaxis	Use hypoallergenic products and obtain detailed allergy history
Aspiration of instruments	Inadequate isolation or reclined positioning	Airway obstruction and pulmonary aspiration	Use throat shields, high-speed suction, and instrument tethers
Misdiagnosis or overtreatment	Incomplete clinical records or overreliance on visual inspection	Unnecessary surgery and poor outcomes	Employ comprehensive diagnostic protocols, radiographic adjuncts, and AI tools
Cross-infection in immunocompromised patients	Inadequate sterilization and failure to screen for systemic risks	Opportunistic infections and systemic dissemination	Strict infection control and antibiotic prophylaxis where indicated
Patient noncompliance with postop care	Inadequate education and unrealistic expectations	Surgical failure and reinfection	Reinforce oral hygiene instruction, deliver written instructions, and schedule follow-ups

12.6 Implant Safety and Peri-implantitis Prevention

Implant treatment has been successful in the majority of instances; however, it must be stated that it can also lead to complications such as peri-implant mucositis or peri-implantitis if patient selection procedures and maintenance protocols are not adequately executed [48]. Safety protocols are the most important here and include the practice of loading the implants only after ensuring a proper osseointegration as supported by resonance frequency analysis. Besides, the application of antibacterial coatings combined with photofunctionalization is required to successfully reduce the risk of early microbial colonization [49]. Additionally, regular supportive periodontal therapy needs to be maintained to assure the long-term stability and health of the implants with the passage of time. In the case of patients having uncontrolled periodontitis or inadequate plaque control, they have to go through disease stabilization prior to placing any implants to prevent possible risks [50, 51].

12.7 Digital Technology and AI for Safety Monitoring

Artificial intelligence (AI) is progressively revolutionizing the practice of periodontics through improved diagnostic accuracy, simplification of clinical workflows, and maintenance of patient safety. In digital transformation in periodontal charting, AI algorithms permit direct data entry and analysis with the incorporation of automated probing systems that provide consistent pocket depth measurements and reduce variability associated with operators [52, 53]. AI-driven risk prediction models, on the contrary, utilize patient-specific information – medical history, lifestyle factors, and clinical results, to assess the risk of periodontal disease and personalize preventive treatment [54]. A very practical use is in radiographic interpretation, where AI systems are able to identify faint indications of early alveolar bone loss that could easily be missed by the human eye. Additionally, the systems are able to segregate anatomical landmarks or zones of vulnerability important to surgical planning such as features including the mental foramen or mandibular canal [55].

AI incorporation into the digital treatment planning workflow also minimizes human error by cross-checking clinical observations, suggesting evidence-based treatment, and highlighting inconsistencies [56]. Beyond diagnosis and planning, AI-powered clinical decision support systems can also dynamically assess drug interactions, highlight contraindications (e.g., anticoagulants or bisphosphonates), and signal alerts for systemic comorbidities such as uncontrolled diabetes or cardiovascular disease. These systems enhance coordinated interdisciplinary treatment and make periodontal therapy safe and individualized to every patient's medical history [57] (Figure 12.3).

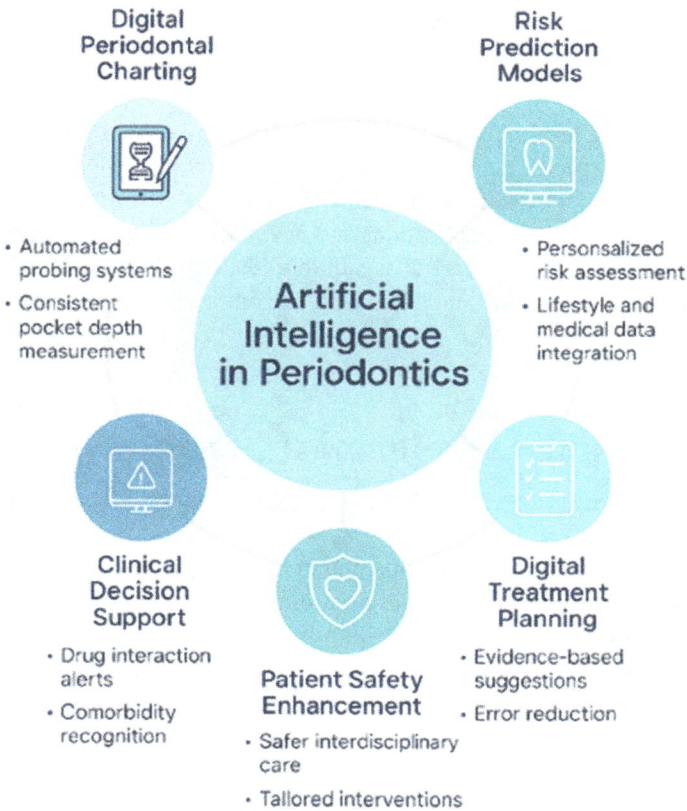

Figure 12.3: Applications of artificial intelligence in periodontics. Core domains include digital periodontal charting (automated probing and pocket depth measurement), risk prediction models (personalized risk assessment and medical data integration), digital treatment planning (evidence-based and error reduction), patient safety enhancement (safer interdisciplinary care and tailored interventions), and clinical decision support (drug interactions and comorbidity recognition).

12.8 Emergency Preparedness in Periodontal Practice

One should anticipate emergencies such as anaphylaxis, syncope, hypertensive crises, or bleeding, especially during surgery or administration of local anesthesia. Precautions consist of having emergency medications and oxygen in the operatory, training of staff in basic life support and AED, and access to protocols for the control of bleeding in anticoagulated patients such as INR testing and the use of local hemostatics [58, 59].

12.9 Patient-Centered Safety: Communication and Consent

Informed consent is not only a legal obligation but also a vital instrument of patient safety. Communication is enhanced, compliance is improved, and shared decision-making is promoted. Consent discussions should clearly cover the advantages and dangers of every procedure, potential complications and how they may be dealt with, and alternatives like not intervening where it is suitable [60, 61]. Visual aids, AI-generated 3D models, and multilingual materials help in comprehension and empower the patient [62, 63].

12.10 Long-Term Safety Through Maintenance and Monitoring

Long-term periodontal safety requires continuous monitoring and prevention of recurrence. Individualized maintenance frequencies according to molecular biomarker profiles such as MMP-8 and IL-1β, and electronic health monitoring via mobile health platforms enable preventive care to become proactive [64, 65]. Systemic conditions such as diabetes, osteoporosis, or cardiovascular disease require interprofessional collaboration in order to optimize safety on the medical-dental interface [66].

12.11 Conclusion

Enhanced patient safety in the framework of periodontal care requires the implementation of a comprehensive and multilayered approach that effectively blends a strong sense of clinical acumen with cutting-edge technology, evidence-based practice compliance, and patient empowerment. As periodontology moves further toward becoming a precision science, safety must also be a fundamental tenet – not merely as a protocol expectation to be followed but rather as a philosophy that supports and guides every clinical decision a practitioner makes. Through judicious use of several risk stratification tools, application of minimally invasive technologies, promotion of antimicrobial stewardship, and utilization of advanced digital surveillance systems, clinicians can effectively minimize the occurrence of adverse events and, concurrently, elevate the overall level of care patients receive. Lastly, safety's meaning cannot be boiled down to merely the lack of harm but rather the intentional and diligent creation of a condition in which the likelihood of harm being suffered is minimized and highly improbable.

References

[1] Renouard, F., Renouard, E., Rendón, A., & Pinsky, H. M. (2023). Increasing the margin of patient safety for periodontal and implant treatments: The role of human factors. Periodontol 2000, 92, 382–398.

[2] The Conceptual Framework for the International Classification for Patient Safety, (2009). World Health Organization: Geneva, https://www.who.int/publications/i/item/the-conceptual-framework-forthe-international-classification.

[3] Darby, I. (2009). Non-surgical management of periodontal disease. Australian Dental Journal, 54, S86–95.

[4] Askar, H., Di Gianfilippo, R., Ravida, A., Tattan, M., Majzoub, J., & Wang, H. L. (2019). Incidence and severity of postoperative complications following oral, periodontal, and implant surgeries: A retrospective study. Journal of Periodontol, 90, 1270–1278.

[5] Wise, R. J., Chen, C. Y., & Kim, D. M. (2018). Treatment of physiologic gingival pigmentation with surgical blade: A 25-year follow-up. International Journal of Periodontics & Restorative Dentistry, 38, s45–s48.

[6] Renouard, F., Renouard, E., Rendón, A., & Pinsky, H. M. (2023). Increasing the margin of patient safety for periodontal and implant treatments: The role of human factors. Periodontol 2000, 92, 382–398.

[7] Ilyes, I., Boariu, M., Rusu, D., Vela, O., Boia, S., Radulescu, V., Șurlin, P., Jentsch, H., Lodin, A., & Stratul, S. (2024). Comparative study of systemic vs local antibiotics with subgingival instrumentation in stage III–IV periodontitis: A retrospective analysis. Antibiotics, 13, 430.

[8] Gray, L. C., Beattie, E., Boscart, V. M., Henderson, A., Hornby-Turner, Y. C., Hubbard, R. E., Wood, S., & Peel, N. M. (2018). Development and testing of the interRAI acute care: A standardized assessment administered by nurses for patients admitted to acute care. Health Service Insights, 11, 1178632918818836.

[9] Toney-Butler, T. J., & Unison-Pace, W. J. Nursing Admission Assessment and Examination. [Updated 2023 Aug 28]. In: StatPearls [Internet]. Treasure Island (FL): StatPearls Publishing; 2025 Jan-. Available from: https://www.ncbi.nlm.nih.gov/books/NBK493211/

[10] Oral Health in America: Advances and Challenges [Internet]. Bethesda (MD): National Institute of Dental and Craniofacial Research(US); 2021 Dec. Section 3A, Oral Health Across the Lifespan: Working-Age Adults. Available from: https://www.ncbi.nlm.nih.gov/books/NBK578294/

[11] Abouleish, A. E., Leib, M. L., & Cohen, N. H. (2015). ASA provides examples to each ASA physical status class. ASA Monitor, 79, 38–39.

[12] Chandra, R. V. (2007). Evaluation of a novel periodontal risk assessment model in patients presenting for dental care. Oral Health and Preventive Dentistry, 5, 39–48.

[13] Sachelarie, L., Stefanescu, C. L., Murineanu, R. M., Grigorian, M., Zaharia, A., Scrobota, I., & Hurjui, L. L. (2025). Role of salivary biomarkers IL-1β and MMP-8 in early detection and staging of periodontal disease. Medicina (Kaunas), 61, 760.

[14] Anju, V. T., Busi, S., Imchen, M., Kumavath, R., Mohan, M. S., Salim, S. A., Subhaswaraj, P., & Dyavaiah, M. (2022). polymicrobial infections and biofilms: Clinical significance and eradication strategies. Antibiotics (Basel), 11, 1731.

[15] Patangia, D. V., Anthony Ryan, C., Dempsey, E., Paul Ross, R., & Stanton, C. (2022). Impact of antibiotics on the human microbiome and consequences for host health. Microbiologyopen, 11, e1260.

[16] Rakic, M., Pejcic, N., Perunovic, N., & Vojvodic, D. (2021). A roadmap towards precision periodontics. Medicina, 57, 233.

[17] Maheaswari, R., Kshirsagar, J. T., & Lavanya, N. (2016). Polymerase chain reaction: A molecular diagnostic tool in periodontology. Journal of Indian Society of Periodontology, 20, 128–135.

[18] Kirakodu, S. S., Govindaswami, M., Novak, M. J., Ebersole, J. L., & Novak, K. F. (2008). Optimizing qPCR for the quantification of periodontal pathogens in a complex plaque biofilm. Open Dentistry Journal, 2, 49–55.

[19] Melander, R. J., Zurawski, D. V., & Melander, C. (2018). Narrow-spectrum antibacterial agents. Medchemcomm, 9, 12–21.

[20] Nair, S. C., & Anoop, K. R. (2012). Intraperiodontal pocket: An ideal route for local antimicrobial drug delivery. Journal of Advanced Pharmaceutical Technology & Research, 3, 9–15.

[21] Singh, G., Gokhale, S. T., Manjunath, S., Al-Qahtani, S. M., Nagate, R. R., Venkataram, V., & Joseph, B. (2021). Evaluation of locally-administered controlled-release doxycycline hyclate gel in smokers and non-smokers in the management of periodontitis: An Indian study. Tropical Journal of Pharmaceutical Research, 20, 1739–1747.

[22] National Health and Medical Research Council (NHMRC). (2019). Australian Guidelines for the Prevention and Control of Infection in Healthcare (2019). Commonwealth of Australia: Canberra, [updated 9 Jan 2024; cited 2025 Jun 7]. Available from https://www.nhmrc.gov.au/health-advice/pub lic-health/preventing-infection.

[23] Centers for Disease Control and Prevention. Interim infection prevention and control recommendations for healthcare personnel during the coronavirus disease 2019 (COVID-19) pandemic. (Available at https://www.cdc.gov/coronavirus/2019-ncov/hcp/infection-control-recommendations.html)

[24] Centers for Disease Control and Prevention. (2011). Immunization of healthcare personnel: Recommendations of the Advisory Committee on Immunization Practices (ACIP). MMWR Recommendations and reports: Morbidity and mortality weekly report Recommendations and reports, 60(RR-7), 1–45, Available at, https://www.cdc.gov/mmwr/pdf/rr/rr6007.pdf [PDF – 48 Pages].).

[25] Abu Dhabi Health Services Company (SEHA). (2023). Patient Assessment Policy: ADM_04-00-003, SEHA: Abu Dhabi.

[26] Asmari, D. A., & Alenezi, A. (2025). Laser technology in periodontal treatment: Benefits, risks, and future directions – a mini review. Journal of Clinical Medicine, 14, 1962.

[27] Ishikawa, I., Aoki, A., & Takasaki, A. A. (2008 Jan). Clinical application of erbium:YAG laser in periodontology. Journal of the International Academy of Periodontology, 10(1), 22–30.

[28] Passanezi, E., Damante, C. A., & Aguiar Greghi, S. L. (2015). Lasers in periodontal therapy. Periodontology 2000, 67, 268–291.

[29] Aoki, A., Mizutani, K., Taniguchi, Y., Lin, T., Ohsugi, Y., Mikami, R., Katagiri, S., Meinzer, W., & Iwata, T. (2024). Current status of Er:YAG laser in periodontal surgery. Japanese Dental Science Review, 60, 1–14.

[30] Jiang, Y., Feng, J., Du, J., Fu, J., Liu, Y., Guo, L., & Liu, Y. (2022). Clinical and biochemical effect of laser as an adjunct to non-surgical treatment of chronic periodontitis. Oral Diseases, 28, 1042–1057.

[31] Hersh, E. V., Moore, P. A., Grosser, T., Polomano, R. C., Farrar, J. T., Saraghi, M., Juska, S. A., Mitchell, C. H., & Theken, K. N. (2020). Nonsteroidal anti-inflammatory drugs and opioids in postsurgical dental pain. Journal of Dental Research, 99, 777–786.

[32] Stiller, O., & Hjemdahl, P. (2022). Lessons from 20 years with COX-2 inhibitors: Importance of dose–response considerations and fair play in comparative trials. Journal of Internal Medicine, 292, 557–574.

[33] Chaiamnuay, S., Allison, J. J., & Curtis, J. R. (2006). Risks versus benefits of cyclooxygenase-2-selective nonsteroidal antiinflammatory drugs. American Journal of Health System Pharmacy, 63, 1837–1851.

[34] Lepelletier, D., Maillard, J. Y., Pozzetto, B., & Simon, A. (2020). Povidone iodine: Properties, mechanisms of action, and role in infection control and Staphylococcus aureus decolonization. Antimicrobial Agents and Chemotherapy, 64, e00682–20.

[35] Csifó-Nagy, B. K., Sólyom, E., Bognár, V. L., Nevelits, A., & Dőri, F. (2021). Efficacy of a new-generation platelet-rich fibrin in the treatment of periodontal intrabony defects: A randomized clinical trial. BMC Oral Health, 21, 580.

[36] Owosho, A. A., Tsai, C. J., Lee, R. S., Freymiller, H., Kadempour, A., Varthis, S., Sax, A. Z., Rosen, E. B., Yom, S. K., Randazzo, J., Drill, E., Riedel, E., Patel, S., Lee, N. Y., Huryn, J. M., & Estilo, C. L. (2017). The prevalence and risk factors associated with osteoradionecrosis of the jaw in oral and oropharyngeal cancer patients treated with intensity-modulated radiation therapy (IMRT): The memorial sloan kettering cancer center experience. Oral Oncology, 64, 44–51.

[37] Goh, E. Z., Beech, N., Johnson, N. R., & Batstone, M. (2023). The dental management of patients irradiated for head and neck cancer. British Dental Journal, 234, 800–804.

[38] Arya, L., & Brizuela, M. Oral Management of Patients Undergoing Radiation Therapy. [Updated 2023 Mar 19]. In: StatPearls [Internet]. Treasure Island (FL): StatPearls Publishing; 2025 Jan-. Available from: https://www.ncbi.nlm.nih.gov/books/NBK587448/

[39] Coropciuc, R., Coopman, R., Garip, M., Gielen, E., Politis, C., Van den Wyngaert, T., & Beuselinck, B. (2023). Risk of Medication-related Osteonecrosis of the Jaw after Dental Extractions in Patients Receiving Antiresorptive Agents – A Retrospective Study of 240 Patients, Bone, vol. 170, 116722.

[40] Wick, A., Bankosegger, P., Otto, S., Hohlweg-Majert, B., Steiner, T., Probst, F., Ristow, O., & Pautke, C. (2022). Risk factors associated with onset of medication-related osteonecrosis of the jaw in patients treated with denosumab. Clinical Oral Investigations, 26, 2839–2852.

[41] Decker, A. M., Taichman, L. S., D'Silva, N. J., & Taichman, R. S. (2018). Periodontal treatment in cancer patients: An interdisciplinary approach. Current Oral Health Reports, 5, 7–12.

[42] Bauer, D. C., & Abrahamsen, B. (2021). bisphosphonate drug holidays in primary care: When and what to do next?. Current Osteoporosis Reports, 19, 182–188.

[43] Diab, D. L., & Watts, N. B. (2013). Bisphosphonate drug holiday: Who, when and how long. Therapeutic Advances in Musculoskeletal Disease, 5, 107–111.

[44] AlRowis, R., Aldawood, A., AlOtaibi, M., Alnasser, E., AlSaif, I., Aljaber, A., & Natto, Z. (2022). Medication-Related Osteonecrosis of the Jaw (MRONJ): A review of pathophysiology, risk factors, preventive measures and treatment strategies. Saudi Dental Journal, 34, 202–210.

[45] Sultan, N., Jafri, Z., Sawai, M., & Bhardwaj, A. (2020). Minimally invasive periodontal therapy. Journal of Oral Biology and Craniofacial Research, 10, 161–165.

[46] Mohan, R., Singh, A., & Gundappa, M. (2011 Jan). Three-dimensional imaging in periodontal diagnosis – utilization of cone beam computed tomography. Journal of Indian Society of Periodontology, 15(1), 11–17.

[47] Acar, B., & Kamburoğlu, K. (2014). Use of cone beam computed tomography in periodontology. Journal of Radiology, 6(5), 139–147.

[48] Rokaya, D., Srimaneepong, V., Wisitrasameewon, W., Humagain, M., & Thunyakitpisal, P. (2020). Peri-implantitis update: Risk indicators, diagnosis, and treatment. European Journal of Dentistry, 14, 672–682.

[49] Kligman, S., Ren, Z., Chung, H., Perillo, M. A., Chang, C., Koo, H., Zheng, Z., & Li, C. (2021). The impact of dental implant surface modifications on Osseointegration and biofilm formation. Journal of Clinical Medicine, 10, 1641.

[50] Schoenmakers, M. G. P., Willems, E. J. S., Slot, D. E., & Van der Weijden, G. A. F. (2022). Success of supportive periodontal therapy in periodontitis patients – a retrospective analysis. International Journal of Dental Hygiene, 20, 318–327.

[51] Zeza, B., Pilloni, A., Tatakis, D. N., Mariotti, A., Di Tanna, G. L., & Mongardini, C. (2017). implant patient compliance varies by periodontal treatment history. Journal of Periodontology, 88, 846–853.

[52] Jundaeng, J., Chamchong, R., & Nithikathkul, C. (2025). Artificial intelligence-powered innovations in periodontal diagnosis: A new era in dental healthcare. Frontiers in Medical Technology, 6, 1469852.

[53] Spartivento, G., Benfante, V., Ali, M., Yezzi, A., Di Raimondo, D., Tuttolomondo, A., Lo Casto, A., & Comelli, A. (2024). revolutionizing periodontal care: The role of artificial intelligence in diagnosis, treatment, and prognosis. Applied Sciences, 15, 3295.

[54] Sarakbi, R. M., Varma, S. R., Muthiah Annamma, L., & Sivaswamy, V. (2025). Implications of artificial intelligence in periodontal treatment maintenance: A scoping review. Frontiers in Oral Health, 6, 1561128.

[55] Tariq, A., Nakhi, F. B., Salah, F., Eltayeb, G., Abdulla, G. J., Najim, N., Khedr, S. A., Elkerdasy, S., Al-Rawi, N., Alkawas, S., Mohammed, M., & Shetty, S. R. (2023). Efficiency and accuracy of artificial intelligence in the radiographic detection of periodontal bone loss: a systematic review. Imaging Science in Dentistry, 53, 193–198.

[56] Karalis, V. D. (2024). The integration of artificial intelligence into clinical practice. Applied Biosciences, 3, 14–44.

[57] Sutton, R. T., Pincock, D., Baumgart, D. C., DC, S., Fedorak, R. N., & Kroeker, K. I. (2020 Feb 6). An overview of clinical decision support systems: benefits, risks, and strategies for success. Nature Partner Journals (npj) Digital Medicine, 3, 17. doi: 10.1038/s41746-020-0221-y.

[58] Resuscitation Council UK. Emergency treatment of anaphylaxis: Guidelines for healthcare providers. London: Resuscitation Council UK; May 2021 [cited 2025 Jun 7]. Available from: https://www.resus.org.uk/library/additional-guidance/guidance-anaphylaxis/emergency-treatment-anaphylaxis

[59] Commins, S. P. (2017). Outpatient emergencies: Anaphylaxis. Medical Clinics of North America, 101(3), 521–536.

[60] Pugh, J. (2020). Autonomy, Rationality, and Contemporary Bioethics [Internet], Oxford University Press: Oxford (UK), Chapter 6, Informed Consent, Autonomy, and Beliefs. Available from: https://www.ncbi.nlm.nih.gov/books/NBK556864/.

[61] Cocanour, C. S. (2017). Informed consent – it's more than a signature on a piece of paper. The American Journal of Surgery, 214, 993–997.

[62] Galmarini, E., Marciano, L., & Schulz, P. J. (2024). The effectiveness of visual-based interventions on health literacy in health care: A systematic review and meta-analysis. BMC Health Services Research, 24(1), 718.

[63] Padmanabhan, V., Islam, M. S., Rahman, M. M. (2024). et al. Understanding patient safety in dentistry: Evaluating the present and envisioning the future – a narrative review. BMJ Open Quality, 13, e002502. doi: 10.1136/bmjoq-2023-002502.

[64] Ramseier, C. A. (2024). Diagnostic measures for monitoring and follow-up in periodontology and implant dentistry. Periodontology 2000, 95, 129–155.

[65] Kinney, J. S., Morelli, T., Oh, M., Braun, T. M., Ramseier, C. A., Sugai, J. V., & Giannobile, W. V. (2014). Crevicular fluid biomarkers and periodontal disease progression. Journal of Clinical Periodontology, 41(2), 113–120.

[66] Fatahzadeh, M., Sabato, E., Singhal, V., Wagner, M., & Fenesy, K. (2025). A novel oral medicine-centered interprofessional curricular initiative to promote collaboration and build oral health capacity. Journal of Dental Education, 89(1), 81–89.

Index

https://doi.org/10.1515/9783112219904-013

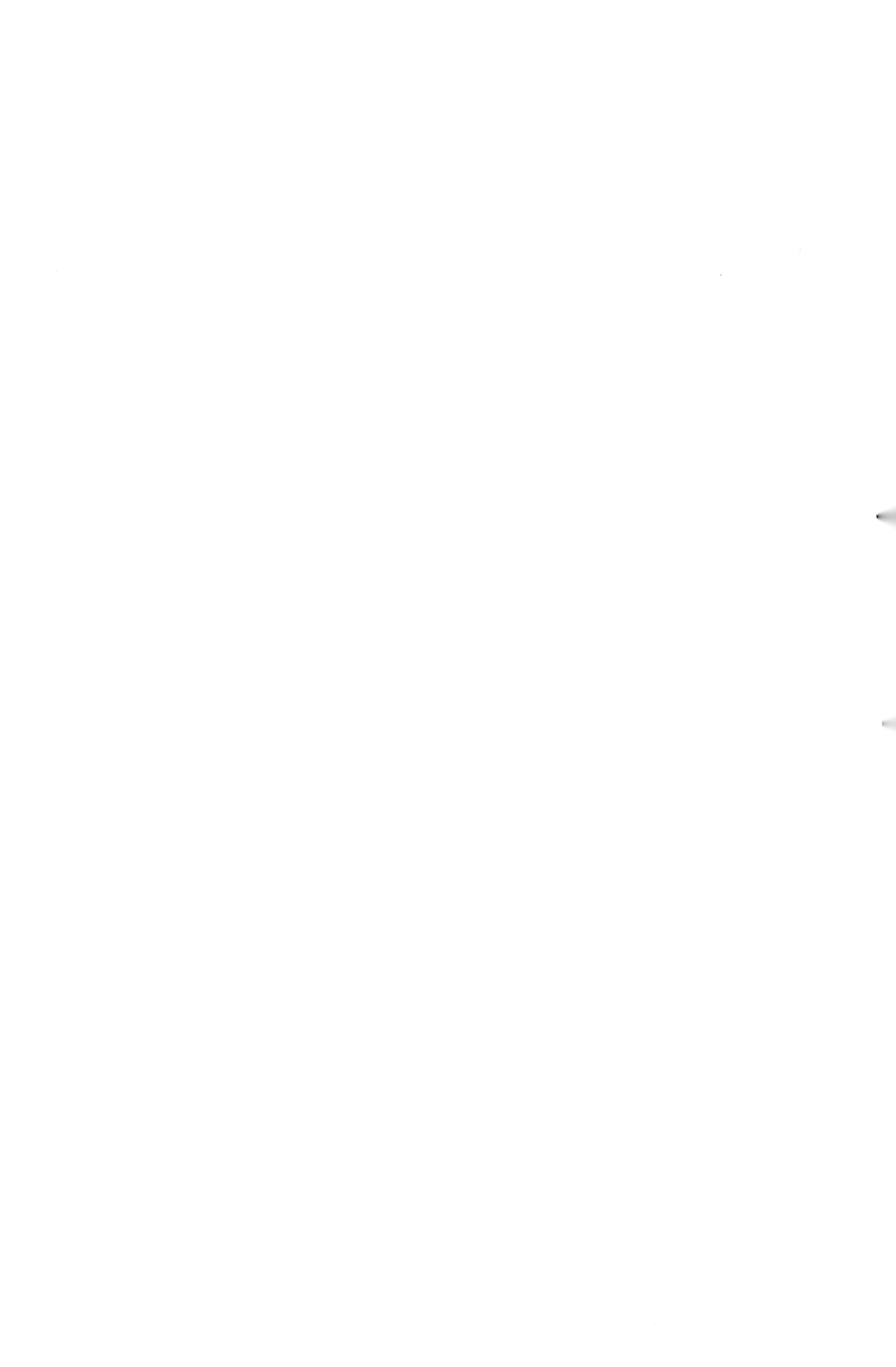

www.ingramcontent.com/pod-product-compliance
Lightning Source LLC
Chambersburg PA
CBHW081515190326
41458CB00015B/5378